NASAL TUMORS
in
ANIMALS
and
MAN

Volume III

Experimental Nasal Carcinogenesis

Editors

Gerd Reznik, D. V. M., Ph.D.

Director
Institute for Pathology and Toxicology
Byk-Gulden Pharmaceuticals
Hamburg, West Germany

Sherman F. Stinson, Ph.D.

Experimental Pathologist
Laboratory of Experimental Pathology
Division of Cancer Cause and Prevention
National Cancer Institute
Frederick, Maryland

CRC Press, Inc.
Boca Raton, Florida

Library of Congress Cataloging in Publication Data
Main entry under title:
Nasal tumors in animals and man.
    Bibliography: p.
    Includes index.
    1. Nose—Tumors.   2. Veterinary oncology.
3. Nose—Tumors—Animal models. I. Reznik,
Gerd. II. Stinson, Sherman F., 1946-
RC280.N6N35 1983   616.99'42107   82-12777

    Direct all inquiries to CRC Press, Inc., 2000 Corporate Blvd., N.W., Boca Raton, Florida, 33431.

© 1983 by CRC Press, Inc.

International Standard Book Number 0-8493-5577-X (Volume I)
International Standard Book Number 0-8493-5578-8 (Volume II)
International Standard Book Number 0-8493-5579-6 (Volume III)
Library of Congress Card Number 82-12777

PREFACE

This monograph brings together within one cover the current knowledge about tumors of the nasal passages in man, in domestic and nondomestic animals, and in the rodents which are commonly employed in carcinogenesis studies in the laboratory. Interest in the experimental induction of tumors of the nasal passages may be said to have begun in the late 1950s and early 1960s with the demonstrations of the carcinogenicity of the polyoma virus, N,N'-2,7-fluorenylenebisacetamide and certain N-nitroso compounds for the upper respiratory tract in mice, rats, and hamsters. These compounds proved to be carcinogenic whether administered orally, subcutaneously, intradermally, intraperitoneally, intravenously, topically, or by inhalation. It soon became evident that, within the nasal passages, different N-nitroso compounds exerted site specific carcinogenic effects. The large amount of diversified experimental observations on laboratory animals that have accummulated over the past 20 odd years have included studies of the cell or cells responsible for the conversion of the N-nitroso compound to the proximate carcinogen and its chemical configuration, the cells on which the proximate carcinogen acts to induce the changes that these cells undergo from their early proliferations through their progression to cancer and the ultimate pattern of spread of the cancers within the area. These observations have been aided by the use of histochemistry and electron microscopy. The considerable progress that has been made in relatively recent years in the precise study of the location and histopathogenesis of the induced tumors of the nasal cavity in laboratory animals can be attributed in large part to the skilled scientific work of those who are the authors of the chapters of the present monograph and those whose works these authors cite in the list of references appended to their chapters. In comparison with man, rodents have infrequently developed spontaneous tumors of the nasal passages, or if they have, comparative pathologists have neglected to find many of them. But with the use of appropriate carcinogens, tumors of various sites and different histologic types are readily reproducible.

The detailed descriptions of the anatomy and histology of the nasal cavity of rodents and the precise directions for the conduct of the autopsy and subsequent trimming of tissue blocks and histologic preparation of the sections, should, if followed, prevent errors that prosectors had made in the past. There have been occasions on which a misdiagnosis of a brain tumor has resulted from an incomplete necropsy of an experimental animal performed by an ill-trained prosector who, following removal of the brain, failed to inspect or provide for later histologic examination of the nasal structures which had, in fact, been the primary source of the tumor. In this instance, a primary tumor of the nasal passages had spread through the cribiform plate to invade the cranial cavity and to infiltrate the brain. Also failure, at the autopsy, to explore properly the nasal cavity in animals with a malignant schwannoma primary at the root of a cranial nerve has resulted in failure to appreciate the considerable distance these tumors may travel as they infiltrate the affected cranial nerve following exit through the foramen and along its course within the walls of the nasal cavity. If, in the future, prosectors carefully follow the procedures described and illustrated in the monograph for the proper methods for the study of primary and secondary tumors of the nasal passages, it is unlikely that such errors, committed in the past, will be repeated in the future.

As experimental pathologists continue their studies of the experimentally induced tumors of laboratory animals, they rely heavily on the publications dealing with these tumors in man. The degree of sophistication possessed by clinical pathologists exceeds that possessed by comparative pathologists whose experience with nasal tumors is of shorter duration and based on smaller numbers. In man, primary tumors may arise from any of the several tissue types that line the nasal cavity. These include epithelium of different types, nervous tissues of different types, lymphoreticular tissues, fibrous tissue, bone, cartilage, and blood and lymph vessels. In man, certain tumors may appear in newborns, may arise more frequently in one sex than the other, may be influenced by hormonal factors and, following a period of growth, may cease to grow or even regress. Clinical pathologists have also observed that certain nasal tumors, while comparable for classification purposes to histologically similar tumors primary at other sites in the body, may look and behave differently. Epidemiologic investigations of the labor force exposed to industrial carcinogens and of domestic animals exposed to environmental carcinogens have revealed a number of agents capable of the induction of tumors of the nasal passages in man and certain domestic animals and information on these matters is presented in the chapters of this monograph.

Comparative pathologists, while they have always profited from the knowledge accummulated by clinical pathologists know very well that tumors of animals may differ in appearance and behavior from tumors of corresponding sites in humans. The exact definitions of the tumors induced in rodents and their histologic typing still await further study for the development of a proper classification and nomenclature. This could be accomplished by following the plan devised by the World Health Organization (WHO) for the classification of human tumors. In brief, the plan if adapted to the present problem would provide for several pathologists knowledgeable about tumors of the nasal passages in rodents to come together with their respective pathologic material and records and carefully work out an acceptable classification. Because of the intermixture of the diverse cell populations of the mucous membrane that lines the nasal cavity, the cell of origin and the criteria for typing the various tumors which arise in this location may not be a simple task.

Those who control the funds available for cancer research will need to be prevailed upon to provide adequate financial support for these and other endeavors related to carcinogenesis of the nasal passages. To paraphrase a saying of Mr. Dooley that ''the supreme court follows the election returns'', those who controlled the purse strings for cancer research have, in the past, favored support for research on cancers common to man such as those of the lung, bowel, breast, and uterus. There is no better example of this favoritism than with cancers of the respiratory tract. Lung tumors are much more common in man than are nasal tumors. Large sums of money have gone into the support of research on tumors of the lung, and comparatively little for the support of tumors of the upper respiratory tract including those of the nasal passages, ethmoturbinals, and maxillary sinuses. Pulmonary tumors of rodents have been a frequently used tool for research ever since Livingood, before the turn of the century, first diagnosed alveologenic tumors of mice, and other investigators in the 1920s, accomplished their induction by the use of carcinogens. The normal anatomy and histology of the lung in different rodent species have, over the years, been carefully worked out as has the classification and histologic typing of the tumors. Moreover, at the autopsy, it is a simple matter to remove the chest plate and examine, the lung for tumors. The situation is different with the structures of the nasal passages. Here either spontaneous tumors arise infrequently in laboratory animals or, if they have been present, prosectors have not exerted themselves to look for them. It is reasonable to believe that failure of prosectors regularly to explore the nasal cavity at necropsy and to fix and prepare properly the structures of this region for subsequent histologic studies account, in part, for the infrequent identification of tumors in this location in untreated rodents. This procedure is more difficult and time consuming than simply removing the chest plate to look for tumors of the lung. Only since the late 1950s were carcinogenic agents discovered that regularly induce nasal tumors and only in the past few years were the anatomy and histology of the nasal cavity structures carefully worked out and the mixture of the various cell types in the mucosa identified.

With all the latest information on these matters contained within the present monograph, it now appears that studies of induced nasal cavity tumors in experimental animals offer challenges for future investigation that exceed those offered by tumors of many other body sites.

Harold L. Stewart, M.D.
1982

INTRODUCTION

Nasal cavity cancer (sinonasal) and nasopharyngeal cancer have been known since ancient days. Nasopharyngeal neoplasms, the major type of human nasal cancer, have been observed in Egyptian mummies which are at least 2000 years old.

During the last 45 years, several studies, mainly from Wales, Canada, Norway, and Russia, have demonstrated an increased epidemiological risk of respiratory tract carcinomas in nickel refinery workers.[1-7] Torjussen[8] showed that carcinomas and possible precancerous histopathological mucosal changes of the nasal cavity were found exclusively in individuals who had been exposed to high concentrations of atmospheric nickel for at least 10 years.

The wood, leather, and some associated industries were selected for a recent review by the International Agency for Research on Cancer (WHO, Lyon)[9] mainly because of a series of reports dating back to 1965 which indicated unusually high relative risks of nasal cancer (in the nasal cavities and sinuses) in certain segments of these industries, in particular the furniture and cabinet-making industry and boot and shoe manufacture and repair. The results of these studies were so striking and so consistent that they strongly suggested the presence of carcinogenic materials in those work environments. The direct causative agents in these occupational environments can often not be identified, are misinterpreted, and cocarcinogenesis cannot be excluded.

As will become clear in the course of this book, nasal cavity cancer has one of the most complex etiologies. The carcinogenic induction can be due to a larger number of agents — chemicals, viruses, radiation, particles, hormones — all of which possible mechanisms of interactions.

Animal experiments have shown that a great number of nitrosamines, bis (chloromethyl)ether, 1,2-Dibromoethane, 1,2-Dibromo-3-chloropropane, 1,4-Dioxane, p-cresidine, formaldehyde, phenacetin, procarbazine, Thio-Tepa, vinylchloride, and many more chemical substances found in the environment induced neoplasms in the nasal cavity of hamsters, mice, rats, monkeys, or other animal species.

Cigarette smoke contains a large number of carcinogenic substances: nitrosonornicotine, formaldehyde, and benzo(a)pyrene are just a few of these. Others include a large number of nitrosamines as well as particulate matter. Thus, cigarette smoke and its products can play an important role in the production of nasal cavity cancer in animals and man.

Human nasopharyngeal carcinomas are far more prevalent in Asian races than in Caucasian races. No causal relationships have been discovered between any environmental agent and this high prevalence of nasopharyngeal carcinoma. Since Chinese all over the world have a similar, high incidence of nasal cancers, current theory suggest that a genetic factor is probably responsible.

Gerd Reznik, D. V. M., Ph.D
1982

REFERENCES

1. **Doll, R., Morgan, L. G., and Speizer, F. E.,** Cancers of the lungs and nasal sinuses in nickel workers, *Br. J. Cancer,* 24, 623, 1970.
2. **Doll, R., Mathews, J. D., and Morgan, L. G.,** Cancers of the lung and nasal sinuses in nickel workers, *Br. J. Ind. Med.,* 34, 102, 1977.
3. **Mastromatteo, E.,** Nickel, a review of its occupational health aspects, *J. Occup. Med.,* 9, 127, 1967.
4. **Pedersen, E., Hogetveit, A. C., and Andersen, A.,** Cancer of respiratory organs among workers at a nickel refinery in Norway, *Int. J. Cancer,* 12, 32, 1973.
5. **Pedersen, E., Andersen, A., and Hogetveit, A. C.,** Second study of the incidence and mortality of cancer of respiratory organs among workers at a nickel refinery, *Ann. Clin. Lab. Sci.,* 8, 503, 1978.
6. **Saknyn, A. V. and Shabynina, N. K.,** Epidemiology of malignant neoplasms in nickel, plants, *Gig. Trud. Prof. Zabol.,* 17, 25, 1973.
7. **Sutherland, R. B.,** Summary report on respiratory cancer mortality at the INCO Port Colborne Refinery, Department of Health, Toronto, Ontario, 1959, 153.
8. **Torjussen, W.,** Nasal Carcinoma in Nickel Workers, A Histopathological, Chemical, Histochemical, Clinical and Epidemiological study, Dissertation, Kristiansand, 1979.
9. IARC Monographs on the evaluation of the carcinogenic risk of chemicals to humans, wood, leather and some associated industries, Vol. 25, International Agency for Research on Cancer, Lyon, 1981.

THE EDITORS

Gerd Reznik, D. V. M., Ph.D., is currently Director of the Institute for Pathology and Toxicology, Byk-Gulden Pharmaceuticals in Hamburg, West Germany. He is also Associate Professor of Experimental Oncology at the Medical School, Hannover, West Germany.

Dr. Reznik received his D. V. M. in 1971 from the University in Giessen, West Germany and a Ph.D. in Veterinary Pathology in 1972 from the Veterinary School in Hannover, West Germany. His Ph.D. thesis dealt with the consequences of different population levels on the interstitial testicular tissue on NMRI mice (histometrical studies). He continued to study medicine in 1977 at Hannover Medical School. He finished the preclinical studies and was Assistant Professor of Experimental Pathology in the Department of Pathology at the Medical School in Hannover from 1972. During this time, he received training in histopathology of animals and humans, worked on the induction of cancer with different carcinogens in different animal species, and investigated special human cases. During this time, Dr. Reznik specialized in cigarette smoke induced changes in the airways of man and animals and published more than 30 papers on this subject. In 1978, he went to the National Cancer Institute, National Institute of Health and Human Services, Bethesda, Md. where he worked in the Bioassay Program as a Veterinary Pathologist. In this time, he researched aging lesions in rats and mice and published many papers on rare tumors. In the years between 1980 and 1981, Dr. Reznik worked as a Veterinary Pathologist in the Tumor Pathology Branch, National Toxicology Program, National Cancer Institute, National Institutes of Health and Human Services. In 1981, Dr. Reznik continued his studies on comparative pathology as a Veterinary Pathologist in the Laboratory of Comparative Carcinogenesis, National Institutes of Health and Human Services, National Cancer Institute, Division of Cancer Cause and Prevention, Frederick, Md. In 1981, he became Deputy Director, Byk-Gulden Pharmaceuticals, Institute for Pathology and Toxicology, Hamburg, West Germany and Director of the same Institute in 1982.

Dr. Reznik has published over 110 works in his field and, in addition to "Nasal Tumors in Animals and Man," has several other book chapters in press.

Sherman F. Stinson, Ph.D., is an experimental pathologist currently affiliated with the Laboratory of Experimental Pathology of the National Cancer Institute, Frederick Cancer Research Facility, Frederick, Md. His research is directed toward mechanisms of epithelial carcinogenesis with particular emphasis on the respiratory tract.

Dr. Stinson received a B.A. in chemistry from California Western University, San Diego, in 1968. From 1968 to 1975 he attended the University of Southern California, Los Angeles, where he received a M.S. and a Ph.D. in pathology. His M.S. and Ph.D. dissertations dealt with a correlation of the biochemical mechanisms and morphologic progression in the pathogenesis of pulmonary oxygen toxicity.

Dr. Stinson continued his interests in the respiratory tract with the Lung Cancer Branch of the National Cancer Institute as a Staff Fellow (1975 to 1978) where he conducted studies on respiratory carcinogenesis and the effects of retinoids on the carcinogenic response in various epithelial tissues. In 1978, he joined the Tumor Pathology Branch of the Carcinogenesis Testing Program, National Cancer Institute, where his responsibilities included supervision of the pathology evaluations of the numerous carcinogenesis bioassays conducted by this program. During his tenure with the Carcinogenesis Testing Program he had the opportunity to study the effects of a wide variety of carcinogenic and toxic agents on the respiratory tract as well as other epithelial tissues.

Dr. Stinson has published over 50 scientific works in his field and has contributed to over 80 Carcinogenesis Technical Reports of the National Cancer Institute.

CONTRIBUTORS

Roy E. Albert, M.D.
Professor and Deputy Director
Institute of Environmental Medicine
New York University Medical Center
New York, New York

V. Balakrishnan
Scientific Officer
Cancer Research Institute
Bombay, India

Thomas R. Bender, M.D., M.P.H.
Director
Alaska Investigations Division
Center for Infectious Diseases
Centers for Disease Control
Anchorage, Alaska

Stephen A. Benjamin, D.V.M., Ph.D.
Professor of Pathology
Professor of Radiation Biology
Director, Collaborative Radiological
  Health Laboratory
College of Veterinary Medicine and
  Biomedical Sciences
Colorado State University
Ft. Collins, Colorado

Morten Boysen, M.D.
ENT Specialist
The Norwegian Radium Hospital and
  Norsk Hydro's Institute for Cancer
  Research
Oslo, Norway

Eva Brittebo, Ph.D.
Department of Pharmacology
Uppsala Biomedical Centre
Uppsala, Sweden

Eva Buiatti, M.D.
Epidemiologist
Centro per lo Studio e la Prevenzione
  Oncologica
Florence, Italy

James J. Butler
Professor of Pathology
The University of Texas System Cancer
  Center
M. D. Anderson Hospital and Tumor
  Institute
Houston, Texas

Francesco Carnevale, M.D.
Assistant
Occupational Medicine Institute
Verona, Italy

Andre Castonguay, Ph.D.
Associate
Division of Chemical Carcinogenesis
American Health Foundation
Valhalla, New York

Dr. Jane C. F. Chang
Postdoctoral Fellow
Chemical Industry Institute of Toxicology
Research Triangle Park, North Carolina

C. N. Chineme, D.V.M., Ph.D.
Professor of Pathology
Department of Veterinary Pathology and
  Microbiology
Ahmadu Bello University
Zaria, Nigeria

Yrjö Collan, M.D.
Professor and Chairman
Department of Pathology
University of Kuopio
Kuopio, Finland

Kamal Ali El-Ghamrawi, M.D., F.F.R.
Professor of Radiation Oncology and Nu-
  clear Medicine
Cairo University
Cairo, Egypt

David Elkon, M.D.
Department of Radiation Oncology
St. Francis General Hospital
Pittsburgh, Pennsylvania

Isaburo Fujimoto, M.D.
Director
Department of Field Research
Center for Adult Disease, Osaka
Osaka, Japan

Keizo Furuya, M.D.
Pathologist
School of Medicine
Tokushima University
Tokushima, Japan
Visiting Pathologist
Naylor Dana Institute
Valhalla, New York

P. Gangadharan
Statistician
Tata Memorial Hospital
Bombay, India

Marco Geddes, M.D.
Epidemiologist
Centro per lo Studio e la Prevenzione
  Oncologica
Florence, Italy

Ronald Glaser
Professor and Chairman
Department of Medical Microbiology and
  Immunology
The Ohio State University
Columbus, Ohio

Aya Hanai, B.Sc.
Vice Director
Osaka Cancer Registry
Department of Field Disease
Center for Adult Disease, Osaka
Osaka, Japan

Dr. John C. Harshbarger
Director
Registry of Tumors in Lower Animals
National Museum of Natural History
Smithsonian Institution
Washington, D.C.

Stephen S. Hecht, Ph.D.
Chief
Division of Chemical Carcinogenesis
Naylor Dana Institute
Valhalla, New York

Dennis K. Heffner, M.D.
Assistant Chairman
Department of Otolaryngic Pathology
Armed Forces Institute of Pathology
Washington, D.C.

Tomohiko Hiyama, M.D.
Department of Field Research
Center for Adult Disease, Osaka
Osaka, Japan

Khang-Loon Ho, M.D.
Senior Pathologist
Department of Pathology
Henry Ford Hospital
Clinical Associate Professor
Department of Pathology
Wayne State University
Detroit, Michigan

Dietrich Hoffmann, Ph.D.
Associate Director and Chief
Division of Environmental Carcinogenesis
American Health Foundation
Naylor Dana Institute for Disease
  Prevention
Valhalla, New York

Naruto Horiuchi, M.D.
Director
Department of Multiphasic Health
  Screening
Center for Adult Disease, Osaka
Osaka, Japan

Marvin Kuschner, M.D.
Dean
Medical School
SUNY at Stony Brook
Stony Brook, New York

Anne P. Lanier, M.D.
Medical Epidemiologist
Alaska Investigations Division
Center for Infectious Diseases
Centers for Disease Control
Anchorage, Alaska

Bruce Mackay, M.D., Ph.D.
Pathologist and Professor of Pathology
University of Texas M.D. Anderson Hos-
  pital and Tumor Institute
Houston, Texas

Per Marton, M.D.
Head
Department of Pathology
The Norwegian Radium Hospital and
  Norsk Hydro's Institute for Cancer
  Research
Oslo, Norway

Dr. Bernard Ph. M. Menco
Lab. v. Medische Fyskia
Psychologie
Utrecht, The Netherlands
Department of Neurobiology and
  Physiology*
Section of Biological Sciences
College of Arts and Sciences
O. T. Hogan Hall
Northwestern University
Evanston, Illinois

Enzo Merler, M.D.
Istituto di Anatomia ed Istologia
  Patologica
Policlinico di Borgo Roma
Verona, Italy

Richard J. Montali, D.V.M.
Head
Department of Pathology
National Zoological Park
Washington, D.C.

Teizo Mukai, M.D.
Director
Oto-rhino-laryngology
Yao City Hospital
Yao City, Japan

**C. O. Njoku, D.V.M., Ph.D.,
  F.R.V.C.S.**
Professor of Veterinary Pathology and
  Head
Department of Veterinary Pathology and
  Microbiology
Ahmadu Bello University
Zaria, Nigeria
Fellow
Royal Veterinary College of Sweden

Akira Oshima, M.D.
Department of Field Research
Center for Adult Disease, Osaka
Osaka, Japan

**Satyendra Dinkerlal Parikh, F.R.C.S.,
  F.I.C.S.**
Head of Ear, Nose, and Throat Unit
Al-Sabah Hospital
Safat, Kuwait

Amiya K. Patnaik, B.V.Sc., M.V.Sc.
Staff Pathologist
The Animal Medical Center
New York, New York

Umapati Prasad, F.R.C.S.E., F.I.C.S.
Professor and Head
Department of Otorhinolaryngology
Faculty of Medicine
University of Malaya
Kuala Lumpur, Malaysia

Dr. Donald F. Proctor
Professor
Environmental Health Sciences, Anesthe-
  siology, Otolaryngology
Johns Hopkins Schools of Hygiene and
  Public Health and of Medicine
Baltimore, Maryland

Dr. Albrecht Reith, M.D., Ph.D.
Head of Laboratory of Electronmicros-
  copy and Morphometry
Department of Pathology
The Norwegian Radium Hospital
Norsk Hydro's Institute for Cancer
  Research
Oslo, Norway
Professor of Cell Biology
University of Constance
West Germany

Gerd Reznik, D.V.M., Ph.D.
Director
Institute for Pathology
  and Toxicology
Byk-Gulden Pharmaceuticals
Hamburg, West Germany

* Present position.

Jean-Paul Riguat, M.D.
Senior Researcher
Laboratoire de Biologie du
 Developpement
U.E.R. Bio-Medicale
Université Paris
Bobigny, France

**Hildegard M. Reznik-Schüller,
D.V.M., Ph.D.**
Veterinary Pathologist
Certified Experimental Oncologist
Group Leader
Ultrastructure Research in Chemical
 Carcinogenesis
Frederick Cancer Research Center
Frederick, Maryland

Abraham Rivenson, M.D.
Director of the Histopathology Laboratory
American Health Foundation
Naylor Dana Institute
Valhalla, New York

Shunichi Sakai, M.D.
Director
Oto-rhino-laryngology
Osaka Kaisei Hospital
Osaka, Japan
Professor*
Department of Oto-rhino-laryngology
Kagawa Medical School
Kagawa, Japan

Dr. Kurt O. Schmid
Associate Professor
Department of Pathology
University of Graz
Graz, Austria

Jay P. Schreider, Ph.D.
Assistant Adjunct Professor
Laboratory for Energy-Related Health
 Research
University of California, Davis
Davis, California

Arthur Sellakumar, D.V.M., M.S.
Associate Professor
Department of Environmental Medicine
New York University Medical Center
Tuxedo, New York

Elvio Silva, M.D.
Assistant Professor of Pathology
M. D. Anderson Hospital and Tumor
 Institute
Houston, Texas

Harold L. Stewart, M.D.,
NIH Scientist Emeritus
Registry of Experimental Cancers
National Cancer Institute
National Institutes of Health
Bethesda, Maryland

Sherman F. Stinson, Ph.D.
Experimental Pathologist
Laboratory of Experimental Pathology
Division of Cancer Cause and Prevention
National Cancer Institute
Frederick, Maryland

Hans Tjälve, D.V.M., Ph.D.
Department of Toxicology
Uppsala University
Uppsala, Sweden

William Torjussen, M.D.
Chief Surgeon ENT
Vest-Agder Sentralsykehus
Kristiansand, Norway

Lee S. Tuckwiller
Postdoctoral Researcher
Department of Medical Microbiology and
 Immunology
The Ohio State University
Columbus, Ohio

Marion G. Valerio, D.V.M.,
Veterinary Pathologist
Litton Bionetics, Inc.
Kensington, Maryland

* Present position.

David Walker
Veterinary Pathologist
Director of Research
Wickham Research Laboratories Ltd.
Wickham, Hampshire
England

Prof. Y. Zeng
Head of Department of Tumor Viruses
Deputy Director of Institute of Virology
Chinese Academy of Medical Sciences
Member of WHO Advisory Panel
Beijing, China

NASAL TUMORS IN ANIMALS AND MAN

Gerd Reznik and Sherman F. Stinson

Volume I

Comparative Anatomy and Physiology of the Nasal Cavity
Comparative Anatomy and Histomorphology of the Nasal and Paranasal Cavities in Rodents
The Ultrastructure of Olfactory and Nasal Respiratory Epithelium Surfaces
Epidemiologic and Etiologic Aspects and Histopathology of Nasal Carcinoma in Finland
Nasal Cavity and Paranasal Sinus Tumors in Woodworkers and
Shoemakers in Italy Compared to Other Countries
Chronic Maxillary Sinusitis and the Epidemiology of Cancer of the Maxillary Sinus
Nasopharyngeal Carcinoma in Man
Cancer of the Nasopharynx in Man: Younger Age Peak and Related Aspects
Cancer of the Nasopharynx in Kuwait and Other Arabian Countries
Nasopharyngeal Carcinoma in Alaskan Natives

Volume II

Histopathologic Classification of Human Sinonasal Tumors
Nasal Cancer in Nickel Workers. Histopathological Findings and Nickel Concentrations in
the Nasal Mucosa of Nickel Workers, and a Short Review of Chromium and Arsenic
Pseudostratified Metaplastic, Dysplastic, and Carcinomatous Nasal Mucosa in Nickel
Workers: A Study by Scanning Electron, Transmission Electron, and Light Microscopy
Nasal Neuroblastomas in Man
Primary Meningioma of the Nasal Cavity and Paranasal Sinuses
Olfactory Esthesioneuroblastoma
Endocrine-Amphicrine Enteric Carcinoma of the Nasal Mucosa in Man
Neoplasms of the Nasal Cavity of Cattle and Sheep
Canine and Feline Nasal and Paranasal Neoplasm: Morphology and Origin
Comparative Aspects of Nasal Passage Carcinoma in Dogs with Man
Tumors of the Nasal Cavity in Nondomesticated Animals

Volume III

Nasal Airway Anatomy and Inhalation Deposition in Experimental Animals and People
The Pathogenesis of Nasal Neoplasia Induced by Alkylating and Aldehyde Compounds
Nitrosamine-Induced Nasal Cavity Carcinogenesis
Experimental Nasal Cavity Tumors Induced by Tobacco-Specific Nitrosamines (TSNA)
Histopathology of the Nasal Cavity in Laboratory Animals Exposed to Cigarette Smoke
and Other Irritants
Radiation-Induced Nasal Cavity Tumors in Animals
Nasal Cavity Cancer in Laboratory Animal Bioassays of Environmental Compounds
Epstein-Barr Virus and Nasopharyngeal Carcinoma
Studies on the Relationship Between Epstein-Barr Virus (EBV) and Nasopharyngeal
Carcinoma (NPC) in China
Nasal Cavity Carcinogens: Possible Routes of Metabolic Activation
Metabolism of N-Nitrosamines by the Nasal Mucosa
Summary and Conclusions

TABLE OF CONTENTS

Volume III

Chapter 1
Nasal Airway Anatomy and Inhalation Deposition in Experimental Animals and
People... 1
Jay P. Schreider

Chapter 2
The Pathogenesis of Nasal Neoplasia Induced by Alkylating and Aldehyde
Compounds 27
A. R. Sellakumar, R. Albert, and M. Kuschner

Chapter 3
Nitrosamine-Induced Nasal Cavity Carcinogenesis 47
Hildegard M. Reznik-Schüller

Chapter 4
Experimental Nasal Cavity Tumors Induced by Tobacco-Specific Nitrosamines
(TSNA) 79
A. Rivenson, K. Furuya, S. S. Hecht, and D. Hoffman

Chapter 5
Histopathology of the Nasal Cavity in Laboratory Animals Exposed to Cigarette Smoke
and Other Irritants.. 115
David Walker

Chapter 6
Radiation-Induced Nasal Cavity Tumors in Animals 137
Stephen A. Benjamin

Chapter 7
Nasal Cavity Cancer in Laboratory Animal Bioassays of Environmental Compounds .. 157
Sherman F. Stinson

Chapter 8
Epstein-Barr Virus and Nasopharyngeal Carcinoma 171
Lee S. Tuckwiller and Ronald Glaser

Chapter 9
Studies on the Relationship between Epstein-Barr Virus (EBV) and Nasopharyngeal
Carcinoma (NPC) in China... 187
Y. Zeng

Chapter 10
Nasal Cavity Carcinogens: Possible Routes of Metabolic Activation 201
Stephen S. Hecht, Andre Castonguay, and Dietrich Hoffmann

Chapter 11
Metabolism of *N*-Nitrosamines by the Nasal Mucosa....................................233
Eva B. Brittebo and Hans Tjälve

Chapter 12
Summary and Conclusions 251
Sherman F. Stinson and Gerd Reznik

Index 253

Chapter 1

NASAL AIRWAY ANATOMY AND INHALATION DEPOSITION IN EXPERIMENTAL ANIMALS AND PEOPLE

Jay P. Schreider

TABLE OF CONTENTS

I.   Introduction 2

II.   Methods of Study 2
       A.   Dissection and Tomography 2
       B.   Casting 2

III.   Nasal Airway Anatomy 4
       A.   Experimental Animals 4
       B.   Man 15

IV.   Aerosol Deposition in the Nasal Cavity 18
       A.   Physical Factors Affecting Deposition and Clearance 18
             1.   Deposition 18
             2.   Clearance 19
       B.   Anatomical Factors Affecting Deposition 20
             1.   Experimental Animals 20
             2.   Man 21
       C.   Deposition in Experimental Animals 21
             1.   Deposition in Positive Casts of the Guinea Pig and Rat 21
             2.   In Vivo Exposures 21
       D.   Deposition in Man 22

V.   Summary 23

Acknowledgments 23

References 25

I. INTRODUCTION

Laboratory animals such as rats, guinea pigs, dogs, and monkeys are commonly used in inhalation toxicology research as surrogates for human exposures. The toxicity of a substance inhaled by these animals depends partially on the extent and loci of deposition in the respiratory tracts. Deposition, in turn, depends on particle characteristics (size, density, and shape), on physical characteristics of the respiratory system, and on the kinetics of gas flow within the system. Differences in deposition characteristics between humans and experimental animals will influence extrapolation of toxicity results obtained with these animals to human beings.

An anatomical model of the respiratory airways is thus necessary for the calculation of the deposition characteristics, for the interpretation of the data from exposure studies, and for the extrapolation of the data found with experimental animals to people. In turn, accurate knowledge of the anatomy of the nasal-pharyngeal airway is essential to the development of an airway model.

II. METHODS OF STUDY

A. Dissection and Tomography

A number of methods are available for studying the anatomy of the nasal airways. Gross dissection and measurement have been used to provide a general picture of the airways of the human being[1] and various laboratory animals, including the rhesus monkey,[2] dog,[3] rat,[4] and guinea pig.[5] Greater detail can be added through the use of transverse sections of the head. This method has been used to some extent in a study of the rat[6] and in a study of European insectivores.[7] Transverse sectioning was used in a very complete fashion in a study of the nasal cavity of the European hamster,[8] in which serial and graded sections were prepared from the fixed heads of a number of male and female hamsters. Although numerical values were not included, a fairly complete picture of the nasal cavity was generated.

Computed tomography was used by Montgomery et al.[9] to generate coronal tomograms of four human cadaver specimens. The tomograms were made at 4-mm intervals from the base of the nostrils to the level of the posterior nasal spine. In addition to providing a picture of the human nasal airways, the tomograms were also used to determine the cross-sectional area of the airways at various positions. This work will be considered later in comparison to the experimental animals.

B. Casting

Casts of the respiratory airways are a valuable aid in the study of anatomical measurements. Precise measurements can be made from replica casts. The casts also assist in the elucidation of the morphologic arrangement of the respiratory tract on a gross level. The respiratory airways should be cast as a single unit; casting the nasal, laryngeal, and lung regions from one animal at the same time obviates scaling problems in relating the dimensions of the regions. In addition, the single cast system establishes the spatial arrangement of the regions and postural effects on their relative positions.

A number of methods have been used to produce casts of excised lungs and in some cases, the nasal region (dog,[10-12] cat,[13] human,[14,15] etc.). Schreider and Hutchens[16] prepared epoxy casts of the nasal region and excised lungs of the guinea pig, the measurements of which will be considered later in this chapter. The brittle nature of these casts necessitated some cast destruction to study the finer details. Phalen et al.[17] produced *in situ* silicone rubber casts of the lungs of hamsters, rats, monkeys, beagles, and humans.

Flexible silicone rubber replica casts of the nasal-pharyngeal airways of rats, beagles, and monkeys were prepared by the method of Schreider and Raabe,[18] using a modified method of Phalen et al.[17] Shrinkage of the casting material is small (less than 0.1%). Silicone rubber was introduced through a tracheal cannula of a freshly killed animal and forced up through the nasal cavity and out through the external nares. In a normal state, the animals have some mucus in the various areas of the nasal cavity. In order to produce complete casts, the mucus was washed out of the nasal cavity prior to casting, so the anatomical information represents a mucus-free state. The silicone rubber was allowed to cure and the surrounding tissue was digested in concentrated potassium hydroxide, leaving a replica cast of the nasal-pharyngeal airways. No respiratory abnormalities were revealed upon dissection of the animals.

The casts used in this study were from two male rats (chronic respiratory disease-free Sprague-Dawley, *Rattus norvegicus,* Albinus, HLA-SD) weighing 250 and 320 g; a male rhesus monkey (*Macaca mulatta,* obtained from the California Primate Research Center, Davis, Calif.) weighing 7 kg; and three adult male beagle dogs (*Canis familiaris,* purebred from the Laboratory for Energy-Related Health Research, Davis, Calif.) weighing 10, 11, and 12 kg. None of the animals had a history of any respiratory or other medical abnormalities.

The gross structures of the whole casts were examined and measured. Special attention was paid to any anatomic structures that might affect airflow or deposition and to differences in structure between the three species, and to any variations in structure in animals of the same species. The flexible nature of the rubber molding compound allowed the more complex parts of the casts to be unfolded and the internal portions to be examined and measured. Linear dimensions were measured using a linear micrometer ocular on a dissecting microscope, a 7× optical comparator, and for the largest structures, a vernier caliper. The angles of curvature of the various passages were measured with a protractor reticule in the optical comparator. The volumes of the nasal cavities (not including the nasopharynx) were estimated by measuring the volume of water displaced by the casts.

A shortcoming of studies of this type involving detailed dissection and measurement of replica airway casts is that it is practical to sufficiently evaluate only a few casts to be used as the basis for a model of the airways. While the procedure for producing replica casts is fairly straightforward,[17,18] morphometric measurements are complex and tedious. Practicality limited the number of specimens that were fully evaluated. Hence, only one representative cast for each species was chosen for detailed measurements.

Following gross examination, cross-sections were made of the most complete cast of each species, including the previously mentioned epoxy cast of the guinea pig nasal cavity, at various points along their length. Each of the these cross-sections was made in a plane perpendicular to the primary local airflow direction. The distance of each section from the anterior tip of the cast was recorded. In all cases, cross-sections were made of the right side of the cast until the two sides joined together to form a single unit, after which the cross-sections were made of the entire cast. The two sides of the nose were treated as mirror images, since examination of the unsectioned casts indicated that the nasal regions were symmetric around the anterior-posterior plane. This method of sectioning allowed each section to be seen in relation to the nasal region as a whole. The cross-sections were made approximately every 5 mm in the dog and monkey, every 1 to 2 mm in the guinea pig, and every 1 mm in the rat. In some cases, it was necessary to support the casts in an epoxy or paraffin matrix prior to sectioning, maintaining the positions of the side pockets relative to the main portion of the casts.

Full-size replicate drawings were made of each of the cross-sections for the dog and monkey. The sections of the dog and monkey casts were large enough to permit accurate tracing of the sections. In some cases, it was possible to lightly ink one side of the cross-section and make an imprint of the section on drawing paper, taking special care to ensure that the sections were not distorted. The small size of the rat and the guinea pig casts precluded tracing or imprinting. The cross-sections were placed on finely ruled graph paper and examined under a dissecting microscope equipped with a linear micrometer ocular. Detailed enlarged (5×) drawings were made of these sections with these measurements.

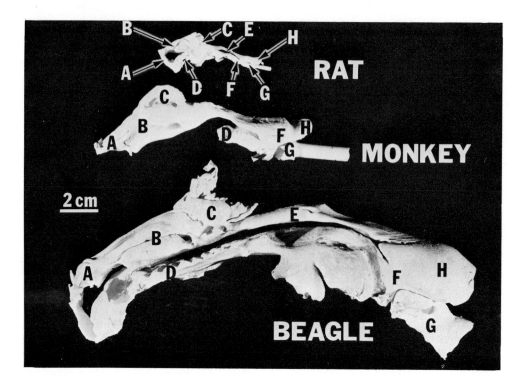

FIGURE 1.   Silicone rubber casts of the nasal-pharyngeal airway of the rat, rhesus monkey, and beagle. (A) external nares; (B) respiratory turbinate region; (C) ethmoturbinate region; (D) mouth and oropharynx; (E) nasopharynx; (F) larynx and laryngopharynx; (G) trachea; (H) laryngopharynx and esophagus.

An image analyzing computer was used to measure the perimeter and area of the diagram of each cross-section. When side pockets were in the same section with the main airway, the perimeters and cross-sectional areas of side pockets and main airways were measured separately. When a section was cut from the right half of the nasal cast, the perimeter and cross-sectional area of both the right and left sides of the nose at that point was estimated by doubling the values for the right side.

III. NASAL AIRWAY ANATOMY

A. Experimental Animals

The casts of the nasal-pharyngeal airway (Figure 1) include the oral cavity of the rat and dog. The cast from the airway of the guinea pig (Figure 2) includes the oral cavity, but stops at the larynx. The positions of the nasal cavities of the rat, monkey, and beagle in relation to the rest of the respective respiratory tract are shown in Figure 3. The differences in the bends of the nasopharynx are clearly demonstrated. These differences are obviously correlated with the differences in the posture of the three animals.

While sections were made from only the right sides of the nasal casts when the two sides were separate, the left sides are drawn as mirror images for clarity in the diagrams of the cross-sections (rat in Figure 4; guinea pig in Figure 5; beagle in Figure 6; and rhesus monkey in Figure 7). The diagrams of each section are numbered correspondingly for reference in both the figures and Tables 1 to 4 (rat, guinea pig, beagle, and monkey, respectively) which give the distance from the anterior end of the nose to the location of each section, the perimeter of the section, and the cross-sectional area of the section. The nasal-pharyngeal airway can be divided into the regions of the nares, maxilloturbinates, ethmoturbinates,

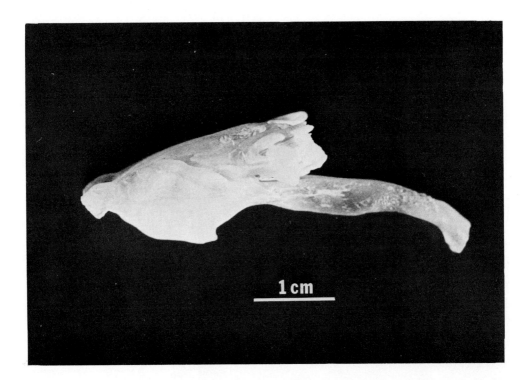

FIGURE 2.   Epoxy cast of the nasal-pharyngeal airway of the guinea pig.

pharynx (including nasopharynx, oropharynx, epiglottis, and laryngopharynx), and larynx; however, the boundaries are not distinct and the regions may overlap.

The most complete cast of the rat was from the 250-g animal. The cast from the 320-g rat was almost identical in structure and gross dimension to that of the 250-g animal. The external naris is 0.5-cm long and encompasses sections 1 through 6 (Figure 4). The naris makes a 40° horizontal bend in sections 4 and 5. This bend brings the two sides of the nose closer together. In sections 4, 5, and 6, the nares become more plate-like and folded. In the respiratory turbinates (sections 7 through 13), the airways become quite scrolled and tortuous. The ethmoturbinate region is made up of sections 14 through 20. In sections 14 and 15, the two sides of the nose make 10° inward bends and join together to form a single unit. The ethmoturbinate region is made up of both a scrolled main structure and a number of air pockets, some of which are the sinuses. The beginnings of the largest pockets can be seen in section 14. When sections have separate air pockets, two sets of values are given in Table 1; one set for the entire section and one set for the main airway alone. The overlapping of regions is evident in sections 17 through 20. The volume of the nasal cavity from nares to, but not including, the nasopharynx is 0.4 cm^3. The nasopharynx begins in section 17, but the pockets of the ethmoturbinate region are still present. The nasopharynx makes a gradual downward bend of 15° in sections 22 through 24. The openings of the Eustachian tubes are seen in section 23. The oropharynx (bottom cavity) begins in section 25. The perimeters and cross-sectional areas of the separated sections of the oropharynx are not included in the values given in Table 1. In section 27, the nasopharynx and oropharynx join and cross in the pharyngeal isthmus. The airway makes a dorsal-ventral bend of 45° in section 27. In the upper portion of section 28, the oropharynx gives rise to the laryngo-pharynx. The epiglottis is found between sections 27 and 28. Since the epiglottis is in a middle position (due to casting material), the laryngopharynx forms a common chamber with the larynx. In section 29 the two passages have separated with the larynx on the bottom

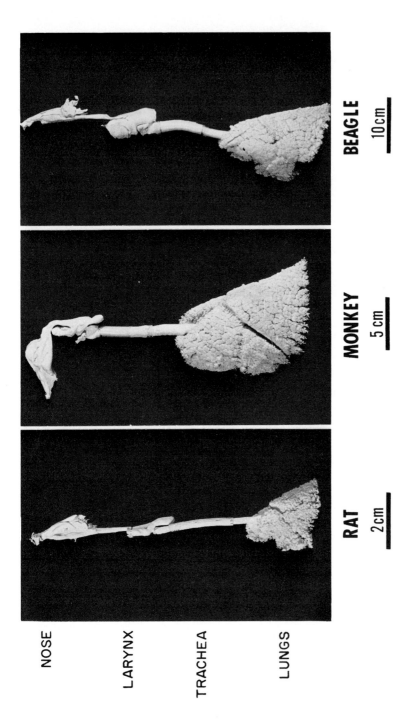

NOSE

LARYNX

TRACHEA

LUNGS

RAT
2 cm

MONKEY
5 cm

BEAGLE
10 cm

FIGURE 3.   Silicone rubber casts of the entire respiratory airway of a rat, monkey, and beagle.

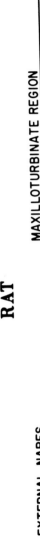

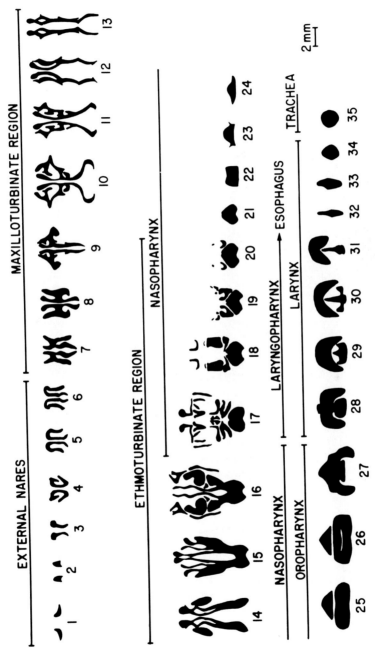

FIGURE 4.   Cross-sections of a cast of the nasal-pharyngeal airway of the rat. The numbers under each diagram correspond to the values in Table 1. (From Schreider, J.P. and Raabe, O.G., *Anat. Rec.*, 200, 195, 1981. With permission.)

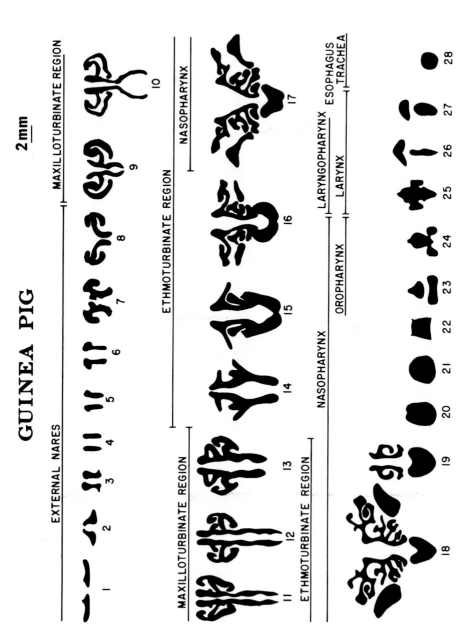

FIGURE 5.   Cross-sections of a cast of the nasal-pharyngeal airway of the guinea pig.   The numbers under each diagram correspond to the values in Table 2. (From Schreider, J.P. and Raabe, O.G., *Anat. Rec.*, 200, 195, 1981. With permission.)

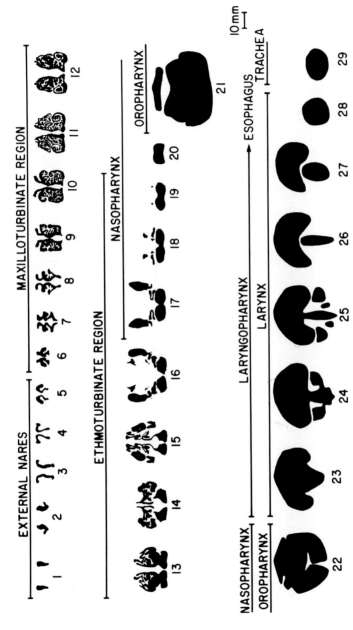

FIGURE 6. Cross-sections of a cast of the nasal-pharyngeal airway of the beagle. The numbers under each diagram correspond to the values in Table 3. (From Schreider, J.P. and Raabe, O.G., *Anat. Rec.*, 200, 195, 1981. With permission.)

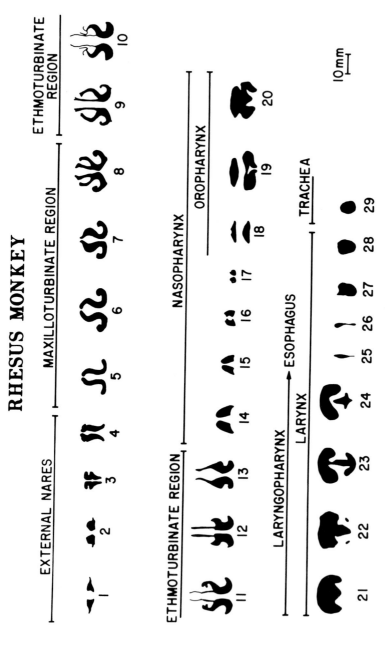

FIGURE 7.   Cross-sections of a cast of the nasal-pharyngeal airway of the rhesus monkey. The numbers under each diagram correspond to the values in Table 4. (From Schreider, J.P. and Raabe, O.G., *Anat. Rec.*, 200, 195, 1981. With permission.)

Table 1
DIMENSIONS OF THE CROSS-
SECTIONS OF THE NASAL CAST OF
THE RAT

Section number	Distance from anterior end of nose (mm)	Perimeter (mm)	Area (mm²)
1	0	8.3	1.4
2	1	5.6	1.3
3	2	11.9	2.0
4	3	21.7	3.5
5	4	23.4	3.8
6	5	27.3	4.5
7	5.5	35.0	7.6
8	7	38.3	9.9
9	8	44.0	9.3
10	10	73.9	13.2
11	12	63.5	10.3
12	14	54.4	10.3
13	16	48.3	8.1
14	17	67.6	16.7
14[a]	17	57.8	13.0
15	18	58.4	21.7
16	19	104.1	25.8
16[a]	19	47.5	14.0
17	20	97.8	17.0
17[a]	20	9.0	5.0
18	21	44.5	12.5
18[a]	21	9.0	5.0
19	22	30.9	7.7
19[a]	22	8.5	4.2
20	23	17.4	5.9
20[a]	23	8.9	4.9
21	25	7.5	3.6
22	32	7.9	3.7
23	35	8.6	2.8
24	37	7.7	2.2
25	40	8.4	3.4
26	41	8.7	3.4
27	42	23.7	15.8
28	43	24.2	14.9
29	44	9.2	3.2
30	44.5	12.8	3.2
31	45	7.6	1.8
32	45.5	7.4	1.9
33	46	7.8	3.1
34	47	6.5	3.0
35	52	7.1	3.8

[a]   Main airway alone. Does not include separate pockets.

and the laryngopharynx on the top (eventually giving rise to the esophagus). The side pockets on the larynx in sections 29 and 30 are the laryngeal ventricles. The larynx makes a reverse ventral-dorsal bend of 45° in sections 30 and 31. The larynx gradually assumes a rounded shape, giving rise to the trachea around section 35.

The cast of the guinea pig that was used for the generation of the cross-sections was from a 600-g animal. The external naris is 0.5-cm long and encompasses sections 1 through 8 (Figure 5). The naris makes an approximately 40° horizontal bend in sections 5 through 8.

Table 2
DIMENSIONS OF THE CROSS-SECTIONS OF THE NASAL CAST OF THE GUINEA PIG

Section number	Distance from anterior end of nose (mm)	Perimeter (mm)	Area (mm²)
1	0	18.0	5.0
2	1	14.0	4.4
3	2	15.3	4.9
4	2.5	12.4	3.6
5	3	13.9	4.2
6	3.5	18.5	5.4
7	4	32.9	13.0
8	5.0	19.8	13.4
9	8	66.4	20.4
10	11	88.0	21.5
11	16	91.5	28.6
12	18	91.2	31.1
13	20	82.0	36.2
14	22	62.7	30.1
15	24	75.1	38.1
16	26	109.4	44.4
16[a]	26	94.3	39.2
17	28	153.5	58.1
17[a]	28	14.9	11.2
18	31	184.6	73.4
18[a]	31	14.5	10.8
19	34	14.2	13.3
19[a]	34	8.2	11.7
20	39	13.9	13.7
21	45	13.2	13.2
22	50	12.0	8.1
23	55	8.0	4.1
24	56	18.9	8.8
25	57	20.7	12.7
26	59	8.9	2.8
27	62	9.1	5.1
28	70	8.6	5.7

[a]   Main airway alone. Does not include side pockets.

The respiratory turbinate region is made up of sections 9 through 13 and assumes a scrolled structure. The ethmoturbinate region is made up of sections 15 through 19. In section 19, the two sides of the nose join to form a single unit. As with the rat, this region is made up of both a scrolled main portion and various side pockets. Portions of the maxillary sinus or recess can be seen in sections 16 through 18. The overlapping of the regions of the ethmoturbinate and the nasopharynx can be seen in sections 17 through 19. The volume of the nasal cavity from the nares to the beginning of the nasopharynx is 0.88 cm^3. The nasopharynx runs from section 17 to section 24. The nasopharynx makes a gradual 30° downward bend in sections 21 through 23. The openings of the Eustachian tubes are seen in section 22. The oropharynx is seen in section 23. In section 24, the oropharynx and nasopharynx join in the pharyngeal isthmus. Between sections 23 and 24, there is a 45° downward bend in the airway. In the upper portion of section 25, the oropharynx gives rise to the laryngopharynx. The epiglottis is found between sections 24 and 25. In section 26, the two portions have separated into the laryngopharynx (top) and the larynx (bottom). The larynx is at its narrowest

Table 3
DIMENSIONS OF THE CROSS-
SECTIONS OF THE NASAL CAST OF
THE BEAGLE

Section number	Distance from anterior end of nose (mm)	Perimeter (mm)	Area (mm^2)
1	0	40.0	33.3
2	5	50.3	42.3
3	10	72.5	44.8
4	15	66.5	32.0
5	20	63.8	37.6
6	25	70.1	49.6
7	30	106.3	75.9
8	35	143.4	95.5
9	40	294.8	155.0
10	43	503.0	205.8
11	50	674.3	228.4
11[a]	50	665.6	227.3
12	55	470.6	267.3
13	60	333.9	312.5
14	65	318.8	240.9
14[a]	65	64.3	91.2
15	70	424.1	277.5
15[a]	70	55.1	68.0
16	75	266.8	289.5
16[a]	75	109.1	143.8
17	80	200.9	272.5
17[a]	80	54.5	113.9
18	90	121.5	138.3
18[a]	90	52.6	105.3
19	100	44.4	95.2
19[a]	100	35.6	92.6
20	120	39.3	88.8
21	150	64.0	139.1
22	160	184.5	1022.5
23	170	131.0	871.3
24	180	210.0	1055.4
25	185	250.9	933.6
25[a]	185	53.1	89.1
26	190	50.8	112.6
27	195	50.6	175.4
28	205	57.5	251.3
29	275	57.0	237.1

[a] Main airway alone. Does not include separate pockets.

point in section 26. The larynx makes a reverse ventral-dorsal bend in section 27. By section 28, the airway has rounded to form the trachea.

The most complete cast of the beagle nasal-pharyngeal airway was from the 10-kg animal. Although the casts from the 11- and 12-kg dogs were less complete, they were almost identical in structure to the cast from the 10-kg dog. The external naris is made up of sections 1 through 5 (Figure 6). The bend of the naris is 30° and takes place in sections 3 and 4. The respiratory turbinate region is made up of sections 6 through 12. The region is quite membranous, infolded, and complex. The ethmoturbinate region runs from sections 13 through 19. There are both folded membranous portions of the main airway (though less complex than the respiratory turbinates) and a number of separate pockets that open into

Table 4
DIMENSIONS OF THE CROSS-SECTIONS OF THE NASAL CAST OF THE RHESUS MONKEY

Section number	Distance from anterior end of nose (mm)	Perimeter (mm)	Area (mm²)
1	0	45.8	55.6
2	3	43.3	51.0
3	8	62.3	61.0
4	13	73.8	86.2
5	18	95.6	105.6
6	23	119.3	161.1
7	25	121.0	155.0
8	28	169.1	180.8
9	33	192.9	165.6
10	38	211.8	165.3
11	40	171.8	164.1
12	43	143.4	161.7
13	48	116.1	152.6
14	53	58.5	91.5
15	58	45.0	53.2
16	63	37.9	38.0
17	68	24.0	18.8
18	73	29.0	27.3
19	78	37.9	66.0
20	80	86.5	224.9
21	83	73.6	253.1
22	88	90.5	263.0
22[a]	88	75.4	256.4
23	90	118.8	257.3
24	93	34.1	43.8
25	95	27.6	15.8
26	98	29.5	18.2
27	103	35.0	72.0
28	105	33.3	75.4
29	110	27.9	56.1

[a]   Main airway alone. Does not include separate pockets.

the main airway through narrow openings. The maxillary recesses begin in section 13 and continue to a point between sections 13 and 14. Portions of the frontal sinuses begin in section 14. The frontal sinuses were not completely cast, and in some cases, it is difficult to distinguish between parts of the frontal sinuses and parts of the ethmoturbinates. The large pockets in sections 16 and 17 are parts of the lateral frontal sinuses. In section 17 the two sides of the nose join and form the nasopharynx. The volume of the nasal cavity from nares to nasopharynx was 20 cm³. As in the rat, parts of the ethmoid pockets are present over the nasopharynx. The pockets end by section 19. In sections 19 and 20, there is a gradual 30° dorsal to ventral bend in the nasopharynx. The nasopharynx flattens in section 21. The oropharynx may also be seen in section 21. In section 22, the two passages cross in the pharyngeal isthmus. In this section, the nasopharynx makes a 50° dorsal to ventral bend and the oropharynx gives rise to the laryngopharynx. The epiglottis is between sections 22 and 23. The laryngeal ventricles can be seen in section 24. In section 25, the posterior portions of these ventricles are seen as distinct pockets. The larynx is at its narrowest state in this section and makes a reverse ventral to dorsal bend of 50°. By section 26, the larynx has separated from the laryngopharynx. The trachea, which begins at section 29, undergoes a gradual 30° dorsal to ventral bend over the anterior half of the trachea.

In the rhesus monkey, the external naris is about 1.3-cm long and is made up of sections 1 through 4 (Figure 7). The horizontal bend of the naris in sections 2 and 3 is 30°. The respiratory turbinate region is composed of sections 5 through 8. This region develops from a single chamber into three connected, flattened chambers with a fairly simple scroll shape. In the ethmoturbinate region (sections 9 through 13), portions of the chambers narrow to a more membranous form. The volume of the nasal cavity from nares to nasopharynx is 8 cm³. Section 14 marks the beginning of the nasopharynx, which continues as two separate airways. The two sides of the nose join to form a single unit between sections 17 and 18 and flatten after joining. The nasopharynx makes an 80° dorsal to ventral bend in sections 16 through 18. The bottom passage in section 18 is the oropharynx. The two passages cross in the pharyngeal isthmus of section 20. The epiglottis is found between sections 20 and 21. In section 21, the nasopharynx makes a 45° dorsal to ventral bend and the oropharynx gives rise to the laryngopharynx. Again, since the epiglottis is in a middle position, the larynx and the laryngopharynx form a common chamber through section 22. In section 22, the two separate pockets are the anterior portions of the laryngeal ventricles, seen more clearly in section 23. In section 23, the airway makes a reverse 45° ventral to dorsal bend. The larynx and laryngopharynx are separated in section 24. The larynx becomes quite narrow in sections 25 and 26, then expands to give rise to the trachea by section 29.

The largest cross-sectional areas for the rat and guinea pig are found in the ethmoturbinate region, followed by the region of the pharyngeal isthmus. In the beagle and rhesus monkey, the largest cross-sectional area is in the region of the pharyngeal isthmus, followed by the turbinate regions. In the rat and guinea pig, the smallest cross-sectional area is found in the areas of the nares and larynx. The monkey has the smallest area in the larynx and nasopharynx, while the beagle has the smallest area in the nares. The greatest perimeters for the rat, guinea pig, and rhesus monkey are found in the ethmoturbinate regions. In the beagle, the largest perimeter is found in the respiratory turbinate region.

B. Man

The position of the human nasal cavity in relation to the rest of the respiratory tract is shown in Figure 8. As expected, this is very similar to the relative positions found with the rhesus monkey. A more detailed view of a sagittal section of the human nasal cavity is shown in Figure 9. Inside the naris is the dilated area of the vestibule. On the wall of the cavity are the superior, medial, and inferior turbinates or conchae, which divide the cavity into air passages or meatuses. The small openings to the paranasal sinuses and ethmoidal air cells are found on the lateral and rear walls of the cavity.

A number of the dimensions of the nasal cavity of an adult are given by Snyder[19] and Anson.[20] In the adult male, the naris is about 2.0-cm long and 0.7- to 0.8-cm wide. The length of the cavity is 7 to 8 cm in length from the most prominent part of the naris to the posterior border of the hard palate. The greatest vertical diameter is 4.0 to 4.5 cm from the nasal floor to the cribriform plate. The width of the roof is 0.1 to 0.3 cm and that of the floor at the widest part of the inferior meatus is 1.2 to 2.3 cm. The post-mortem value for the widths may have been much greater due to the shrinkage of the mucosa. The choana or posterior opening to the nasopharynx is 2.0- to 3.0-cm high, 1.2- to 1.7-cm wide at the floor, and 0.7- to 1.0-cm wide at the roof. The surface area of both vestibules is 21 cm². The surface area of the turbinates and nasal passages on both sides of the nose is 160 cm². The distance from the epiglottis to the trachea is 7.0 cm. The vertical diameter of the larynx is about 4.4 cm, the transverse diameter about 4.3 cm, and the anterior-posterior diameter about 3.6 cm. The anterior-posterior diameter of the trachea ranges from 1.3 to 2.3 cm and the transverse diameter ranges from 1.2 to 1.8 cm. The volume of the nasal cavity is given as 8 to 9 cm³ per side.

Using the previously mentioned computed tomograms of the nasal airway, Montgomery

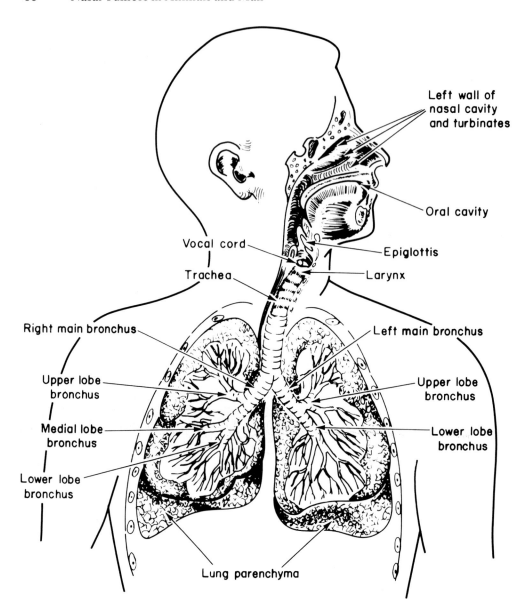

FIGURE 8.   The respiratory airways of man. (From Raabe, O. G., in *Mechanisms in Respiratory Toxicology,* Vol. I, CRC Press, Boca Raton, Fla., 1982, 27.)

et al.[9] generated a series of tracings of the nasal airway. The tracings were generated for four different human cadavers. Figure 10 shows the tracings of one of the specimens. In this specimen, the inferior turbinates started in section 1 and ended in section 11, while the medial turbinates began in section 2 and ended in section 10. Post-mortem shrinkage of the mucosa could have led to a larger than normal air passage. Table 5 gives the distance from the base of the nostrils at which each tomogram was made and the cross-sectional area of the airway at that point. These values were estimated from a graph of the cross-sectional areas of the airways. The volume of the right side was 11.5 cm³ and that of the left was 13.5 cm³. These volumes do not include the sinuses and are only for that region encompassed by the tomograms.

The region encompassed by the human sections is approximately equivalent to sections

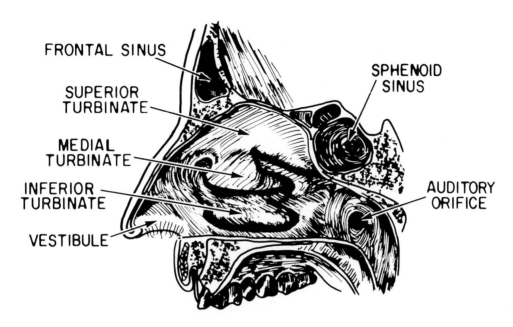

FIGURE 9. Sagittal section of the human nasal cavity showing the left lateral wall.

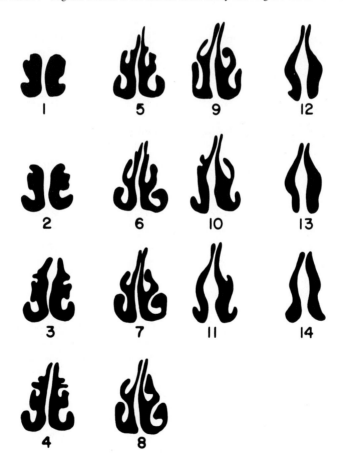

FIGURE 10. Tracing of tomograms of the human nasal airway. (From Montgomery, W., Vig, P., Staab, E., and Matteson, S., *Am. J. Orthodon.*, 76, 366, 1979. With permission.)

Table 5
DIMENSIONS OF THE TOMOGRAMS OF
THE NASAL CAVITY OF A HUMAN CADAVER

Section	Distance from base of nostrils (mm)	Area (mm²)	
		Left side	Right side
1	0	2.3	2.4
2	4	2.4	2.5
3	8	2.8	2.8
4	12	2.8	2.7
5	16	2.5	2.3
6	20	2.8	2.3
7	24	2.7	2.3
8	28	3.0	2.5
9	32	3.2	2.5
10	36	2.9	2.2
11	40	2.8	2.0
12	44	2.3	1.7
13	48	2.3	1.6
14	52	2.2	2.0

5 through 13 in the rhesus monkey (Figure 7). A comparison between the cross-sections of the human-nasal airway and that of the rhesus monkey shows a great deal of similarity. While the human sections do not include the regions of the external nares, pharynx, or larynx, the similarity between the turbinate regions suggests that the nasal cavity of the rhesus monkey would be an acceptable model for the human nasal cavity.

IV. AEROSOL DEPOSITION IN THE NASAL CAVITY

A. Physical Factors Affecting Deposition and Clearance

1. Deposition

The deposition of inhaled airborne particles in the respiratory airways will depend on the physical characteristics of the particles (size, density, and shape), on the physical characteristics of the airways, and on the kinetics of gas flow within the airways. There are five primary processes leading to particle deposition in the airways: electrostatic attraction, interception, impaction, gravitational settling, and Brownian diffusion (Figure 11). These processes are covered in detail in a recent review.[21] In all these cases, contact of the particle with the moist walls of the airways will result in the removal of the particle from the airstream.

Electrostatic forces on a particle may cause that particle to be attracted to and contact the walls of an airway. This process is probably a minor cause of particle deposition in the nasal airway. Fraser[22] found that if the particles in an aerosol had an average of 1000 electronic units of charge per particle, the inhalation deposition would be doubled. Melandri[23] found that the deposition of monodisperse aerosols in people would be enhanced if the particles were charged. The charge-to-mass ratio of a particle will determine the importance of electrostatic attraction on the extent of deposition.

Deposition by interception is caused by the noninertial incidental contact of a particle and the wall of an airway. This process will depend on the physical size of the particle and will be the most important for particles with large aspect ratios, such as long fibers. Deposition by this process would not take place if the particles were points rather than extended bodies.

As the velocity of an airstream changes direction or magnitude in, e.g., a bend or eddy, inertia will prevent a suspended particle from following exactly the path of the airstream.

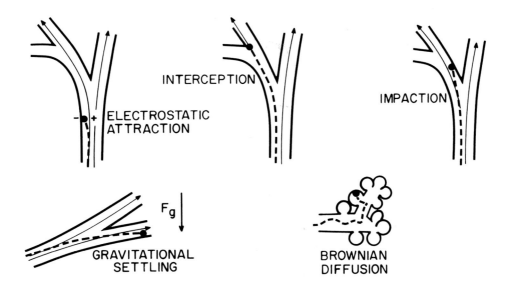

FIGURE 11.   Representation of five major mechanisms of deposition of inhaled airborne particles in the respiratory tract. (From Raabe, O. G., in *Mechanisms in Respiratory Toxicology,* Vol. I, CRC Press, Boca Raton, Fla., 1982, 27.)

If the inertia is great enough, the particle will impact on the walls of the airway. The extent of deposition due to impaction will depend on the initial velocity of the particle, the aerodynamic diameter of the particle, the dimensions of the airway, and the degree of the change in direction of the airstream.

Particles will settle downward under the influence of the earth's gravity. Deposition by this process can occur in any airway that is not exactly vertical. The extent of deposition due to gravitation will depend on the diameter of the airway, the inclination of the airway with respect to gravity, the velocity of the particle in the airway (and thus the residence time of the particle in the airway), and the aerodynamic diameter of the particle.

Small particles suspended in air are in constant random motion (Brownian motion) caused by bombardment of the particles by the gas molecules in air. The magnitude of the motion is described by the diffusion coefficient of the particle, which is determined by the physical diameter of the particle. If the motion of the particle is great enough, the particle will contact the walls of the airway. Diffusion primarily affects the deposition of particles with physical diameters less than 0.5 μm.[21]

Deposition by diffusion, electrostatic attraction, and interception depends on the physical size of the particle, while deposition by impaction and gravitational settling depends on the aerodynamic diameter of the particle. The physical and aerodynamic diameters of a particle can be quite different, depending on the shape and density of the particle. Since diffusion is the major process affecting the deposition of particles with physical diameters less than 0.5 μm, and impaction and settling are the most important processes for particles with aerodynamic diameters larger than 0.5 μm, 0.5 μm is often used as the boundary between the region of deposition regulated by physical diameter and the region regulated by aerodynamic diameter.[21]

2. Clearance

Particles deposited in the nasal cavity may be cleared by ciliary mucus flow or may be absorbed by the blood. The extent of clearance will depend on the characteristics of the deposited particles and on the sites of deposition. Particles that are freely soluble in body fluids may be absorbed by the blood before they are cleared by mucus flow. Less soluble particles may be partially absorbed by the blood. This partial absorption, which can have important consequences, may occur in the nasal turbinates even for only moderately soluble particles.[21]

The anterior third of the nose clears only by extrinsic means (blowing, sneezing, wiping, etc.), and particles deposited in this area may remain for one or more days after deposition.[21] In the posterior regions of the nose, mucociliary clearance averages 6 mm/min.[15,24,25] The International Commission on Radiological Protection (ICRP) Task Group[26] adopted a 4-min half-time as the mucociliary clearance rate from the nasal-pharyngeal region.

B. Anatomical Factors Affecting Deposition

1. Experimental Animals

Many of the structural similarities and differences between the nasal cavities of the four species reported on here have an important effect on the airflow and, as a result, on the deposition of particles from air flowing through these airways. The bend in the nares is the first change in direction of airflow in the nasal cavity and is a major site of deposition of larger particles.

The respiratory regions are the sites of the most obvious differences between the animals. This region in the rhesus monkey is a fairly simple scroll with relatively wide chambers, while in the dog it is extremely complex, with thin membranous chambers. Due to its complex and membranous nature, this region of the dog should be more effective than that of the monkey in removing many of the particles that penetrate the nares. The large surface area of the turbinates of the dog might be expected to be more effective in absorbing soluble gases than the relatively simple monkey turbinates. The complexity of the respiratory turbinates of the rat and guinea pig lie between that of the dog and monkey, and the particle deposition and gas uptake efficiency for this region of the nose might also be expected to lie between that for the monkey and the dog. In the dog, rat, and guinea pig much of the air is forced to flow through the complex turbinates. While there is a membranous portion in the ethmoturbinate region of the rhesus monkey, the air probably passes this portion by following a more direct path through the lower, wider portion of the region.

Due to the narrow openings and the airflow characteristics, it is improbable that there would be a significant amount of air exchange in the various sinuses and air pockets. In the ethmoid area, the airflow will change direction, passing down to the nasopharynx. Incoming air might not readily enter the pockets, but the change in direction and the structure around the openings to the pockets could result in the formation of eddies in the region.

The large bend of the nasopharynx of the monkey is due to the more erect posture of the monkey. Since the two sides of the nasopharynx join at this bend, this could be the site of additional particle deposition. In all the animals, the rapid expansions and contractions during breathing in the pharynx and larynx should result in some degree of turbulence in the airflow, leading to increased deposition. In addition, the structures of the larynx could be the site of considerable deposition by impaction for mouth breathing, in which case the particle-laden air would not have been previously depleted by passage through the nose. The rat and guinea pig are obligate nose breathers, while the dog and monkey will switch to mouth breathing at higher respiratory rates.

Using the anatomical measurements and the breathing characteristics of the animals, the Reynolds number (a dimensionless parameter partially describing airflow characteristics) can be calculated, assuming uniform flow, for each cross-section. The calculations suggest that turbulent flow will not take place in the nasal region of the rat or guinea pig but will take place in the nasopharynx and larynx of the rhesus monkey, and in the nares, nasopharynx and larynx of the beagle. The airflow in the nares of the monkey should be disturbed, but nonturbulent.

2. Man

Since the anterior nares in man have the smallest cross-sectional area of any section of the upper airway (see the previously presented dimensions), the velocity through this area will be the greatest. According to the work of Proctor et al.[27] and Proctor and Swift,[28] the airstream will bend and widen just posterior to this point and develop turbulence in the flow. The main airflow will then continue between the middle meatus and the septum at a reduced velocity. Just beyond the naris, a portion of the air is deflected downward and continues along the middle meatus. This air stream develops a number of eddies. The airstreams will converge in the region of the choana and continue into the nasopharynx. During normal inspiration, there will be some convergence of airstreams passing through the vocal cords, but turbulence will develop only below the larynx in the trachea. Under conditions of higher flow rates, the turbulence will develop higher but not above the larynx.[28] According to Proetz,[29] the airflow will not enter the sinuses.

Because of the turbulence and sharp bends, deposition by impaction would be expected to occur in the regions of the nares, the sharp bend in the nasopharynx, and in the laryngeal region. It is also expected that the low air velocity through (and thus long residence time in) the nasal cavity, coupled with the large diffusing area, would lead to a fairly efficient removal of soluble gases. While less than the removal is found with the more complex turbinate structure of some of the previously considered experimental animals, this removal should still be significant.

C. Deposition in Experimental Animals
1. Deposition in Positive Casts of the Guinea Pig and Rat

Acrylic molds of the nasal cavity of guinea pigs and rats were used to study particle deposition in these animals.[30-32] Briefly, a low melting metal alloy was used to produce a cast of the nasal cavity. The cast was then encased in casting acrylic and the metal melted out, leaving a positive cast or mold of the nasal cavity. The larynx was not included in this preparation. Monodisperse aerosols of unit density spherical particles of methylene blue, ranging in size from 1 to 7 μm, were pulled through the mold at a rate equivalent to the normal resting inhalation rate of the animal in question. The amount of material depositing in the cast was measured colorimetrically and compared to the amount deposited on a filter behind the cast to give the fraction of "inhaled" material that was deposited in the cast. The results of the deposition measurements are given in Figure 12. All the deposited material was found in the front third of the nose. The highest concentration was found just posterior to the nares, with the material fanning out in a posterior direction, in decreasing concentration, supporting the supposition that impaction is the main deposition process in the nasal cavity for the larger particles. No material was ever recovered in the sinuses or smaller air pockets, suggesting little or no air exchange into these pockets.

The use of acrylic nasal molds for deposition measurements has the advantages of yielding reproducible results and allowing easy visualization of the deposition sites. Like the previously discussed silicone rubber casts, the metal casts and the resulting acrylic molds were made from saline-rinsed, mucus-free noses. In addition, the walls of the mold were inflexible and devoid of nasal hairs. Because of the lack of mucus and nasal hairs, the deposition values should be treated as the lower limits of nasal deposition. It should also be noted that these deposition values do not include laryngeal deposition.

2. In Vivo Exposures

The small number of studies involving exposures to well-characterized aerosols of a series of particle sizes makes interspecies comparison of particle deposition very difficult. Raabe et al.[33] exposed hamsters and rats to a series of well-characterized, monodisperse, radiolabeled aluminosilicate aerosols. The deposition was measured for the entire nasal-pharyngeal

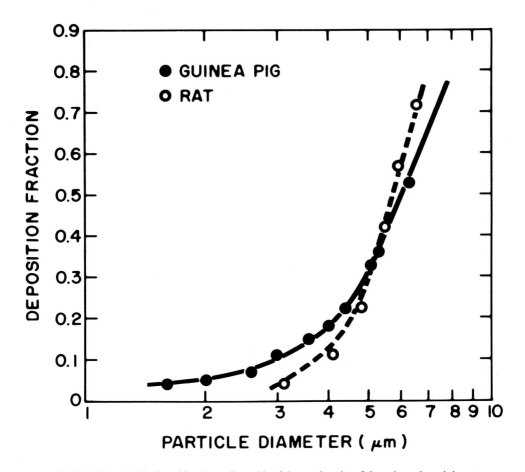

FIGURE 12.   Particle deposition in acrylic molds of the nasal cavity of the guinea pig and the rat.

region. Cuddihy et al.,[34] again using radiolabeled, monodisperse aerosols, measured deposition in the beagle nasal-pharyngeal region. Fairchild et al.[35] used a radiolabeled polydisperse aerosol of streptococcus to measure deposition in the nose and the nasopharynx. The results of these various exposures are shown in Figure 13. Frank et al.[36] found that up to 99% of SO_2 inhaled by the dog was taken up by the nose. Cameron et al.,[37] using rabbits and monkeys, found that up to 90% of inhaled mustard gas was taken up by the nose, while only 25% of inhaled phosgene was taken up by the nose.

D. Deposition in Man

Selected data[38-40] from experimental measurements of particle deposition in the nasal-pharyngeal region of man are presented in Figure 14. Also included are the values calculated by the ICRP Task Group on Lung Dynamics for 15 breaths per minute (BPM) and a tidal volume (TV) of 1450 cm³. The deposition fraction is plotted against the characteristic term (D_{ar}^2Q) that controls inertial impaction, where D_{ar} is the aerodynamic resistance diameter,[41] and Q is the minute volume. Speizer and Frank[42] have shown that virtually all the inhaled SO_2 is removed by the nasal-pharyngeal region of man.

While the scarcity of animal data and the high degree of intraexperimental variation make such comparisons equivocal, a comparison of Figures 13 and 14 indicates that the deposition data for experimental animals fall within the same range of values for man. This may be due to the number of factors, sometimes competing, that control deposition in this region. While the turbinates of the beagle, and to a lesser extent the rodents, are more complex

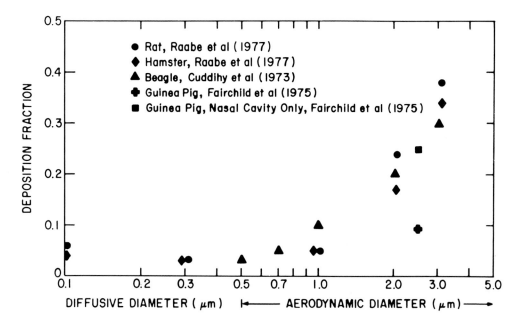

FIGURE 13.   Selected data[33-35] for the deposition of inhaled aerosols in experimental animals.

than those of the rhesus monkey and man, the bend in the nasopharynx of man and the rhesus monkey is much sharper than that of the beagle and rodents. In addition, the airflow in the nares of man, the beagle, and to a lesser extent the monkey, should be disturbed if not turbulent. Since the animals studied all have a sharp bend in the nares, and impaction is the principal means of deposition of the larger particles, it is not surprising that these larger particles are deposited to a similar extent in the various animals.

V. SUMMARY

The anatomical characteristics of the various experimental animals and man are summarized in Table 6. The surface areas of the nasal cavity of the experimental animals were estimated in a segmental calculation using the perimeter and thickness of the appropriate sections of each animal nasal cast (Tables 1 to 4). These surface areas do include the sinuses and air pockets, while the surface area of the human nasal cavity does not. The rest of the values were taken directly from the text and tables. The dimensions listed for the nasal cavity of man are those given by Snyder[19] and Anson.[20]

The anatomical characteristics of the nasal cavities of various experimental animals and man have been presented along with particle deposition considerations. There are a number of differences and similarities between the species. Perhaps one of the most obvious examples of anatomical differences is in the structure of the turbinate regions. Some of the differences could affect deposition of various sized particles in the nasal cavities. A degree of caution, therefore, has to be exercised in extrapolating the nasal deposition characteristics from one species to another. Simple scaling calculations may not be sufficient.

ACKNOWLEDGMENTS

The author is indebted to Drs. Steven Book, Wesley Harris, Leon Rosenblatt, and Otto Raabe for beneficial advice and assistance; Dr. Marvin Goldman for leadership as director of the Laboratory for Energy-Related Health Research; Shirley Coffelt for the preparation of the photographs; Ken Shiomoto for preparation of the illustrations; Charles Baty for

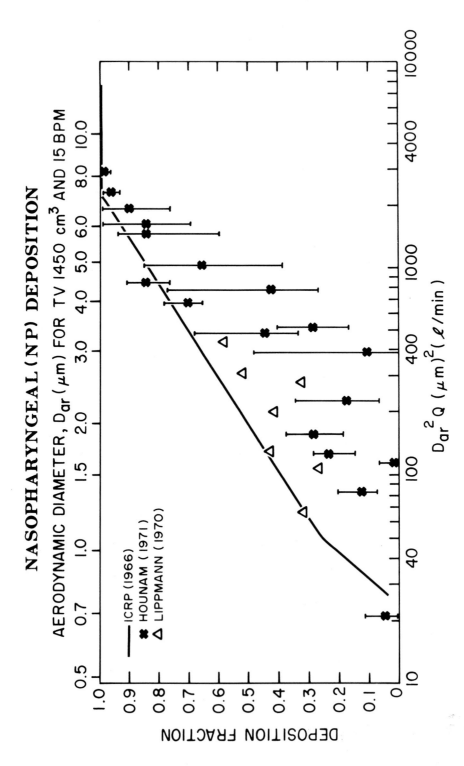

FIGURE 14.   Selected data[38-40] reported for the deposition fraction of monodisperse aerosols in the nasal-pharyngeal (NP) region of the respiratory tract are plotted against the characteristic term $(D_{ar}^2Q)^{39}$ that controls inertial impaction; for reference, the calculated value[24] is shown for 15 breaths per minute (BPM) at 1450 cm^3 tidal volume (TV). (From Raabe, O. G., in *Mechanisms in Respiratory Toxicology*, Vol. I, CRC Press, Boca Raton, Fla., 1982, 27.)

Table 6
INTERSPECIES COMPARISON OF NASAL CAVITY CHARACTERISTICS

	Rat	Guinea pig	Beagle	Rhesus monkey	Man
Weight	250 g	600 g	10 kg	7 kg	~70 kg
Naris cross-section	0.7 mm^2	2.5 mm^2	16.7 mm^2	22.9 mm^2	140 mm^2
Bend in naris	40°	40°	30°	30°	NA
Length	2.3 cm	3.4 cm	10 cm	5.3 cm	7—8 cm
Greatest vertical diameter	9.6 mm	12.8 mm	23 mm	27 mm	40—45 mm
Surface area (both sides of nasal cavity)	10.4 cm^2	27.4 cm^2	220.7 cm^2	61.6 cm^2	181 cm^2
Volume (both sides)	0.4 cm^3	0.9 cm^3	20 cm^3	8 cm^3	16—19 cm^3 (does not include sinuses)
Bend in nasopharynx	15°	30°	30°	80°	~90°
Turbinate complexity	Complex scroll	Complex scroll	Very complex membranous	Simple scroll	Simple scroll

Note: NA, not available.

preparation of the typescript; and Marion Lundquist for supervision of the clerical activities. This report was made possible by the support of the Office of Health and Environmental Research (OHER) of the U.S. Department of Energy (DOE) under contract DE-AMO3-76SF00472 with the University of California, Davis and has been assigned document number UCD 472-504.

REFERENCES

1. **Goss, C.,** *Anatomy of the Human Body by Henry Gray,* Lea & Febiger, Philadelphia, 1973.
2. **Hartman, C. and Strauss, W.,** *The Anatomy of the Rhesus Monkey,* Hafner, New York, 1933.
3. **Miller, M.,** *Anatomy of the Dog,* W. B. Saunders, Philadelphia, 1964.
4. **Hebel, R. and Stromberg, M.,** *Anatomy of the Laboratory Rat,* William & Wilkins, Baltimore, 1976.
5. **Cooper, G. and Schiller, A.,** *Anatomy of the Guinea Pig,* Harvard University Press, Cambridge, 1975.
6. **Leibich, H.,** Zum Bau der oberen Luftwege der weiblichen Ratte, *Anat. Anz.,* 138, 170, 1979.
7. **Wohrmann-Repenning, A.,** Zur vergleichenden makro- und mikroskopischen Anatomie der Nasenhöhle europäischer Insectivoren, *Gegenbaurs Morphol. Jahrb.,* 121, 698, 1975.
8. **Reznik, G. and Jensen, K.,** Anatomy of the nasal cavity of the European hamster, *Z. Versuchstierk,* 21, 321, 1979.
9. **Montgomery, W., Vig, P., Staab, E., and Matteson, S.,** Computed tomography: a three-dimensional study of the nasal airway, *Am. J. Orthodon.,* 76, 363, 1979.
10. **Rahn, H. and Ross, B.,** Bronchial tree casts, lobe weights and anatomical dead space measurements in the dog lung, *J. Appl. Physiol.,* 10, 154, 1957.
11. **Tucker, J. and Krementz, E.,** Anatomical corrosion specimens. II. Bronchopulmonary in the dog, *Anat. Rec.,* 127, 667, 1957.
12. **Eisman, M.,** Lung models, hollow flexible reproductions, *J. Appl. Physiol.,* 29, 541, 1970.
13. **Frank, N. and Yoder, R.,** A method of making a flexible cast of the lung, *J. Appl. Physiol.,* 21, 1925, 1966.
14. **Thompsett, D.,** *Anatomical Techniques,* E. S. Livingstone, London, 1970.
15. **Proctor, D. F. and Wagner, H. N.,** Mucociliary clearance in the human nose, in *Inhaled Particles and Vapours II,* Davies, C. N., Ed., Pergamon Press, Oxford, 1967, 25.

16. **Schreider, J. and Hutchens, J.,** Morphology of the guinea pig respiratory tract, *Anat. Rec.,* 196, 313, 1980.
17. **Phalen, R., Yeh, H., Raabe, O., and Velasquez, D.,** Casting of the lungs *in situ, Anat. Rec.,* 177, 255, 1973.
18. **Schreider, J. and Raabe, O.,** Replica casts of the entire respiratory airways of experimental animals, *J. Environ. Pathol. Toxicol.,* 4, 427, 1980.
19. **Snyder, W. S. (Chairman),** *International Commission on Radiological Protection (ICRP) Task Group on Reference Man,* Pergamon Press, Oxford, 1975, 151.
20. **Anson, B.,** *Morris' Human Anatomy,* McGraw-Hill, New York, 1966, 1394.
21. **Raabe, O. G.,** Deposition and clearance of inhaled aerosols, in *Mechanisms in Respiratory Toxicology,* Vol. I, CRC Press, Boca Raton, Fla., 1982, 27.
22. **Fraser, D. A.,** The deposition of unipolar charged particles in the lungs of animals, *Arch. Environ. Health,* 13, 152, 1966.
23. **Melandri, C., Prodi, V., Tarroni, G., Formignani, M., DeZaiacomo, T., Bompane, G. R., Maestri, G., and Giaconelli-Malton, G. G.,** On the deposition of unipolarly charged particles in the human respiratory tract, in *Inhaled Particles IV,* Walton, W. H., Ed., Pergamon Press, Elmsford, N.Y., 1977, 193.
24. **Proctor, D. F., Andersen, I., and Lundquist, G.,** Clearance of inhaled particles from the human nose, *Arch. Intern. Med.,* 131, 132, 1973.
25. **Proctor, D. F. and Wagner, H. N.,** Clearance of particles from the human nose, *Arch. Environ. Health,* 11, 366, 1965.
26. **Morrow, P. E. (Chairman),** International Commission on Radiological Protection (ICRP) Task Group on Lung Dynamics, Deposition and retention models for internal dosimetry of the human respiratory tract, *Health Phys.,* 12, 173, 1966.
27. **Proctor, D. F., Swift, D. L., Quinlan, M., Salman, S., Takagi, Y., and Evering, S.,** The nose and man's atmospheric environment, *Arch. Environ. Health,* 18, 671, 1969.
28. **Proctor, D. F. and Swift, D.,** The nose — a defense against the atmospheric environment, *Inhaled Particles III,* Vol. 1, Walton, W. H., Ed., Unwin Brothers Ltd., Surrey, England, 1971, 59.
29. **Proetz, A.,** Air currents in the upper respiratory tract and their clinical importance, *Ann. Otol. Rhinol. Laryngol.,* 60, 439, 1951.
30. **Schreider, J.,** Lung Anatomy and Characteristics of Aerosol Retention of the Guinea Pig, Ph.D. thesis, Division of Biological Sciences, Department of Pharmacological and Physiological Sciences, University of Chicago, 1977.
31. **Schreider, J. and Hutchens, J.,** Particle deposition in the guinea pig respiratory tract, *J. Aerosol Sci.,* 10, 599, 1979.
32. **Hutchens, J. and Schreider, J.,** unpublished data, 1977.
33. **Raabe, O., Yeh, H., Newton, G., Phalen, R., and Velasquez, D.,** Deposition of inhaled monodisperse aerosols in small rodents, in *Inhaled Particles IV,* Walton, W., Ed., Pergamon Press, Elmsford, N.Y., 1977, 3.
34. **Cuddihy, R., Brownstein, D., Raabe, O., and Kanapilly, G.,** Respiratory tract deposition of inhaled polydisperse aerosols in beagle dogs, *J. Aerosol Sci.,* 4, 35, 1973.
35. **Fairchild, G., Stultz, S., and Coffin, D.,** Sulfuric acid effect on the deposition of radioactive aerosol in the respiratory tract of guinea pigs, *Am. Ind. Hyg. Assoc. J.,* 36, 584, 1975.
36. **Frank, N. R., Yoder, R., Brain, J., and Yokoyama, E.,** SO_2 (^{35}S labeled) absorption by the nose and mouth under conditions of varying concentration and flow, *Arch. Environ. Health,* 18, 315, 1964.
37. **Cameron, G., Gaddum, J., and Shorf, R.,** The absorption of war gases by the nose, *J. Pathol.,* 58, 449, 1946.
38. **Hounam, R., Black, A., and Walsh, M.,** The deposition of aerosol particles in the nasopharyngeal region of the human respiratory tract, in *Inhaled Particles III,* Walton, W., Ed., Unwin Brothers Ltd., Surrey, England, 1971, 71.
39. **Hounam, R., Black, A., and Walsh, M.,** The deposition of aerosol particles in the nasopharyngeal region of the human respiratory tract, *J. Aerosol Sci.,* 2, 47, 1971.
40. **Lippmann, M.,** Deposition and clearance of inhaled particles in the human nose, *Ann. Otol.,* 79, 519, 1970.
41. **Raabe, O. G.,** Aerosol aerodynamic size conventions for inertial sampler calibration, *J. Air Poll. Control Assoc.,* 26, 856, 1976.
42. **Speizer, F. and Frank, N.,** The uptake and release of SO_2 by the human nose, *Arch. Environ. Health,* 12, 725, 1966.

Chapter 2

THE PATHOGENESIS OF NASAL NEOPLASIA INDUCED BY ALKYLATING AND ALDEHYDE COMPOUNDS

A. R. Sellakumar, R. Albert and M. Kuschner

TABLE OF CONTENTS

I.   Introduction 28

II.   Carcinogenicity of Dimethylcarbamoyl Chloride (C_3H_6ONCl).................. 28

        A.   Inhalation Studies with Rats 28
        B.   Pathology of Hamsters.. 29
        C.   Differences in Species Susceptibility to DMCC 33

III.   Nasal Tumors Induced by Epichlorohydrin..................................... 33

IV.   Nasal Tumors Induced by Bis(Chloromethyl)Ether............................. 34

V.   Carcinogenicity of Aldehydes 36

VI.   Discussion 40

Acknowledgments... 42

References.. 44

I. INTRODUCTION

Various segments of the respiratory system manifest different patterns of susceptibility to any given carcinogen. There seems to be a general pattern of response of the respiratory tract with regard to different classes of carcinogens, distinctly affecting certain portions of the respiratory tract and inducing morphologically different types of lesions and tumors. The response also varies when different species of animals are used.

In past studies involving the respiratory tract, major importance was usually placed on the lower respiratory tract, specifically the bronchi and lungs. Many investigators quite often failed to examine changes in the nasal epithelium. Lately, a number of important chemicals have shown preneoplastic and neoplastic lesions in the nasal area. Nitroso compounds have shown various types of tumors in the nose of several species,[1-4] but little data are available on nonnitroso compounds. This chapter will focus primarily on the different direct-acting alkylating and acylating agents and aldehydes and their mode of action in the nasal epithelium, based upon our studies with dimethylcarbamoyl chloride (DMCC), epichlorohydrin (ECH), bis(chloromethyl)ether (BCME), and formaldehyde (HCHO) which were tested by inhalation.[5] This chapter will discuss some of the interesting lesions which were produced in the nasal cavity and the differences in species susceptibility which were encountered.

II. CARCINOGENICITY OF DIMETHYLCARBAMOYL CHLORIDE (C_3H_6ONCl)

A. Inhalation Studies with Rats

DMCC is a derivative of carbamic acid which is used as an intermediate in the production of some carbamate pesticides and in the synthesis of three drugs: pyrodistigmine bromide, neostigmine bromide, and neostigmine methosulfate. It is an extremely reactive material which rapidly hydrolyzes to form dimethylamine, hydrochloric acid, and carbon dioxide. In order to determine a level suitable for a chronic study, groups of 100 Sprague-Dawley rats (8-week-old males, from Blue Spruce Farms, Altamont, N.Y.) were subjected to 30 exposures (6 hr/day, 5 days/week) at levels of 100, 30, 10, and 1 ppm. The 14-day LC_{50} following a single, 6-hr exposure was found to be 180 ppm. Due to very high mortality, exposures were stopped short of 30 days for all but the group exposed to 1 ppm. Only animals from the 10- (15 exposures) and 1-ppm group (30 exposures) survived to be held for lifetime observation. In addition, two groups of 100 male Sprague-Dawley rats received chronic exposure to 1 and 0.3 ppm (6 hr/day, 5 days/week for life). Another group of 50 were sham-exposed to conditioned fresh air and another 50 were maintained as untreated controls. All exposures were performed in 1.3 m^3 chambers which are described elsewhere.[6]

A high mortality, shortening of life span, and weight depression were seen in the group surviving the highest dose of 10 ppm, reflecting the toxicity of the compound. In a chronic study at 1 ppm, the mortality rose sharply by 40 weeks, with 77% of the animals dead; by the 50th week, 100% of the animals had died. In the lower dose group receiving 0.3 ppm, 50% of them died by 52 weeks and 100% by the time they reached 120 weeks. Nasal tumors were found in all four treated groups, whereas none were observed in either the air-sham or colony controls. The highest incidence of respiratory tract tumors was seen in the group receiving 1 ppm for life (96 of 98) followed by the group receiving 10 ppm for 15 exposures (17 of 57). In all cases the nasal cavity was the most susceptible organ to the carcinogenic effect.

The incidences, induction times, and segmental distribution of the tumors in the respiratory tract and the morphological classification of the individual tumors are reported in Tables 1 and 2. The probabilities for nasal tumor-bearing deaths are plotted for the four groups in Figure 1. These probabilities were derived from actuarial computation methods[7] and used to correct for animals actually at risk. A clear dose-response relationship with respect to the

Table 1
NUMBER AND MORPHOLOGICAL TYPES OF TUMORS FOUND
FOLLOWING INHALATION OF DMCC

Respiratory tract	Treatment			
	10 ppm × 15	1 ppm × 30	1 ppm × life	0.3 ppm × life
Larynx	1 Papilloma	1 Papilloma	2 Papillomas	1 Squamous cell carcinoma
Trachea	3 Papillomas 4 Squamous cell carcinomas	1 Polyp	—	—
Bronchi	1 Squamous cell carcinoma	—	—	—
Lungs	—	—	—	—
Nasal cavity	8 Squamous cell carcinomas	2 Papillomas 10 Squamous cell carcinomas	94 Squamous cell carcinomas	3 Papillomas 7 Squamous cell carcinomas

Table 2
CARCINOMA INCIDENCE AND
INDUCTION TIME FOLLOWING
INHALATION OF DMCC

Concentration × time ppm × mean exposure day	Respiratory carcinoma[a] (%)	Mean induction time
177 (1 ppm × 177)[b]	96	262
150 (10 ppm × 15)	21	329
30 (1 ppm × 30)	10	554
112 (0.3 ppm × 372)	8	568

[a]   Corrected for survival.
[b]   1 ppm for life.

incidence of cancer was seen. A marked decrease in the induction time of cancer with an increase in concentration was also noted (see Table 2). At 1 ppm for life, deaths were largely accompanied by tumors. Since no deaths occurred before 185 days (the first tumor seen at 196 days), the entire group was considered to be at risk. However, since two rats were inadvertently discarded, the calculations of tumor incidence for this group was based on a group of 98 animals. Of the 98 animals, 96 developed tumors in the nasal cavity. The tumors were noted just a few weeks before death with distortion of the face and nasal swelling (Figure 2). Sagittal sections of the skull showed a friable, opaque, grey-white mass which usually filled the nasal cavity and expanded, and occasionally perforated the bones of the skull (Figure 3). All tumors were classified as squamous cell carcinomas. The earliest stages in the transformation appeared to be a type of nodular atypical basal overgrowth in which cells lost their polarity and acquired large hyperchromatic nuclei (Figure 4). This was followed by invasive downgrowth, filling the nasal cavity and involving the nasoturbinates, ethmoturbinates, and eroded bone, occasionally involving the nerves (Figure 5). To our knowledge, these changes are very similar to the ones found during the induction of squamous cell carcinoma of the bronchus.

B. Pathology of Hamsters
The significant findings with DMCC in rats prompted the initiation of a comparative study

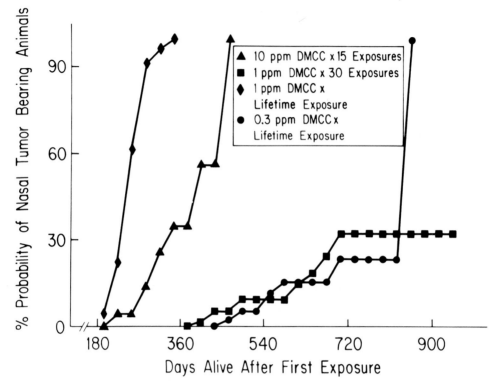

FIGURE 1.   Percent probability of nasal tumors from animals exposed to various dose levels of dimethylcarbamoyl chloride.

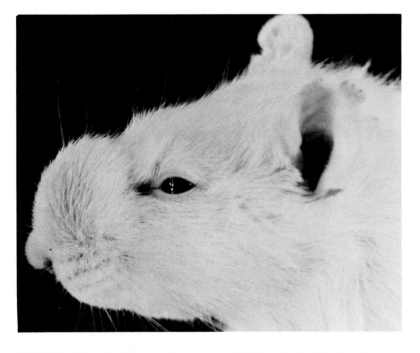

FIGURE 2.   Deformity of the nose in a rat dying at 218 days after the initiation of exposure to dimethylcarbamoyl chloride.

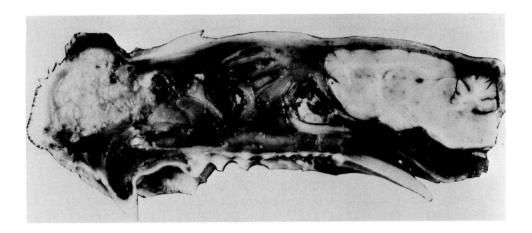

FIGURE 3.   Saggital section through the skull of the rat shown in Figure 2. The grey-white mass, a squamous cell carcinoma, fills the anterior portion of the nasal cavity and has perforated the nasal bones.

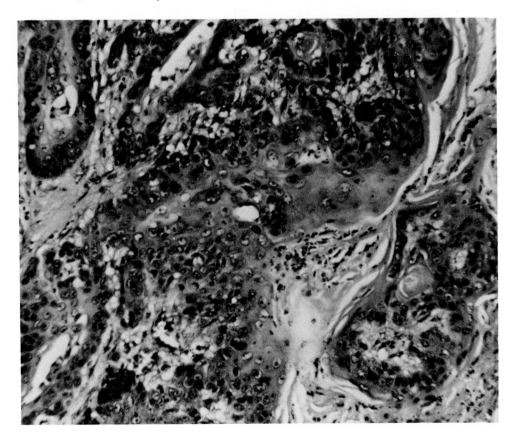

FIGURE 4.   Squamous cell carcinoma with areas of atypical squamous metaplasia. (H and E, ×220.)

with Syrian Golden hamsters. One hundred male 6-week-old Syrian Golden hamsters (Charles River, Wilmington, Mass.) were exposed to 1 ppm DMCC for life (6 hr/day, 5 days/week). The survival of the hamsters was excellent until 56 weeks; 50% survived until 72 weeks and 10% were still alive after 92 weeks of exposure. The major pathological changes were found in the nasal cavity.[8] As in the rats, nasal swelling was seen, but in much lower

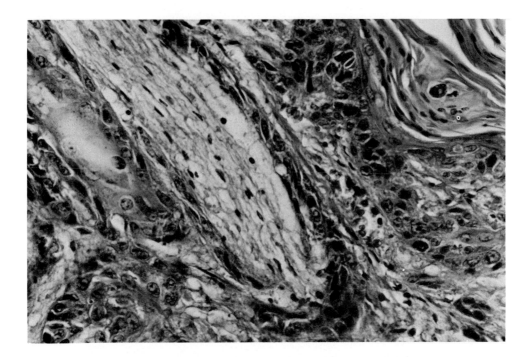

FIGURE 5.   Nerve trunk surrounded and invaded by squamous cell carcinoma. (H and E, ×410.)

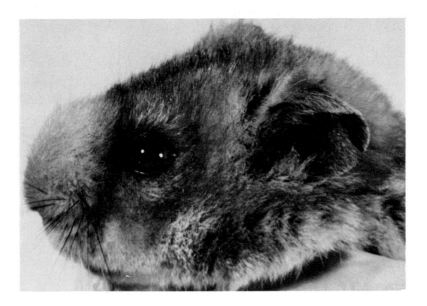

FIGURE 6.   Nasal deformity in a hamster dying at 547 days after the initiation of exposure to dimethylcarbamoyl chloride.

incidences. The first swelling was not seen until 533 days (Figure 6) and only six hamsters showed this gross abnormality. Sagittal sections of the head, however, revealed lesions similar to those seen in the rats — a greyish-white mass filling the nasal cavity (Figure 7). Of the 99 animals at risk (one test animal was cannabalized and, therefore, removed from the pool), 50/99 or 50% developed nasal tumors and 1/99 or 1% developed a laryngeal

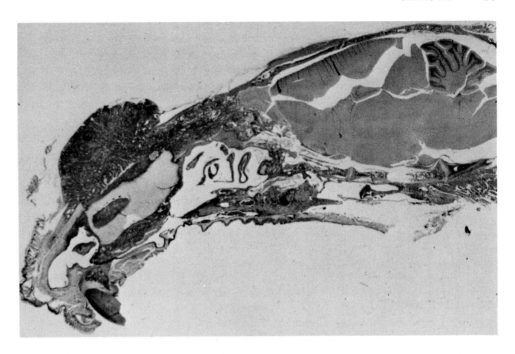

FIGURE 7. Saggital section through the skull shows the tumor penetrates the nasal bone and extends into the surrounding areas.

tumor. All of the tumors were classified as moderately to well-differerentiated squamous cell carcinomas, often with highly keratinized pearls. The tumors perforated the nasal turbinates and infiltrated the submucosal areas, however, none extended to the brain or metastasized to other organs.

C. Differences in Species Susceptibility to DMCC

Spontaneous tumors of the nasal cavity are very rare in both rats and hamsters. Hamsters have repeatedly shown a lower response than the rat when exposed to respiratory tract irritants and carcinogens.[9] In comparing the response of rats and hamsters to 1 ppm DMCC, the rats show increased sensitivity in all areas. The rate of mortality was higher in rats; 77% dead by 40 weeks compared to only 4% mortality in the hamster at the same time. Rat deaths were primarily due to tumors. Tumors appeared earlier in the rats; 195 days compared to 406 days for the first hamster tumor. The rat tumors more often appeared with gross nasal swelling; 61% compared to only 7% in the hamsters. Tumors not only appeared earlier, but were in much higher incidences in the rats; 98% compared to only 51% in the hamsters. This suggests some resistence in hamsters to the potent carcinogenic effects of DMCC. Percent probability tumor incidence curves for both rats and hamsters are shown in Figure 8. When corrected for early mortality by the use of actuarial table analysis, the percentage tumor-bearing hamsters reached 77% after 625 calendar days compared to 100% for rats by 360 calendar days. Except for the one hamster which developed a laryngeal tumor, both rats and hamsters showed tumors only in the nasal cavity and all tumors were classified as squamous cell carcinomas.

III. NASAL TUMORS INDUCED BY EPICHLOROHYDRIN

Epichlorohydrin (ECH) is a bifunctional alkylating agent with a number of industrial applications. ECH (1-chloro-2,3-epoxypropane) has the following structure:

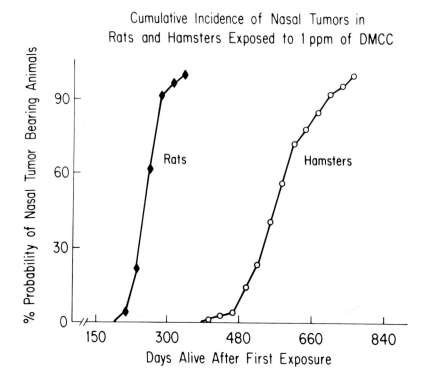

FIGURE 8.   Percent probability of nasal tumor-bearing rats and hamsters following exposure to dimethylcarbamoyl chloride.

$$CH_2CHCH_2Cl$$

A detailed description of the toxic and carcinogenic properties of ECH is given elsewhere.[10] A single, 6-hr exposure to ECH, with follow-up to 14 days, showed the lethal median concentration to be about 360 ppm. Further inhalation studies, where rats received 30 exposures at 100 ppm for 6 hr/day, 5 days/week, were also carried out. Malignant, squamous cell carcinomas were seen in 15 of the 140 or 11% test rats. The site and morphological type of tumor were very similar to the ones observed with DMCC. In another study with 100 rats which received chronic exposures to 30 ppm ECH, 1 nasal squamous cell carcinoma and 1 nasal papilloma were seen. A second chronic study with exposure to 10 ppm ECH showed no neoplastic lesions in any segment of the respiratory tract (see Table 3).

IV. NASAL TUMORS INDUCED BY BIS(CHLOROMETHYL)ETHER

Among the chlorinated ethers, bis(chloromethyl)ether (BCME) represents the most interesting compound, based on its once widespread industrial use, extreme reactivity, and its implication as a carcinogen following skin, subcutaneous, and epidemiological studies.[11] A lifetime study was initiated originally with 70 male Sprague-Dawley rats at a level of 0.1 ppm of BCME. Inhalation studies showed tumors in the olfactory and nasal epithelium.[12] By the time they had received 80 expsoures, 50% of the group had died. Of those remaining, 20 were removed from the exposure regimen and held for lifetime observation while the remainder continued to receive exposures. Further details of this study are given elsewhere.[12] In other studies with BCME, a total of 200 rats were exposed to levels of 0.1 ppm BCME

Table 3
EFFECT OF DOSE RATE UPON
INHALATION CARCINOGENESIS BY
EPICHLOROHYDRIN

	Concentration (ppm)		
	100	**30 (Lifetime)**	**10 (Lifetime)**
Number of exposures	30	290[a]	250[a]
Total dose (ppm/ days)	3000	8700	2500
Nasal cancer incidence	14/140	1/100	0/100

[a]   Based upon median survival time.

Table 4
CANCERS AND INDUCTION TIME SEEN IN 200 RATS
FOLLOWING 0.1 PPM OF BCME EXPOSURE

Origin and type of cancer	Total number cancers	Mean cancer time (days)	Range (days)
Nose			
Esthesioneuroepitheliomas	17	447	260—853
Malignant olfactory tumor (unclassified)	1	405	405
Ganglioneuroepithelioma	1	334	334
Squamous cell carcinoma	1	594	594
Poorly differentiated epithelial tumors	4	462	253—676
Adenocarcinoma	2	696	652—738
Lung			
Squamous cell carcinoma	13	411	215—578
Adenocarcinoma	1	877	877

for either 10, 20, 40, 60, or 100 exposures and then held for lifetime observation. The data from the 20 animals removed from the chronic study above at 30 exposures were included here in the calculation of dose response curves and tumor incidences.

In the chronic study, two carcinomas were seen in the nasal cavity. These were an esthesioneuroepithelioma and a squamous cell carcinoma and were seen at 383 and 578 days, respectively.

In the dose response study, in which animals were exposed for various short terms and held for lifetime observation, the tumor yield was impressive. A total of 40 cancers of the respiratory tract (both nasal cavity and lung) were seen in the 200 test animals. The morphologic type and induction times are shown in Table 4.

The tumors seen in the nasal cavity in this study were of some interest. The predominant type of tumor seen in these groups was classified as esthesioneuroepithelioma (sometimes referred to as olfactory neuroblastomas by some investigators). For the most part, the tumors were made up of sheets and cords of fairly uniform cuboidal to columnar cells that replaced normal olfactory epithelium. The nasal bone was destroyed and the tumor extended caudally

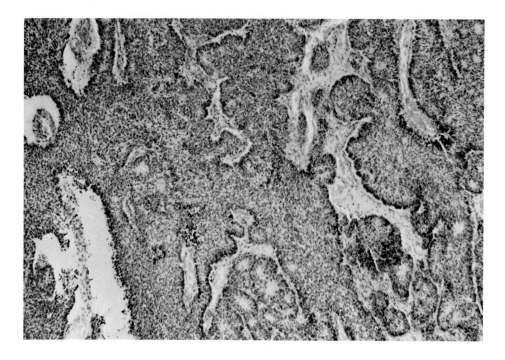

FIGURE 9.   Esthesioneuroepithelioma showing sheets and anastomosing cords of tumor cells replacing nasal epithelium and destroying bones. Areas of rosette formation may be seen. (H and E, ×72.)

to invade the brain (Figure 9). The nuclei were fairly uniform and the characteristic "rosette" formation was prominent (Figure 10). In one case, the nasal tumor was made up of large elongated, often multinucleated cells, that were interpreted as neoplastic ganglion cells. Nests of immature cells were interspersed among the largest cells (Figure 11). One tumor was interpreted as a ganglioneuroepithelioma. In addition to these tumors, one squamous cell carcinoma, two adenocarcinomas, four poorly differentiated, and one unclassified epithelial tumor were observed in the nasal cavity. The number of cancers of each type at each exposure level is shown in Table 5. The highest incidence involving the nose occurred at 80 exposures and the highest incidence involving the lung occurred at 100 expsoures. The magnitude of the tumor response from such a relatively low level of exposure shows the great tumorigenic property of this compound. Later human epidemiological studies substantiated these findings by identifying atypical cells in human sputum[13] and lung cancer incidences in exposed workers.[14]

V. CARCINOGENICITY OF ALDEHYDES

Very few studies have been done on the carcinogenicity of aldehydes. In general, only formaldehyde (HCHO) and acetaldehyde (CH_3CHO) have been tested in a few systems. There is evidence that both formalin and hexamethylenetetramine (which releases HCHO in vivo) cause sarcomas in rats at the injection site.[15,16] When rabbits were exposed to formalin in the oral mucosa, preneoplastic lesions and carcinomas *in situ* were seen.[17] Long-term exposure by inhalation produced nasal tumors in rats with hexamethylphosphoramide.[18] Neoplastic transformation of mouse BALB/3T3 cells in culture has been demonstrated.[19] Recently, the CIIT group has shown that HCHO is a potential carcinogen in the nasal mucosa of rats.[20] There is only one study which showed that high level exposures to acetaldehyde induced a few nasal tumors and laryngeal tumors in Syrian hamsters.[21]

Hydrogen chloride (HCl) and formaldehyde (HCHO) are both highly irritating, extensively

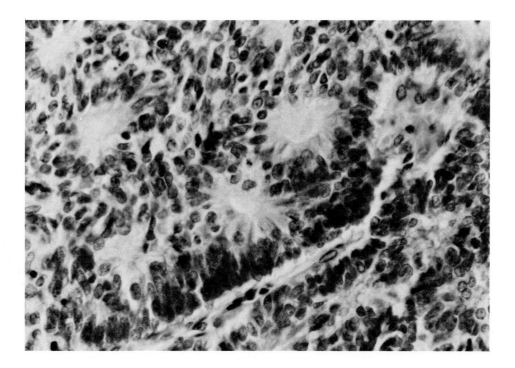

FIGURE 10. Esthesioneuroepithelioma of olfactory epithelium with striking rosette formation by fairly uniform cuboidal to columnar cells. (H and E, ×544.)

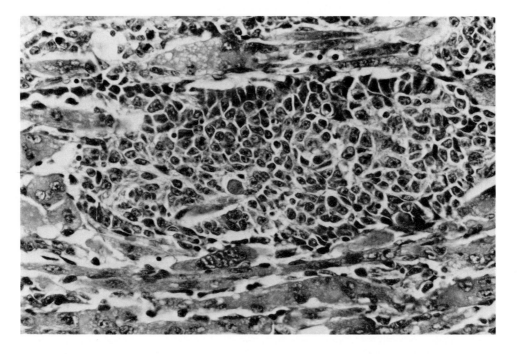

FIGURE 11. Large, bizarre, polygonal and elongated cells with one or more prominent vesicular nuclei. These are interpreted as neoplastic ganglia cells. Nodular masses of immature cells, possibly neoplastic neuroblasts, are encompassed by larger cells. (H and E, ×352.)

Table 5
CANCERS IN RATS FOLLOWING LIMITED
EXPOSURES OF 0.1 PPM OF BCME

Origin and type of cancer	Number of exposures					
	100 (30)	80 (50)	60 (20)	40 (20)	20 (50)	10 (50)
Nose						
Esthesioneuroepitheliomas	3	9	2	2	1	0
Malignant olfactory tumor (undescribed)	1	0	0	0	0	0
Ganglioneuroepithelioma	0	1	0	0	0	0
Squamous cell carcinoma	0	1	0	0	0	0
Poorly differentiated epithelial tumor	1	1	0	1	1	0
Adenocarcinoma	0	0	0	0	1	1
Lung						
Squamous cell carcinoma	8	3	2	0	0	0
Adenocarcinoma	0	0	0	1	0	0

used industrial chemicals which, when combined, could form a low level of bis(chloromethyl)ether (BCME).[22]

$$2CH_2O + HCl \rightarrow ClCH_2O^- + H^+CH_2O \rightarrow$$

$$ClCH_2OCH_2OH + HCl \rightarrow ClCH_2OCH_2Cl$$

Because of this positive chemical reaction in forming BCME when these two chemicals are used in close proximity, a pilot study was initiated with 99 8-week-old Sprague-Dawley rats (Blue Spruce Farms, Altamont, N.Y.). They were exposed to a mixture of HCl and HCHO at average concentrations of 10.6 and 14.7 ppm, respectively. HCHO vapors were generated by passing air over a slurry of paraformaldehyde (Purified Trioxymethylene, Fischer Scientific). The HCl was metered from a tank of concentrated hydrogen chloride gas (Matheson Gas Products, East Rutherford, N.J.). Formaldehyde levels of 800 to 1500 ppm and HCl levels of 5000 to 8000 ppm were required in the reaction vessel to maintain the chamber concentrations at nominal levels of 15 ppm HCHO and 10 ppm HCl. Trace amounts of BCME (less than 1 ppb) were detected but not quantitated in the inhalation chamber. The animals were exposed 6 hr/day, 5 days/week for life. A high proportion of the lesions were found to be in the nasal mucosa.[23] These included hyperplasia and squamous metaplasia and were seen in higher incidences in the test group than in the controls. Of the exposed animals, 28 showed tumors of the nasal cavity, of which 25 were squamous cell carcinomas and 3 were papillomas (Table 6). The temporal pattern of the carcinoma response is shown in the mortality-corrected cumulative incidence curve with respect to elapsed time after the onset of exposure. The first tumor of any type was a papilloma seen in an animal dying at 195 days and the first carcinoma was seen at 223 days. Similar to the other alkylating agents, DMCC and ECH, the tumors were located only in the nasal cavity and were classified as squamous cell carcinomas. There were two animals dying at 552 and 560 days which had nasal cancers with metastatic lesions in the lungs. No primary tumors were detected in other segments of the respiratory tract. Tumors were primarily located in the anterior portions of the nasal cavity, involving the nasal and maxillary turbinates, but did not extend to the brain as had been seen in the BCME experiments. Since this study was limited to the combined effects of HCHO and HCl, the study did not include groups receiving HCHO and HCl alone.

Table 6
LESIONS FOUND IN THE NASAL
MUCOSA OF RATS[a] EXPOSED TO
HYDROGEN CHLORIDE AND
FORMALDEHYDE

	Exposed	Controls
Number of rats examined	99	50
Number with		
Rhinitis	65	41
Epithelial hyperplasia and hyperplasia with atypia	71	8
Squamous metaplasia	64	0
Squamous papilloma	3	0
Squamous cell carcinoma	25	0

[a]   Includes colony controls.

In previous studies with BCME, the tumors induced were predominantly esthesioneuroe-pitheliomas of the nasal cavity and squamous cell carcinomas of the lower respiratory tract.[12] The lack of induction of esthesioneuroepitheliomas or lower respiratory tract carcinomas with the mixture of HCHO and HCl seems to indicate that BCME may not have been the only causative factor in the initiation of the tumors. Since the original experiment did not include groups exposed to HCHO or HCl alone, it was unknown whether the irritant effects of these compounds alone could have contributed to the carcinogenesis. In order to explore the exact mechanism involved, a second study was initiated to determine whether the combined exposures were necessary to produce cancers or whether HCl or HCHO alone were carcinogenic. This study was also designed to determine whether the carcinogenic response would occur if the HCl and HCHO were introduced into the inhalation chamber separately so that they could mix at low concentrations, preventing the formation of alkylating agents.

In this second study, 600 9-week-old Sprague-Dawley rats (Charles River, Wilmington, Mass.) were used. The groups of 100 rats each were exposed as follows: combined exposure to HCHO and HCl where the gases were premixed at high concentration before dilution, as in the previous pilot study; combined exposure to HCHO and HCl, not premixed, but fed separately into the inlet air supply of the exposure chamber; HCHO alone; HCl alone; air sham-exposed controls; and untreated controls. All exposures were performed in the usual pattern of 6 hr/day, 5 days/week for life.

The rate of survival was excellent up to the first year in all treated groups and at 588 days, the highest mortality was seen in the combined exposures to HCHO and HCl (45 to 49%) with only 38% mortality in the HCHO alone group and 29% in the HCl alone group. Thus far, the preliminary results reveal that the relative damage in the nasal epithelium has varied from one treatment group to the other. The groups receiving the combined exposures developed more lesions than HCHO alone or HCl alone. Mild to severe rhinitis was seen along with hyperplastic and squamous metaplastic lesions of the respiratory epithelium of the turbinates (Figure 12). The group treated with HCl showed only one squamous metaplastic lesion so far. Nasal tumors were found in both groups receiving combined exposures and with HCHO alone. The results of this experiment confirm the carcinogenic response with HCHO in rats as reported by the Chemical Industry Institute of Toxicology.[20] There were 21 tumors in the premixed group, 7 tumors in the nonpremixed group, and 18 in the HCHO alone group. No tumors have yet been observed in the groups exposed to HCl or fresh air or in the untreated controls. All tumors were located in the nasal cavity. They first appeared as a nasal swelling and the tumors were observed in all three groups after 430 days and

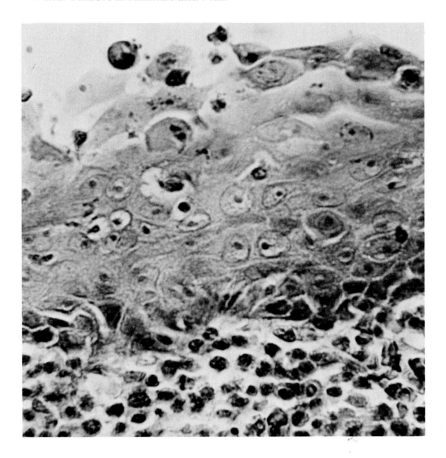

FIGURE 12.   Atypical squamous metaplasia of the nasal turbinate in a rat exposed to formaldehyde vapor. (H and E, ×880.)

there is no significant time difference between groups as far as the appearance of the first tumors is concerned. With the exception of one tumor, an adenocarcinoma in the nonpremixed group, all tumors were squamous cell carcinomas (Figure 13) showing various differentiation; some were localized, arising from the turbinate (Figure 14), or sometimes very invasive (Figure 15), and most of the time highly keratinized.

It is clear, up to this point in the study, that much of the carcinogenic response is from HCHO exposures since the HCl exposure did not produce any tumors. So far, there is no difference between the premixed and the HCHO alone group in the induction of tumors. However, the nonpremixed group seems to be showing a lesser incidence suggesting that the HCl has played some suppressing role on tumor formation by HCHO.

VI. DISCUSSION

Spontaneous nasal tumors in hamsters and rats are very rare. However, several investigators, using a variety of chemicals, have been able to induce tumors in greater incidences in rats than in hamsters (Table 7). The tumors primarily arise from the nasal cavity, deriving from the respiratory, olfactory, and submucosal glands. The tumor types are squamous cell carcinomas, adenocarcinomas, and esthesioneuroepitheliomas. The occurrence of these tumor types depends upon the chemical and the mode of administration. We also found species differences in susceptibility and tumor type induced in the nasal cavity.[6,8] For example, BCME administered by inhalation produced 17 esthesioneuroepitheliomas and 1 squamous

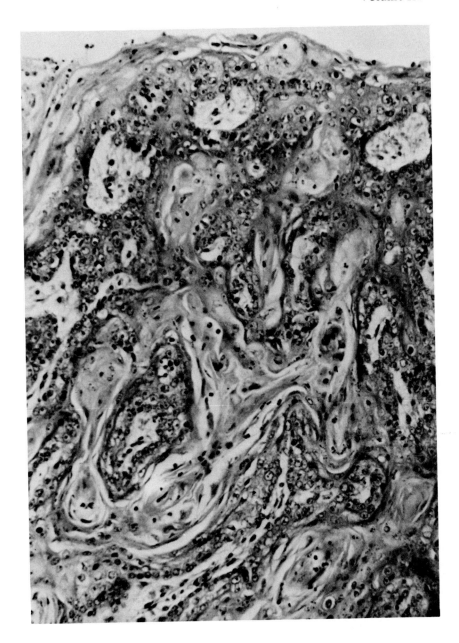

FIGURE 13. Nasal squamous cell carcinoma with areas of squamous metaplasia in a rat exposed to formaldehyde vapor. (H and E, ×250.)

cell carcinoma compared to none in hamsters.[12] DMCC induced a high tumor incidence in rats (98%) and hamsters (51%), but the same type (squamous cell carcinomas) in both species. This would appear to depend upon some unexplained differences in the target cells affected by these two chemicals even though the mode of administration was the same (inhalation) for both studies. Subcutaneous injection of various compounds has induced different types of tumors in the nasal cavity of rats and hamsters (Table 7) suggesting that there are several factors such as irritation, metabolism, pharmacokinetics, physiological, and repair mechanisms involved in the induction of tumors. In the case of direct-acting alkylating agents and aldehyde, irritation was one of the factors taken seriously in the

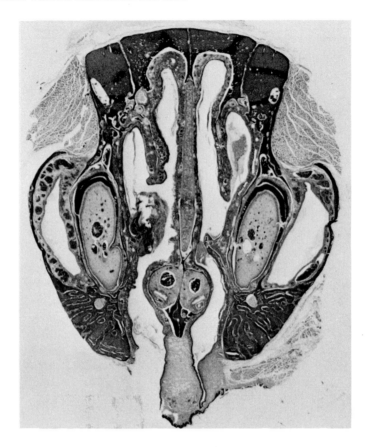

FIGURE 14.   Squamous cell carcinoma arising from the nasoturbinate of a rat
exposed to formaldehyde vapor.

induction of tumors. Since the tumors were found in the anterior portion of the cavity, where
there was maximum deposition during exposure, the changes being due to constant irritation
is possible. However, in our ongoing HCl and HCHO studies, the preliminary results indicate
that the addition of HCl does not enhance the carcinogenic effect of formaldehyde. It is
quite possible that the level of HCHO given, by itself, was on a plateau of irritation response
and that the HCl alone was not tested long enough or at a high enough concentration. Due
to the complex problems involved in knowing the mechanisms involved in the carcinogenesis,
additional studies, such as the role of cytotoxic effects of the chemicals, the DNA interaction
of these chemicals in the nasal mucosa, and even the role of hyperplasia as a promoter,
should be investigated.

ACKNOWLEDGMENTS

These investigations were supported by contract N01 CP 33260 from the National Cancer
Institute and by a center Grant ES 00260 and Grant ES 002270 from the National Institutes
of Environmental Health Sciences.

The authors wish to acknowledge Dorothy Natalizio and Fred Blanchard for technical
assistance and Maureen Freitag for typing services.

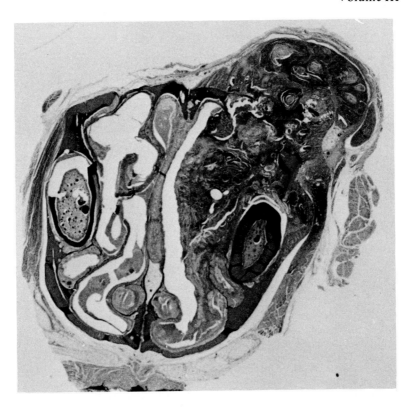

FIGURE 15.   Invasive squamous cell carcinoma arising from the respiratory turbinate and infiltrating the surrounding areas.

Table 7
SELECTED REFERENCES FOR POSITIVE NASAL TUMOR INDUCTION WITH NONNITROSO COMPOUNDS

		Ref.
By inhalation		
Bis(chloromethyl)ether	Rat	12
Dimethylcarbamoyl chloride	Rat	6
	Hamster	8
Epichlorohydrin	Rat	9
Hydrogen chloride + formaldehyde	Rat	23
Formaldehyde	Rat	20
Hexamethyl phosphoramide	Rat	18
Acetaldehyde	Hamster	21
1,2, Dibromo-3-chloropropane	Rat	24
1,2 Dibromoethane	Rat	24
By systemic administration		
Thio-TEPA	Rat	25
Procarbazine	Rat	26
P-cresidine	Rat	27
Phenacetin	Rat	28
1,4 Dioxane	Rat	29

REFERENCES

1. **Hoffman, E. and Graffi, A.,** Carcinoma der Nasenhöhle bei Mäusen nach Tropfung der Rückenhaut mit Diäthylnitrosamin, *Acta Biol. Med. Gdansk,* 12, 623, 1964.
2. **Thomas, C.,** Zur Morphologie der Nasenhöhlentumoren bei der Ratte, *Z. Krebsforsch.,* 67, 1, 1965.
3. **Montesano, R. and Saffiotti, U.,** Carcinogenic response of respiratory tract of Syrian Golden hamsters to different doses of diethylnitrosamine, *Cancer Res.,* 28, 2197, 1978.
4. **Herrold, K. M.,** Induction of olfactory neuroepithelial tumors in Syrian hamsters by diethylnitrosamine, *Cancer,* 17, 114, 1964.
5. **Van Duuren, B. L., Goldschmidt, B. M., Katz, G., Seidman, I., and Paul, J. S.,** Carcinogenic activity of alkylating agents, *J. Natl. Cancer Inst.,* 33, 695, 1974.
6. **Sellakumar, A., Laskin, S., Katz, G., Rusch, G., and Kuschner, M.,** Dose response studies following inhalation of dimethylcarbamoyl chloride in rats, *Am. Ind. Hyg. Conf.,* Abstr., New Orleans, La., May 1977.
7. **Kaplan, E. S. and Meir, P.,** Non-parametric estimation from incomplete observations, *J. Am. Stat. Assoc.,* 53, 457, 1964.
8. **Sellakumar, A. R., Laskin, S., Kuschner, M., Katz, G. V., Rusch, G. M., Snyder, C. A., and Albert, R. E.,** Inhalation carcinogenesis by dimethylcarbamoyl chloride in Syrian Golden hamsters, *J. Environ. Pathol. Toxicol.,* 3, 107, 1980.
9. **Laskin, S., Kuschner, M., and Drew, R. T.,** *Studies in Pulmonary Carcinogenicity,* Inhalation Carcinogenesis Conf. 691001, Hanna, M. G., Jr., Nettesheim, P., and Gilbert, J. R., Eds., Clearing House for Federal Scientific and Technical Information, Springfield, Va., 1970.
10. **Laskin, S., Sellakumar, A., Kuschner, M., Nelson, N., LaMendola, S., Rusch, G., Katz, G., Dulak, N., and Albert, R.,** Inhalation carcinogenicity of epichlorohydrin in noninbred Sprague-Dawley rats, *J. Natl. Cancer Inst.,* 65, 751, 1980.
11. **Van Duuren, B., Sivak, A., and Goldschmit, B.,** Carcinogenicity of halo-ethers, *J. Natl. Cancer Inst.,* 43, 481, 1969.
12. **Kuschner, M., Laskin, S., Drew, R., Cappiello, V., and Nelson, N.,** Inhalation carcinogenicity of alfa halo-ethers. III. Lifetime and limited period inhalation studies with bis(chloromethyl)ether at 0.1 ppm, *Arch. Environ. Health,* 30, 73, 1975.
13. **Wagoner, J.,** Epidemiology program of NIOSH. Read before the American Public Health Association Annual Meeting Symposium on Occupational Carcinogenesis, Boston, November 1972.
14. **Skababe, H.,** Lung cancer due to exposure to bis(chloromethyl)ether, *Ind. Health,* 11, 145, 1973.
15. **Watanabe, R., Matsunago, T., Soejima, T., and Iwata, Y.,** Study on the aldehyde carcinogenicity. Communication. I. Experimentally induced rat sarcomas by repeated injection of formalin, *Gann,* 45, 451, 1954.
16. **Watanabe, F. and Sugimoto, S.,** Studies on the carcinogenicity of aldehydes. II. Seven cases of transplantable sarcomas on rats developed in the area of repeated subcutaneous injections of Urotropin (hexamethylenetetramine), *Gann,* 46, 365, 1955.
17. **Mueller, R., Daebe, G., and Schumann, D.,** Leukoplakia induced by repeated deposition of formalin in rabbit oral mucosa. Long-term experiments with a new "oral tank", *Exp. Pathol.,* 16, 36, 1978.
18. **Zapp, J. A.,** HMPA: a possible carcinogen, *Science,* 90, 422, 1975.
19. **Brusick, D., Myhr, B., Stetba, D., and Rundell, J.,** *Genetic and Transforming Activity of Formaldehyde,* Litton Bionetics Report, Kensington, Va., April 1980.
20. **Swenberg, J., Kerns, W., Mitchell, R., Ardle, E., and Pavkav, K.,** Induction of squamous cell carcinoma of the rat nasal cavity by intubation exposure to formaldehyde vapor, *Cancer Res.,* 40, 3398, 1980.
21. **Feron, V. and Woutensen, R.,** Respiratory tract tumors in hamsters exposed to acetaldehyde vapour alone or simultaneously to benzo(a)pyrene, Abstr., Symposium on Co-carcinogenesis and Biological Effects of Tumor Promoters at Elman Castle, Klais, Bavaria, Germany, October 1980.
22. **Frankel, L. S., McCallum, K. S., and Collier, L.,** Formation of bis(chloromethyl)ether from formaldehyde and hydrogen chloride, *Environ. Sci. Technol.,* 8, 356, 1974.
23. **Sellakumar, A. R., Albert, R. E., Rusch, G., Katz, G. V., Nelson, N., and Kuschner, M.,** Inhalation carcinogenicity of formaldehyde and hydrogen chloride, *Proc. Am. Assoc. Cancer Res.,* 21, 106, 1980.
24. **Reznik, G., Reznik-Schüller, H., Ward, J. M., and Stinson, S. F.,** Morphology of nasal tumors in rats after chronic inhalation of 1,2-dibromo-3-chloropropane, *Br. J. Cancer,* 42, 772, 1980.
25. DHEW, PHS, NIH, NCI, Bioassay of Thio-Tepa for Possible Carcinogenicity, Tech. Rep. Ser. No. 58, U.S. Government Printing Office, Washington, D.C., 1978, 168.
26. DHEW, PHS, NIH, NCI, Bioassay of Procarbazine for Possible Carcinogenicity, Tech. Rep. Ser. No. 19, U.S. Government Printing Office, Washington, D.C., 1979, 124.
27. DHEW, PHS, NIH, NCI, Bioassay of P-Cresidine for Possible Carcinogenicity, Tech. Rep. Ser. No. 142, U.S. Government Printing Office, Washington, D.C., 1979, 63.

28. **Isaka, H., Yashii, Otsuji, A., Koike, M., Najai, Y., Koura, M., Sugiyasaw, K., and Kanabaya Shi, T.,** Tumor of Sprague-Dawley rats induced by long-term feeding of phenacetin, *Gann,* 70, 29, 1979.
29. DHEW, PHS, NIH, NCI, Bioassay of 1,4-Dioxane for Possible Carcinogenicity, Tech. Rep. Ser. No. 80, U.S. Government Printing Office, Washington, D.C., 1978, 108.
30. DHEW, PHS, NIH, NCI, Bioassay of 1,2 Dibromoethane for Possible Carcinogenicity, Tech. Rep. Ser. No. 206, U.S. Government Printing Office, Washington, D.C., 1980, 100.

Chapter 3

NITROSAMINE-INDUCED NASAL CAVITY CARCINOGENESIS

Hildegard M. Reznik-Schüller

TABLE OF CONTENTS

I.   Introduction 48

II.   Nitrosamine-Induced Nasal Cavity Tumors in Rats 48

III.   Nitrosamine-Induced Nasal Cavity Tumors in Syrian Golden Hamsters 56

IV.   Nitrosamine-Induced Nasal Cavity Tumors in European Hamsters 67

V.   Nitrosamine-Induced Nasal Cavity Tumors in Chinese Hamsters and Gerbils ... 70

VI.   Nitrosamine-Induced Nasal Cavity Tumors in Mice 72

VII.   Nitrosamine-Induced Nasal Cavity Tumors in Nonhuman Primates and Dogs... 72

References 74

I. INTRODUCTION

A wide variety of chemicals has been found to induce tumors of the nasal cavities in various animal species. In the majority of such studies, histopathology has been used for diagnosis, with only a few reports on the ultrastructure of neoplasms in this organ system. It is for this reason that, even today, the pathogenesis of nasal cavity tumors is not clear and the classification of these tumors is often a matter of debate. This holds especially true for those tumors located in the olfactory region. Tumors in this area could have grown from the respiratory epithelium that coats the respiratory portion (maxilloturbinals, nasoturbinals, nasal septum) of the nose into the olfactory region. In that case, they should be addressed as adenocarcinomas, squamous carcinomas, or a mixture of the two. Were they derived from the olfactory epithelium, they could have originated from any of its cell types (olfactory sensory cells and their precursors, sustentacular cells, basal cells). Yet another possibility was raised by Pour and co-workers[1] who considered the epithelia of Bowman's gland as a probable site of origin of tumors of the olfactory region. Neuroblasts of the olfactory bulb are also among the cells which have been suggested as a possible source of neoplasms in this area.

The lack of system reflects the inadequacy of light microscopy in diagnosing neurogenic tumors. Neurosecretory granules, and neurotubules, which are distinct and unmistakable characteristics of neurogenic cells,[3-5] can only be discerned by electron microscopy (EM). In contrast, the typical growing pattern (formation of rosettes and pseudorosettes) of neurogenic tumors as well as the presence of dentritic processes and small uniform nuclei, which represent the basis for light microscopic diagnosis, are not present in all neurogenic tumors.[4]

Nitrosamines are a class of chemicals of which a number can induce a high incidence of nasal cavity tumors in laboratory animals. Since it is well-established that nitrosamines must first be metabolically activated[6,7] before their carcinogenic effect is seen, one might speculate that certain cell types in the nasal cavity can perform this metabolism. This in turn might explain the pronounced organotrophy of such compounds for the nasal cavities. Unfortunately, no attempts have yet been made to identify such target cell types in this organ system. The mechanisms of nasal cavity carcinogenesis are, therefore, far from being understood. Pathological studies can add significantly to our knowledge if attempts are made to identify the nature and site of early lesions and to follow the development of induced tumors sequentially. Moreover, it is vital to identify the affected cell types by EM to avoid misdiagnoses.

II. NITROSAMINE-INDUCED NASAL CAVITY TUMORS IN RATS

Since rats have been used extensively in experimental carcinogenesis, abundant data are available on induced nasal cavity tumors in this species. A large number of nitrosamines have been found to exert a carcinogenic effect in this region in rats (Table 1). Unfortunately, some of the reports are not very specific about the diagnosis, which makes it difficult to review the data comparatively. Some authors simply state that "nasal cavity tumors" were induced without giving a histopathological diagnosis or description, while others do not mention in which anatomical part of the nose they found the neoplasms. To make the situation worse, in not one of these studies was EM applied for diagnosis. With respect to the diagnostic problems outlined in the introduction, this puts these diagnoses of neurogenic tumors into question. In addition, there appears to be considerable confusion about the nomenclature of neoplasms in the olfactory region (Table 1). To the critical reviewer of the literature, it appears that every laboratory has created its own nomenclature and very often a profound lack of knowledge of the anatomy of the rodent nasal cavity is apparent.

Since nitrosamines must first be metabolically activated in the host organism, it would

Table 1
SOME NITROSAMINES WHICH INDUCE NASAL CAVITY TUMORS IN RATS

Chemical	Carcinogenicity	Diagnosis of induced tumors in nasal cavities	Ref.
N-Nitrosodimethylamine (inhalation)	Strong	Carcinomas of ethmoturbinal region	23, 26
N-Nitrosomethylethylamine	Medium	Not specified	9
N-Nitrodimethylamine	Medium	Adenocarcinomas, squamous cell carcinomas	15
N-Nitrosomethylvinylamine	Strong	Squamous epithelium carcinomas	23
N-Nitrosomethylallylamine	Medium	Squamous cell carcinomas, neuroblastomas, esthesioneuroepitheliomas	23
N-Nitrosomethyl-n-amylamine	Medium	Squamous cell papillomas, squamous cell carcinomas	10
N-Nitrosodiethylamine	Weak	Adenocarcinomas, esthesioneuroepitheliomas, poorly differentiated carcinomas, squamous carcinomas	10, 20, 23
N-Nitroso-O,N-diethylhydroxylamine	Strong	Carcinomas of paranasal sinuses	22
N-Nitrosodi-n-propylamine	Medium	Adenocarcinomas, poorly differentiated carcinomas of endoturbinal region, squamous cell carcinomas of endoturbinal region; squamous cell carcinomas, squamous cell papillomas	10, 26
N-Nitrosodi-isopropylamine	Medium	Adenocarcinomas	10
N-Nitroso-hydroxypropyl-n-propylamine	Strong	Squamous cell carcinomas, squamous cell papillomas, poorly differentiated carcinomas of endoturbinal region	26
N-Nitroso-bis(2-hydroxypropyl)amine	Strong	Adenocarcinomas in olfactory region; squamous cell carcinomas	28
N-Nitrosomethyl-n-propylamine	Medium	Squamous cell papillomas, squamous cell carcinomas, poorly differentiated carcinomas of endoturbinal region	26
N-Nitroso-di-isopropanolamine	Strong	Adenocarcinomas, squamous cell carcinomas, papillomas, adenomas	21
N-Nitrosoethyl-n-butylamine	Weak	Adenocarcinomas of ethmoturbinals	23
4-(N-methyl-N-nitrosamino)-1-(3-pyridyl)-1-butanone	Strong	Not specified	15
N-Nitrosomorpholine	Strong	Carcinomas of ethmoid cells, squamous cell carcinomas, esthesioneuroepitheliomas	23, 24, 29
N-Nitroso-2,6-dimethylmorpholine	Strong	Malignant tumors arising from epithelium in olfactory region	29

Table 1 (continued)
SOME NITROSAMINES WHICH INDUCE NASAL CAVITY TUMORS IN RATS

Chemical	Carcinogenicity	Diagnosis of induced tumors in nasal cavities	Ref.
N-Nitrosopiperidine	Strong	Adenocarcinomas, squamous cell carcinomas, olfactory carcinomas, ethmoid carcinomas, cholesteatomas	7, 17, 23, 24
N-Nitroso-3-piperidinol	Strong	Adenocarcinomas, squamous cell carcinomas	7
N-Nitroso-4-piperidinol	Strong	Adenocarcinomas, squamous cell carcinomas	7
N-Nitroso-4-piperidinone	Strong	Adenocarcinomas, squamous cell carcinomas	7
N-Nitroso-3,4-dichloropiperidine	Medium	Squamous cell carcinomas, adenocarcinomas	12
N-Nitrosopiperazine	Medium	Esthesioneuroblastomas, squamous cell carcinomas, adenocarcinomas	16
N,N'-Dinitrosopiperazine	Weak	Esthesioneuroepitheliomas, adenocarcinomas, squamous cell carcinomas	23, 24
N-Nitrosomethylpiperazine	Strong	Carcinomas of olfactory region; squamous cell carcinomas	30
N,N'-Dinitroso-2,6-dimethylpiperazine	Strong	Squamous cell carcinomas, adenocarcinomas	13
N-Nitrosopyrrolidine	Weak	Olfactory carcinomas	19
N-Nitroso-3,4-dichloropyrrolidine	Strong	Olfactory carcinomas	21
N-Nitroso-3-pyrroline	Weak	?	26
N-Nitrosohexamethyleneimine	Medium	Adenocarcinomas, squamous cell carcinomas, undifferentiated carcinomas, neuroepithelial tumors	11, 20
N-Nitrosoheptamethyleneimine	Strong	Squamous cell carcinomas	29
N-Nitrosonornicotine	Strong	Adenocarcinomas of olfactory epithelium, olfactory neuroblastomas, papillomas, polyps, rhabdomyosarcomas of nasal mucosa	15, 16
N-Nitroso-bis(2-chloroethyl)amine	Weak	Olfactory adenocarcinomas	13

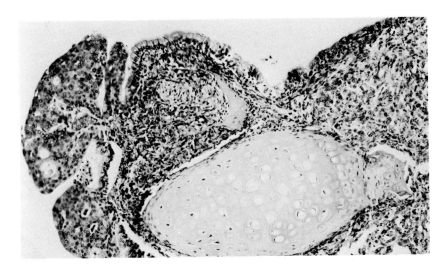

FIGURE 1. Histopathology of papilloma at the nasal septum of a rat. The neoplasm consists of squamous cells and demonstrates a well-developed short stalk. No infiltrative growth into the subepithelial tissue is detectable. (H and E; × 130.)

be helpful to look for a correlation between chemical structure and the type of cells that they affect when reviewing their carcinogenic effect in the nasal cavities. However, in view of the insufficiencies in the pathology reports mentioned above, this is impossible. This review will, therefore, merely give a general description of the types of tumors induced by nitrosamines in the rat nasal cavities.

Generally, the induced neoplasms may be divided into two categories: those that arise in the anterior part of the nose and those that originate in the posterior portion. As outlined in Chapter 2, Volume I, the atrioturbinals of the anterior nose are coated with squamous epithelium, while the maxillo- and nasoturbinals, nasal septum, and the maxillary sinuses are lined with respiratory epithelium. Therefore, epithelial tumors in the anterior portion of the nose can originate from squamous, basal, mucous, or ciliated cells. The benign tumors found in this region are papillomas (Figure 1) and papillary adenomas (Figure 2) and only rarely adenomas, while their malignant counterparts are squamous cell carcinomas (Figure 3) and adenocarcinomas (Figure 4).[8,11,12,23,25,26,28,30,37] Papillomas and papillary adenomas are usually multiple or occur coincidentally with the carcinomas. These lesions are generally accompanied by multiple focal hyperplasia and/or squamous metaplasia. Apparently, such "precancerous" changes do not always develop into neoplasms. This view is supported by a study on the pathogenesis of *N*-nitrosodiethylamine-induced nasal cavity tumors in Wistar rats.[33] The author reports that papillomas grew directly from the respiratory epithelium after proliferation of basal cells without first going through a stage of squamous metaplasia. Multiple proliferations of basal cells (Figure 5) in the respiratory epithelium were also found as precursor lesions of squamous cell carcinomas in Fischer 344 rats treated with nitrosomethylpiperazine in our laboratory. In this serial sacrifice study, however, such hyperplastic foci underwent squamous metaplasia (Figure 6) before they transformed into squamous cell carcinomas. The same experiment revealed that hyperplasia of basal cells in the squamous epithelium of the atrioturbinals developed later than the corresponding lesions in the respiratory epithelium. Unlike the early changes in the respiratory epithelium, hyperplasia in the atrioturbinals did not develop further into neoplasms. This demonstrates that although the same cell types (basal cells) react to treatment with the nitrosamine, the grade of their response may differ at different locations in the nasal cavity. An explanation for this phenomenon might be that the amount of active metabolite available in the two regions

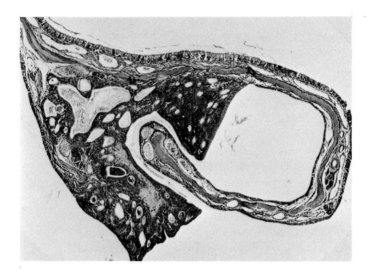

FIGURE 2.   Histopathology of papillary adenoma in nasoturbinals of rat; in contrast to the papilloma of Figure 1, this neoplasm exhibits a somewhat glandular growth pattern and contains mucous cells. (H and E; ×54.)

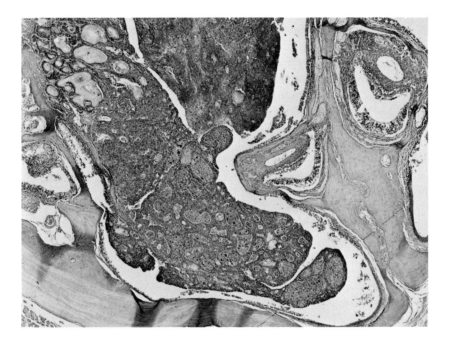

FIGURE 3.   Histopathology of squamous cell carcinoma in the maxilloturbinal of rat nasal cavity. The neoplasm invades the bone and forms keratin. (H and E; ×35.)

is different. The basal cells themselves are unlikely to activate nitrosamines to any great extent because they have very little endoplasmic reticulum, the major source of oxidative enzymes believed to be involved in nitrosamine activation. Mucous cells, which are found in the respiratory epithelium and Bowman's glands, are the more likely sites for this task. These cell types possess abundant rough endoplasmic reticulum and have been shown by histochemistry to be rich in cytochrome P450-dependent enzymes.[34] If these cells can metabolize and/or secrete the nitrosamines in the nasal cavities, the concentration of active

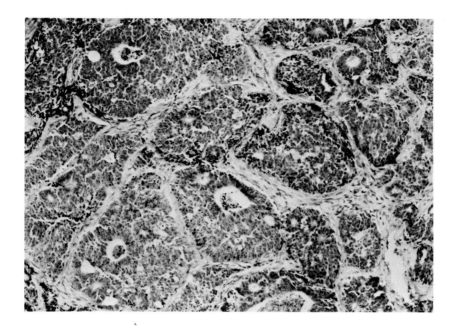

FIGURE 4. Histopathology of adenocarcinoma in respiratory portion of rat nasal cavity; the neoplasm exhibits a gland-like growth pattern. Acini with central lumina are surrounded by a sparse stroma. (H and E; ×130.)

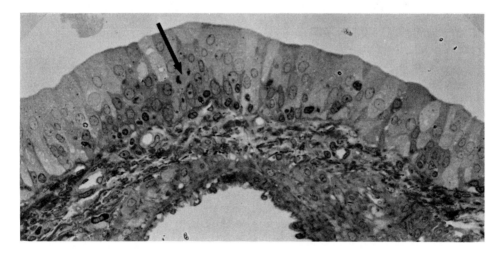

FIGURE 5. Histopathology of epithelium in nasoturbinal of Fischer 344 rat treated with nitrosomethylpiperazine for 10 weeks; focal proliferation of basal cells with 1 mitosis (arrowed) in basal portion of epithelium. The surface layer still looks normal except for a lack in ciliated cells. (Semithin section, toluidine blue; ×240.)

metabolite would of course be highest in and around the cells, while the atrioturbinals whose squamous epithelium is lacking mucous cells would have a substantially lower concentration. This interpretation is supported by the finding of Kraft and Tannenbaum[33] who investigated the distribution of *N*-nitrosomethylbenzylamine (MBN) by whole-body autoradiography and densitometry in Sprague-Dawley rats. They found the highest levels of the radioactively labeled carcinogen and/or its metabolites in the target organs of MBN-induced tumorigenesis, nasal cavities, lung, and esophagus. Although the authors fail to mention this in the text, it is apparent from their illustrations that the atrioturbinals did not contain detectable amounts of radioactivity while the respiratory portion contained high concentrations.

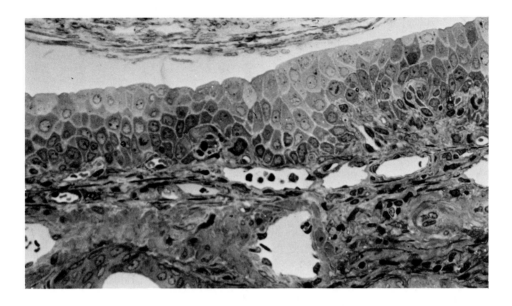

FIGURE 6.   Histopathology of epithelium in maxilloturbinal of Fischer 344 rat treated with nitrosomethylpi-perazine for 14 weeks; pronounced hyperplasia and early squamous metaplasia in basal part of epithelium while most of the nonciliated cells at the surface are still tall columnar. (Semithin section, toluidine blue; × 240.)

The squamous cell carcinomas which are induced by chronic nitrosamine treatment usually demonstrate pronounced keratinization (Figure 3). The neoplastic squamous cells tend to be arranged in clusters. Their nuclei contain little heterochromatin. EM (Figure 7) reveals bundles of cytoplasmic filaments and keratohyalin granules in their cytoplasm. Cells are linked by numerous desmosomes which at the light microscopic level appear as prominent "intracellular bridges". Squamous cell carcinomas tend to invade the bony skeleton of the nose and may then eventually lead to ulcerations of their exterior surfaces. In some cases, this tumor type may grow into the posterior part of the turbinal apparatus, and after penetrating the cribriform plate, invade the brain.

The pathogenesis of adenocarcinomas in the respiratory portion of the nose has not yet been described. These tumors generally demonstrate gland-like elements (e.g., formation of acini, Figure 4, and secretion of mucus). They are usually composed of all the cell types present in the respiratory epithelium. Occasionally they may exhibit focal areas of squamous metaplasia indicating they they might differentiate into squamous carcinomas at a later stage.

The nasal cavity tumors of the second category arise in the posterior portion of the nose. This area is occupied by the ethmoturbinal apparatus which is lined with olfactory epithelium. This type of epithelium consists of olfactory sensory cells and their precursors (neuroblasts) and sustentacular cells with their precursors (basal cells). In addition, Bowman's glands are found in the subepithelial layer. All of these different cell types could, in theory, give rise to the tumors induced by nitrosamines in this region. Pathogenesis studies would appear to be the best way to follow the development of this group of neoplasms. Since the only investigation of this type was one recently conducted in the author's laboratory, it shall now be described in some detail.

The histopathological diagnosis of neoplasms found in the literature (Table 1) includes adenomas, well- and poorly differentiated adenocarcinomas, neurogenic tumors, and squa-mous cell carcinomas. The benign neoplasms grow within the epithelial lining of the turbinals or along their lumina, while the malignant tumors invade through the cribiform plate into the brain (Figure 8) and/or infiltrate the bony skeleton of the skull. While the diagnosis of squamous cell carcinomas does not generally pose any problems (due to the presence of

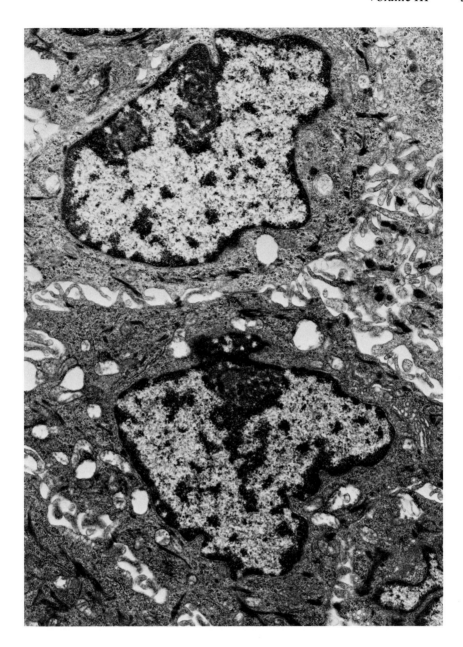

FIGURE 7. Electron micrograph of squamous cell carcinoma induced by nitrosomethylpiperazine in a Fischer 344 rat; the tumor cells have prominent bundles of cytoplasmic tonofilaments and are linked together by numerous desmosomes. (Uranyl acetate, lead citrate; × 12,250.)

typical characteristics such as keratin formation), the classification of the neurogenic neoplasms and adenocarcinomas is still a matter of considerable debate. We therefore conducted a serial sacrifice study in Fischer 344 rats treated with nitrosomethylpiperazine to study, by light and electron microscopy, the pathogenesis of tumors arising in the olfactory region. The earliest change found in this study was severe toxic degeneration of the olfactory sensory cells (Figure 9) which led to multiple focal areas depleted of this cell type. With continuous nitrosamine treatment, proliferation of cells in the basal layer of the olfactory epithelium was observed (Figure 10). These cells were identified by EM as basal cells and neuroen-

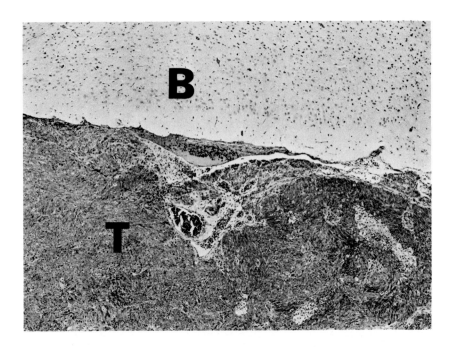

FIGURE 8.   Histopathology of adenocarcinoma in olfactory region which has grown through the cribiform plate and is invading the brain. B, brain. T, tumor. (H and E; ×54.)

docrine cells (Figure 11). These proliferating cells formed multiple focal hyperplasias and tended to form intraepithelial rosette-like structures (Figure 12). Such altered areas increased in size and grew through the basement membrane into the subepithelial tissue layer, thus giving rise to malignant neoplasms which on the basis of their pathogenesis were diagnosed as adenocarcinomas.

III. NITROSAMINE-INDUCED NASAL CAVITY TUMORS IN SYRIAN GOLDEN HAMSTERS

Of the three different hamster species (European, Chinese, Syrian Golden) most commonly used in research, the Syrian Golden hamster has been utilized most frequently as a model in nitrosamine-induced respiratory tract carcinogenesis. The upper respiratory tract (nasal cavities and trachea) of this species appears to be highly sensitive to the carcinogenic effects of nitrosamines. The earliest information on morphology and pathogenesis of nitrosamine-induced nasal cavity carcinogenesis derives from experiments with *N*-nitrosodiethylamine (DEN).[34-38] This compound induces up to 100% nasal cavity tumors in Syrian Golden hamsters in both the respiratory and olfactory portion. The tumors in the anterior region of the nose were diagnosed as papillomas,[38] squamous call carcinomas,[36,38] polyps,[39] adenomas,[39] and adenocarcinomas,[36,39] while the neoplasms in the posterior area were reported as olfactory neuroepithelial tumors[36,39] and adenocarcinomas.[36,37,39] The squamous cell papillomas arise from the respiratory epithelium of the maxillo- and nasoturbinals as well as the nasal septum and naso-lacrimal duct.[40] As their malignant counterparts, the squamous cell carcinomas, they are usually accompanied by multiple squamous metaplasia. The pathogenesis of DEN-induced squamous cell papillomas and carcinomas has not yet been defined at the cellular or subcellular level. Therefore, it is not yet known if — as in the rat — these arise from proliferated basal cells or if other cell types contribute to their formation. The morphology and pathogenesis of DEN-induced adenocarcinomas in the anterior and posterior part of the hamster nasal cavity have been studied by Stenback.[37] He found hyperplasia and

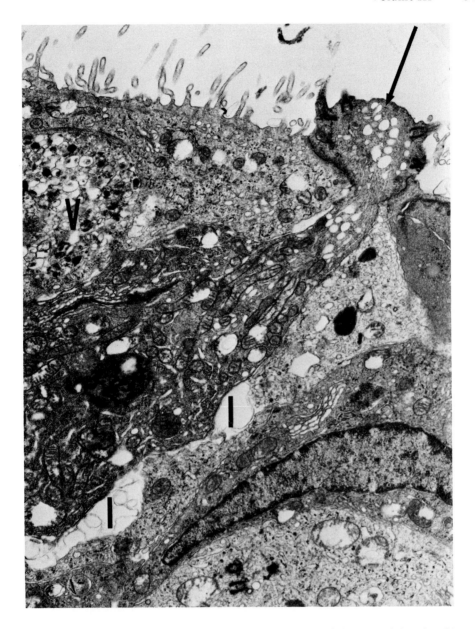

FIGURE 9. Electron micrograph of olfactory epithelium in Fischer 344 rat treated 5 weeks with nitrosomethylpiperazine; an olfactory bulb (arrowed) is vacuolized; mitochondria are swollen; intercellular spaces (I) are wide; cytoplasmic vacuole (V) filled with cellular debris. (Uranyl acetate, lead citrate; ×10,000.)

squamous metaplasia after initial epithelial necrosis in all parts of the nasal cavities. Subsequently, adenomatous hyperplasia of the columnar epithelium featuring increased cell size and loss of cilia developed from such lesions and later gave rise to polyploidal tumor masses. Such tumors grew in a glandular pattern. They contained mucin and exhibited focal areas of squamous metaplasia. The submucous glands of the anterior nasal cavity were identified as an additional site of origin of adenocarcinomas. After initial epithelial dysplasia they gave rise to acinar or tubular adenocarcinomas. While the acinar variety of these neoplasms exhibited pronounced production of mucin as well as areas of osseous and fibrous metaplasia, the tubular adenocarcinomas were only faintly mucin-positive. In the posterior region of the

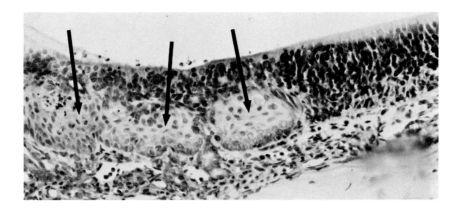

FIGURE 10.   Histopathology of olfactory epithelium in Fischer 344 rat treated with nitrosomethylpiperazine for 8 weeks; in the basal epithelial portion small, pale staining cells have proliferated
(arrowed). (H and E; ×100.)

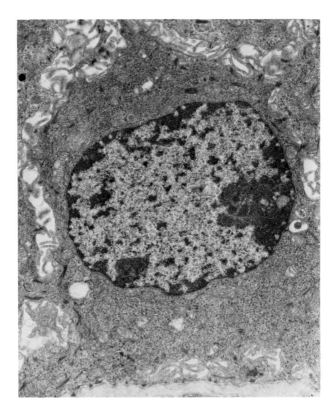

A

FIGURE 11.   Electron micrograph of proliferated cells in basal part of
olfactory epithelium shown in Figure 11; these cells are (A) basal cells
and (B) neuroendocrine cells. (Uranyl acetate, lead citrate; ×9000; ×6000.)

nasal cavities, the adenocarcinomas arose from the tubuloalveolar mucous glands (Bowman's
glands) beneath the olfactory epithelium. They contained abundant mucous material. A
detailed histopathological description of DEN-induced olfactory neuroepithelial tumors in

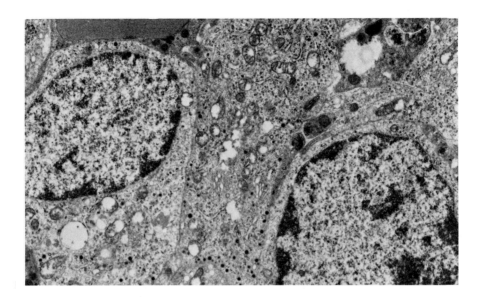

FIGURE 11B

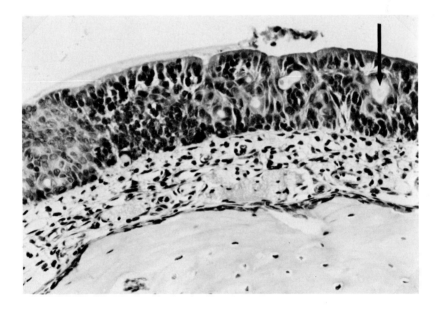

FIGURE 12. Histopathology of olfactory epithelium in Fischer 344 rat after 15 weeks of treatment with nitrosomethylpiperazine; rosette-like structures (arrowed) have developed in the hyperplastic basal portion. (H and E; ×130.)

Syrian hamsters was given by Herrold.[34] She described these tumors as highly cellular with small round-to-oval neoplastic cells exhibiting hyperchroatism. Formation of rosettes and pseudorosettes as well as fibrils extending from the cytoplasm of tumor cells were also reported. Based on their histological features Herrold[34] classified these neoplasms as olfactory neuroblastomas derived from the olfactory epithelium.

The only EM study on nitrosamine-induced nasal cavity tumors in Syrian Golden hamsters has been conducted in my laboratory,[37] in which DEN-induced tumors in the olfactory region of Syrian Golden hamsters were investigated. Histopathologically, the neoplasms resembled the neurogenic tumors reported in the literature after treatment with DEN[36,38] and other

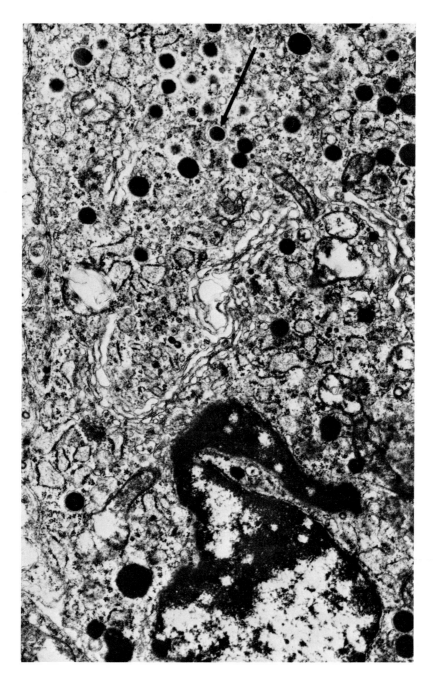

FIGURE 13.   Electron micrograph demonstrating neoplastic neuroblast of DEN-induced tumor
in the olfactory region of a Syrian Golden hamster; numerous dense-cored cytoplasmic granules
(arrowed). (Uranyl-acetate, lead citrate; × 14,000.)

nitrosamines.[41-47] EM revealed that the tumors consisted of two cell types which exhibited
various degrees of differentiation. The first cell type contained membrane-bound, dense-
cored granules (100 to 280 nm in diameter) in their cytoplasm (Figures 13 and 14) and
occasionally exhibited slender cytoplasmic extensions, most of which appeared degenerate.
Mitotic cells of this type were a common finding (Figure 14). When bordering the luminal
edges of rosette-like structures, such cells occasionally demonstrated a short cilium with a

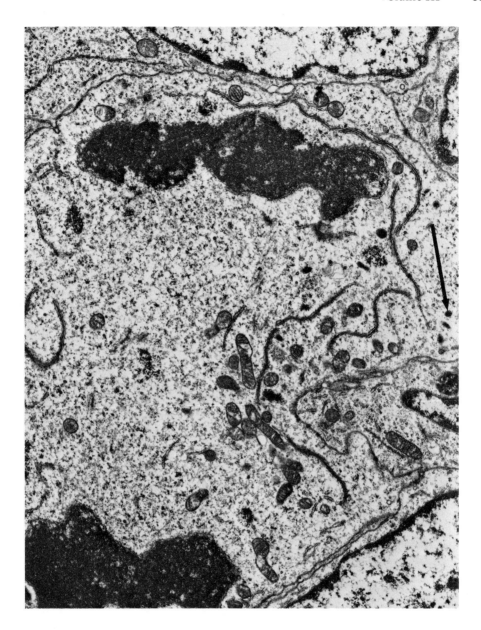

FIGURE 14.   Electron micrograph exemplifying mitotic neuroblast of DEN-induced tumor in olfactory region of Syrian Golden hamster; dense-cored granules (arrowed). (Uranyl acetate, lead citrate; ×9200.)

thick base and attenuated tip. Neither neurotubules nor neurofibrils were found in any of the tumor cells. Based on its morphology this cell type was classified as a neuroblast.

The second cell type found in the olfactory neoplasms was characterized by numerous cytoplasmic ribosomes and polyribosomes as well as occasional branched microvilli (Figure 15) at their luminal edges. Some of these cells also demonstrated bundles of perinuclear filaments (Figure 16) which is an early marker for squamous metaplasia. These cells, some of which exhibited mitosis, were classified as basal cells and their poorly differentiated derivatives (sustentacular cells). These EM data demonstrate that one of the two cell types involved in the development of DEN-induced carcinomas in the olfactory region is of neurogenic origin. Dense-cored cytoplasmic granules are one of the characteristic features

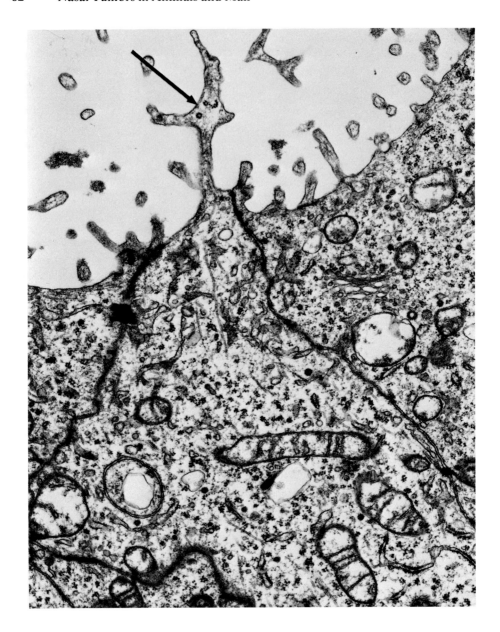

FIGURE 15.   Electron micrograph exhibiting neoplastic sustentacular cells of DEN-induced tumor in olfactory region of Syrian Golden hamster; the cells possess characteristic branched microvilli (arrowed) and their cytoplasm contains numerous polyribosomes. (Uranyl acetate, lead citrate; ×20,000.)

of neuroblasts which are usually preserved in neuroblastomas while the neoplastic cells may have lost their other morphological markers (e.g., neurotubules, axons). Neuroblasts are supposedly the precursor cells from which olfactory sensory cells differentiate during embryonic development,[49] a process which appears to be mimicked in the DEN-induced tumors. However, differentiation into olfactory sensory cells obviously remains at a rather poorly developed stage, since axon-like structures were scanty and dentritic bulbs were not found. The degeneration of axon-like cytoplasmic processes in conjunction with their rarity coincides with the reports on atrophia and toxic degeneration of olfactory sensory cells after treatment with DEN[50] and other nitrosamines.[42] It seems possible that such damage to the olfactory sensory cells could create a stimulus for their stem cells (neuroblasts) to proliferate.

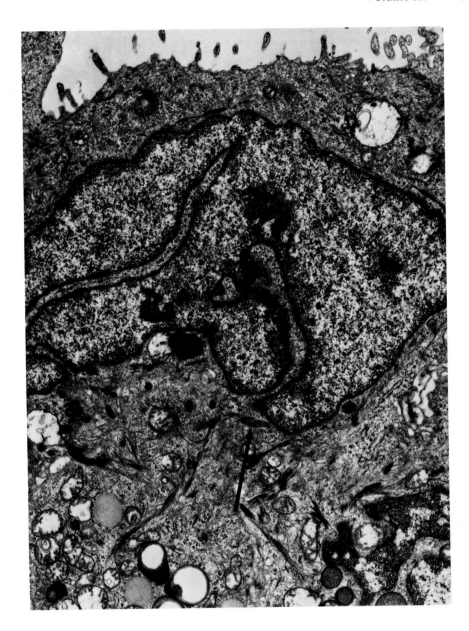

FIGURE 16.   Electron micrograph of tumor cell in olfactory region of DEN-treated Syrian Golden hamster; perinuclear bundles of tonofilaments (arrowed) indicate early squamous metaplasia. (Uranyl acetate, lead citrate; × 14,000.)

The second cell type which contributed to the formation of DEN-induced carcinomas in the olfactory region resembled the basal cells of normal olfactory epithelium[51,52] in its contents of ribosomes and polyribosomes, as well as in their small size and scarcity of other cytoplasmic organelles. In the normal olfactory epithelium, basal cells serve as stem cells for the renewal of sustentacular cells.[51,52] The presence of branched microvilli (a morphological marker for mature sustentacular cells)[52,53] indicates that at least some of the neoplastic basal cells still follow this pathway of normal differentiation. The presence of perinuclear bundles of filaments demonstrates that some of these cells had started undergoing squamous metaplasia. Focal areas of squamous cell differentiation have consistently been reported in neurogenic and adenoid neoplasms induced in the Syrian hamster olfactory region by a variety

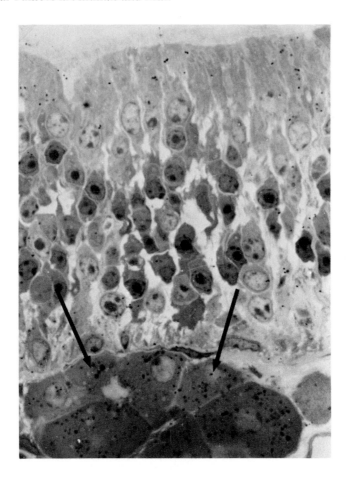

FIGURE 17.   Light microscopic autoradiogram of olfactory region in Syrian
Golden hamster 1 hr after 1-g administration of [³H]-DEN; most autoradiographic grains are concentrated in Bowman's glands (arrowed), indicating
its epithelia are the principle site of bound radioactivity. (Semithin section
Kodak® NTB 2-emulsion, toluidine blue; × 1000.)

of nitrosamines.[36,39,42-48,50,54-56] From our EM data from DEN-induced tumors, it appears
that such foci derive from the basal cells of the olfactory epithelium. Since no other laboratory
did any EM studies on nitrosamine-induced nasal cavity tumors in hamsters, generalizations
as to whether all such neoplasms in the olfactory region derive from neuroblasts and basal
cells are of course somewhat speculative. On the other hand, the histopathology of these
neoplasms is very similar in all studies regardless of the type of nitrosamine used (Table
2). Moreover, the pathology reports are generally more detailed than the respective descriptions in rats, so that data from different laboratories are easier to compare. The histopathological description of Syrian hamster nasal cavity tumorigenesis induced by di-*n*-
propylnitrosamine and related compounds in the olfactory region[42] is one of the best reports
in this area. In accordance with our EM data with DEN, the authors found focal atrophy of
olfactory sensory cells followed by proliferation of "sustentacular cells intermingled with
a small cell type" which was frequently located near the basal lamina of the epithelium. In
view of our findings, these small cells are most probably basal cells. When the nitrosamine
treatment was continued, the hamsters developed squamous metaplasia, which is also in
agreement with our results with DEN. From such early lesions, malignant neoplasms developed which demonstrated formation of rosettes and pseudorosettes which are considered

Table 2

SOME NITROSAMINES WHICH INDUCE NASAL CAVITY TUMORS IN SYRIAN GOLDEN HAMSTERS

Chemical	Carcinogenicity	Diagnosis of nasal cavity tumors	Ref.
N-Nitrosodimethylamine	Weak	Esthesioneuroepithelial tumors	55
N-Nitrosodiethylamine	Strong	Olfactory neuroepithelium tumors; in carcinomas derived from neuroblasts; adenocarcinomas derived from basal cells and sustentacular cell carcinomas; neuroepithelial tumors; squamous cell papillomas	34—38
N-Nitrosodiethanolamine	Medium	Poorly differentiated adenocarcinomas	56
N-Nitroso-di-*n*-propylamine	Medium	Carcinomas originating in the olfactory epithelium (composed of basal cells and sustentacular cells); mucoepidermoid carcinomas	40
N-Nitroso-β-hydroxypropyl-*n*-propylamine	Weak	Carcinomas originating in the olfactory epithelium (composed of basal cells and sustentacular cells); mucoepidermoid carcinomas	40
N-Nitroso-β-oxopropyl-*n*-propylamine	Medium	Carcinomas originating in the olfactory epithelium (composed of basal cells and sustentacular cells); mucoepidermoid carcinomas	40
N-Nitrosomethyl-*n*-propylamine	Medium	Carcinomas originating in the olfactory epithelium (composed of basal cells and sustentacular cells); mucoepidermoid carcinomas	40, 43
N-Nitroso-*1*-oxopropylpropylamine	Medium	?	53
N-Nitroso-bis(2-hydroxypropyl)amine	Strong	Papillomas, mucoepidermoid tumors, squamous cell carcinomas, adenocarcinomas	53
N-Nitroso(2-hydroxypropyl)(2-oxopropyl)amine	Medium	Squamous cell papillomas, mucoepidermoid tumors, squamous cell carcinomas, adenocarcinomas	43
N-Nitrosomethyl-*n*-propylamine	Strong	Adenocarcinomas and poorly differentiated carcinomas of posterior region of nasal cavity	43
N-Nitrosomorpholine	Medium	Olfactory neuroepitheliomas, mixed tumors, adenocarcinomas, anaplastic adenocarcinomas, squamous carcinomas, squamous papillomas	57
N-Nitroso-2,6-dimethylmorpholine	Strong	Adenocarcinomas in posterior region of nasal cavity papillomas, papillary polyps in anterior region of nasal cavity	45, 46

Table 2 (continued)
SOME NITROSAMINES WHICH INDUCE NASAL CAVITY TUMORS IN SYRIAN GOLDEN HAMSTERS

Chemical	Carcinogenicity	Diagnosis of nasal cavity tumors	Ref.
N-Nitrosopiperidine	Weak	Adenocarcinomas, squamous carcinomas, olfactory neuroepitheliomas	57
N-Nitrosopyrrolidine	Weak	Not specified	58
N-Nitrosohexamethyleneimine	Medium	Adenocarcinomas, squamous carcinomas, esthesio-neuroepitheliomas, papillomas	54
N-Nitrosoheptamethyleneimine	Medium	Polyps, adenocarcinomas, adenosquamous carcinomas	59
N-Nitrosonornicotine	Weak	Papillomas, adenocarcinomas	60, 61
N-Nitrosodiallylamine	Strong	Adenocarcinomas, papillary polyps	54

to be a typical feature of neurogenic tumors by many investigators. In addition to the described pathway which closely resembles our findings with DEN, Pour and colleagues[42] also report that epithelia of Bowman's glands contributed to the formation of nasal olfactory carcinomas induced by di-*n*-propylnitrosamine and three structurally related nitrosamines. The authors conclude that the induced tumors derived from basal cells and sustentacular cells of the olfactory epithelia, and from epithelia of Bowman's gland, and that neurogenic elements did not participate in the neoplastic development. At first glance, this conclusion seems to contradict some of our results with DEN (undifferentiated neuroblasts were one of the cell types contributing to DEN-induced nasal cavity tumors). However, considering the fact that Pour's group did not use EM for diagnosis, it does seem quite possible that the undifferentiated neuroblasts were just not recognized.

The data we have reviewed on nitrosamine-induced nasal cavity carcinogenesis in Syrian Golden hamsters demonstrate that of the many cell types present in this organ apparently only a few react to treatment with nitrosamines by proliferation and neoplastic transformation. Neuroblasts and basal cells of the olfactory epithelium, which were found to be the source of nitrosamine-induced tumors in the olfactory region, are both stem cells which are known to have a low level of metabolic competence. Since nitrosamines need to be metabolically activated, one would expect a metabolically more active cell type to serve as the source of nitrosamine-induced tumors. It does seem possible, however, that the metabolic activation takes place in other cells which are close enough to the "susceptible" stem cells. Autoradiographic studies with radioactively labeled nitrosamines would seem to be the best method for solving this problem. However, the only investigation of this nature is a preliminary experiment conducted in my laboratory. Three Syrian Golden hamsters were given a single dose of [³H]-DEN by gavage. The animals were killed 1 hr later and their nasal cavities processed for light microscopic autoradiography. We found that in the olfactory portion of the nose most bound radioactivity was concentrated in the cytoplasm of Bowman's gland epithelia (Figure 17), while the olfactory epithelium itself was only slightly labeled. In the respiratory portion of the nose, most bound radioactivity was found in the mucous cells of the respiratory epithelia as well as in the submucous glands. These data suggest that DEN may be activated in Bowman's glands and mucous cells but nevertheless the metabolites can travel to other cells in the neighborhood which then produce tumors.

IV. NITROSAMINE-INDUCED NASAL CAVITY TUMORS IN EUROPEAN HAMSTERS

The European hamster has not been used in carcinogenesis studies in the U.S., but has been studied extensively at the Medical University of Hannover, West Germany. An outbred strain EGH MHH was developed there and has been used in research for over 10 years. The respiratory tract (nasal cavity and lungs) has proved to be even more sensitive to the effects of nitrosamines than that of the Syrian Golden hamster (Table 3). Unlike the Syrian Golden hamster, the European hamster develops nasal cavity tumors only in the respiratory portion,[62-69] with no neoplastic growths being reported in the olfactory region. The benign tumors that are induced by nitrosamines are papillomas and papillary polyps while their malignant counterparts are squamous cell carcinomas and adenocarcinomas. No neurogenic tumors were diagnosed in nitrosamine-treated European hamsters. The benign neoplasms (papillomas, papillary polyps) are usually located in the most apical parts of the nose (atrioturbinals and rostral portion of maxillo- and nasoturbinals). Occasionally, they may be fairly large and obstruct the nasal airways with reactive inflammation. The malignant tumors (adenocarcinomas and squamous cell carcinomas) are found mostly in the region of the maxillo- and nasoturbinals and may at times also involve the maxillary sinus. They tend to grow agressively, destroying the nasal bones and infiltrating the olfactory region, olfactory

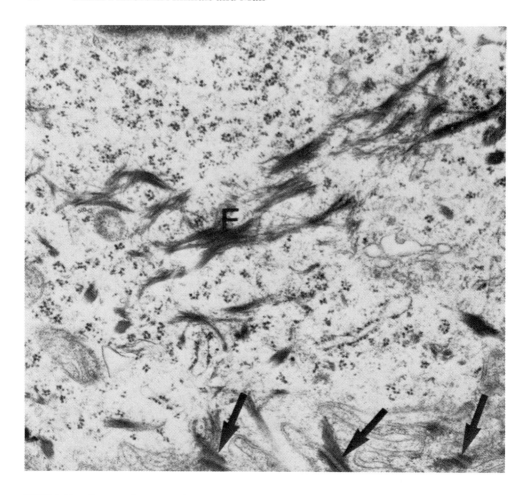

FIGURE 18.   Electron micrograph of tumor cell in DBN-induced squamous cell carcinoma in the maxilloturbinals of a European hamster; prominent bundles of tonofilaments (F) are typical of an early squamous metaplasia; desmosomes (arrowed). (Uranyl acetate, lead citrate; ×32,800.)

bulb, and brain. Since none of the nitrosamines that have been tested in this species is carcinogenic only in the nasal cavities, the nasal cavity tumors are generally accompanied by neoplasms in other organs, and especially the lung. EM studies of squamous cell and adenocarcinomas induced by N-nitrosodiethylamine (DEN)[65] and N-nitrosodibutylamine (DBN)[66] have confirmed that they are derived from cells of the respiratory epithelium. In animals treated with DBN, the squamous cell carcinomas consist of cells exhibiting early stages of squamous metaplasia (Figure 18). Moreover, their abundance of ribosomes, paucity of other cytoplasmic organelles as well as a high nucleus/cytoplasm ratio suggest that they are derived from basal cells. The tumor cells constituting DEN-induced adenocarcinomas demonstrated abundant rough and smooth endoplasmic reticulum as well as secretory granules but no tonofilaments or other indicators of squamous metaplasia. Judged by these morphological features, they were assumed to have arisen from mucous cells. The ultrastructure of DBN-induced nasal adenocarcinomas and squamous cell carcinomas resembled that of their DEN-induced counterparts. In contrast with the DEN-study, however, some mucous cells in the DBN-induced adenocarcinomas demonstrated early squamous metaplasia (Figure 19). This indicates that tumors of squamous differentiation may represent a development from preexisting adenocarcinomas.

Table 3
SOME NITROSAMINES WHICH INDUCE NASAL CAVITY TUMORS IN EUROPEAN HAMSTERS

Chemical	Carcinogenicity	Diagnosis of nasal cavity tumors	Ref.
N-Nitrosodiethylamine	Strong	Papillomas and squamous cell carcinomas originating from respiratory epithelium in atrio-, naso- and maxilloturbinals	62—64
N-Nitrosodibutylamine	Strong	Papillomas, papillary polyps, squamous cell carcinomas, adenocarcinomas	64—66
N-Nitrosodi-isopropanolamine	Strong	Papillomas, squamous cell carcinomas originating in atrioturbinals, maxilloturbinals, and nasal septum	62, 67
N-Nitrosomorpholine	Strong	Papillary polyps, papillomas, squamous cell carcinomas, adenocarcinomas	62, 68
N-Nitrosopiperidine	Strong	Squamous cell papillomas, squamous cell carcinomas originating in respiratory epithelium of naso- and maxilloturbinals, Jakobson's organ, squamous cell carcinomas of meatus nasopharyngeus	62, 68
N-Nitrosoheptamethyleneimine	Strong	Papillomas, squamous cell carcinomas, adenocarcinomas	62, 69

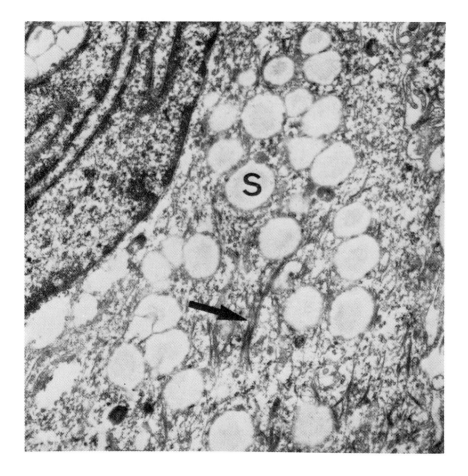

FIGURE 19.   Electron micrograph demonstrating tumor cell with secretion granules (S) and tonofilaments (arrowed) in DBN-induced squamous cell carcinoma of European hamster nasoturbinal.
(Uranyl acetate, lead citrate; × 14,000.)

V. NITROSAMINE-INDUCED NASAL CAVITY TUMORS IN CHINESE HAMSTERS AND GERBILS

Relatively few nitrosamines have been reported to produce nasal cavity carcinogens in Chinese hamsters and gerbils (Table 4). Neither of these speices has been used much in nitrosamine carcinogenesis, a factor which might explain the paucity of data. In none of the studies with Chinese hamsters were the nasal cavities the main target organ. The majority of the induced neoplasms were found in lung,[71] upper digestive tract,[70,72] and liver,[70] while the coincident carcinogenic effects in the nasal cavities were not very great. As with the findings in Syrian Golden hamsters, the induced nasal cavity tumors were found in the respiratory and olfactory portion of the nose. In general, neoplasms with squamous differentiation (papillomas, squamous cell carcinomas) were located in the respiratory part (maxillo- and nasoturbinals, maxillary sinus), while in the olfactory region mainly adenocarcinomas developed. The squamous cell tumors were usually multiple and obstructed the nasal passages, thus leading to secondary inflammation. The adenocarcinomas tended to grow aggressively through the cribriform plate and olfactory bulb to invade the brain. In no case were any neurogenic elements reported in nitrosamine-induced nasal cavity tumors in Chinese hamsters.

Gerbils have been used to an even smaller extent than Chinese hamsters, and, so far,

Table 4
SOME NITROSAMINES WHICH INDUCE NASAL TUMORS IN CHINESE HAMSTERS AND GERBILS

Chemical	Species	Carcinogenicity	Diagnosis of nasal cavity tumors	Ref.
N-Nitrosodimethylamine	Chinese hamster	Weak	Adenocarcinomas in endoturbinal region	70
N-Nitrosodiethylamine	Chinese hamster	Medium	Squamous cell papillomas and squamous cell carcinomas of maxilloturbinals, nasoturbinals, maxillary sinus, and endoturbinals	70
N-Nitrosodibutylamine	Chinese hamster	Weak	Not specified	71
N-Nitrosomorpholine	Chinese hamster	Medium	Papillomas, squamous cell carcinomas in apical region of nasal cavity adenocarcinomas in region of endoturbinals	72
N-Nitrosopiperidine	Chinese hamster	Strong	Adenocarcinomas	72
N-Nitrosodiethylamine	Gerbil	Strong	Mixed carcinomas in respiratory region, olfactory region, adenocarcinomas	73—75

Table 5
SOME NITROSAMINES WHICH INDUCE NASAL CAVITY TUMORS IN MICE

Chemical	Carcinogenicity	Diagnosis of nasal cavity tumors	Ref.
N-Nitrosodiethylamine	Medium	Squamous cell carcinomas	76—78
N-Nitrosodipropylamine	Strong	Squamous cell papillomas, squamous cell carcinomas, adenocarcinomas in endo- and ectoturbinals	79
N-Nitrosomethylpropylamine	Strong	Squamous cell papillomas, squamous cell carcinomas, papillary polyps, adenomas, adenocarcinomas	79
N-Nitroso-*N*-bis(2-hydroxypropyl)amine	Medium	Adenomas, adenocarcinomas, squamous cell carcinomas	80
N-Nitroso-*N*-bis(2-acetoxypropyl)amine	Medium	Squamous cell carcinomas in anterior part of nasal cavity	80

only diethylnitrosamine[73-75] has been reported to induce nasal cavity tumors. The induced tumors were described as mixed carcinomas of the respiratory and olfactory region and as adenocarcinomas. The mixed carcinomas consisted of large cuboidal cells, nonciliated columnar cells, ciliated columnar cells, small cells, and squamous cells, while the adenocarcinomas, which were found predominantly at the respiratory-olfactory junction, consisted mainly of nonciliated and ciliated columnar cells.[73] Although formation of rosette-like structures were observed in some cases there was no other evidence for neurogenic elements contributing to the tumors.

VI. NITROSAMINE-INDUCED NASAL CAVITY TUMORS IN MICE

Relatively few nitrosamines have been reported to induce nasal cavity tumors in mice (Table 5). The first studies in this area were done in 1964.[76,77] They demonstrated that DEN induces up to 87% nasal cavity tumors in mice when administered by skin painting or instillation into the nostrils. Subcutaneous treatment with this compound also resulted in the development of nasal cavity tumors, but at a lower incidence.[78] In all of these experiments the induced neoplasms were described as squamous cell carcinomas. Their exact anatomical location in the nose was, unfortunately, not reported.

Experiments aimed at comparing the carcinogenic effects of *N*-nitrosodipropylamine (DPN) and its β-metabolites[79,80] in mice rats and hamsters revealed that DPN and *N*-nitrosomethylpropylamine (MPN) induced up to 93% nasal cavity tumors in mice, while *N*-nitrosobis-(2-hydroxypropylamine (BHP) and *N*-bis(2-acetoxypropyl-nitrosamine (BAP) were less potent carcinogens for the nasal cavity in this species. With DPN and MPN, the benign neoplasms (papillomas) tended to occur in the anterior portion of the nose, while most of the malignant tumors (squamous cell carcinomas, adenocarcinomas) were found in the posterior portion (endo- and ectoturbinals). BHP induced adenomas, adenocarcinomas, and squamous cell carcinomas in all parts of the nasal cavities while BAP induced only squamous cell carcinomas in the anterior region. With none of these nitrosamines were neurogenic tumors induced in the nasal cavities of mice. However, since the lesions were only diagnosed by light microscopy, neurogenic elements may well have not been recognized.

VII. NITROSAMINE-INDUCED NASAL CAVITY TUMORS IN NONHUMAN PRIMATES AND DOGS

The only information available on nitrosamine-induced nasal cavity tumors in nonhuman primates (Table 6) derives from a comprehensive review of the use of several monkey species in chemical carcinogenesis.[81] Of the four nitrosamines tested, DEN induced nasal cavity tumors at an incidence of 100% in bushbabies *Galago crassicaudatus)*. The authors describe sneezing, audible nasal respiratory sounds, lacrimation, and serous nasal discharge as the first clinical symptoms. Neoplastic growth then became apparent in the anterior portion of the nose and progressed from there to the posterior region invading the cibriform plate, brain, and/or postorbital sinus. The tumors were diagnosed as mucoepidermoid carcinomas and anaplastic adenocarcinomas by histopathology.

Studies of this nature are extremely valuable because they faciliate extrapolation of carcinogenesis data to humans. Since nitrosamines require metabolic activation in the host organism, interspecies differences in metabolic pathways complicate extrapolation of data elaborated in rodent experiments to man. A number of metabolic pathways involved in drug metabolism in nonhuman primates resemble those in man more closely than those in rodents.[82] In addition, the relatively long lifespan of nonhuman primates permits the administration of the compounds at a dose level more comparable with that of human exposure. Since DEN induces nasal cavity tumors in rodents, nonhuman primates, and dogs (see below), it seems highly unlikely that the compound does not exert a similar effect in man.

Table 6
SOME NITROSAMINES WHICH INDUCE NASAL CAVITY TUMORS IN NONHUMAN PRIMATES AND DOGS

Chemical	Species	Carcinogenicity	Diagnosis of nasal cavity tumors	Ref.
N-Nitrosodiethylamine	*Galago crassicaudatus* (bushbabies)	Strong	Mucoepidermoid carcinomas, anaplastic adenocarcinomas	81, 83
N-Nitrosodiethylamine	Dogs	Medium	Mucoepidermoid carcinomas, squamous cell carcinomas	84, 85
N-Nitrosopiperidine	Dogs	Weak	Squamous cell carcinomas, papillary adenocarcinomas	85

In dogs, DEN and nitrosopiperidine have been reported to induce nasal cavity tumors.[84,85] Both nitrosamines induced mainly tumors of squamous differentiation (squamous cell carcinomas, mucoepidermoid carcinomas), some of which metastasized to the lungs. In addition, one papillary adenocarcinoma was described.

REFERENCES

1. **Pour, P., Cardesa, A., Althoff, J., and Mohr, U.,** Tumorigenesis in the nasal olfactory region of Syrian Gold hamsters as a result of Di-*n*-propylnitrosamine and related compounds, *Cancer Res.,* 34, 16, 1974.
2. **Frisch, D.,** Ultrastructure of mouse olfactory mucosa, *J. Anat.,* 121, 87, 1967.
3. **Mackay, B., Luna, M. A., and Butler, G. J.,** Adult neuroblastoma. Electron microscopic observations in nine cases, *Cancer,* 37, 1334, 1976.
4. **Yamamoto, M.,** An electron microscopic study of the olfactory mucosa in the bat and rabbit, *Arch. Histol. Jpn.,* 38, 359, 1976.
5. **Magee, P. N.,** Activation and inactivation of chemical carcinogens and mutagens in the mammal, *Essays Biochem.,* 10, 105, 1974.
6. **Lijinsky, W.,** Significance of in vivo formation of *N*-nitroso compounds, *Oncology,* 37, 223, 1980.
7. **Lijinsky, W. and Taylor, H. W.,** Tumorigenesis by oxygenated nitrosopiperidines in rats, *J. Natl. Cancer Inst.,* 55, 705, 1975.
8. **Lijinsky, W. and Reuber, M. D.,** Carcinogenicity in rats of nitrosomethylethylamines labeled with deuterium in several positions, *Cancer Res.,* 40, 19, 1980.
9. **Lijinsky, W. and Taylor, H. W.,** Carcinogenicity of methylated derivatives of *N*-nitrosodiethylamine and related compounds in Sprague-Dawley rats, *J. Natl. Cancer Inst.,* 62, 407, 1979.
10. **Bulay, O. and Mirvish, S. S.,** Carcinogenesis in rat esophagus by intraperitoneal injection of different doses of methyl-*n*-amylnitrosamine, *Cancer Res.,* 39, 3644, 1979.
11. **Lijinsky, W. and Taylor, H. W.,** Relative carcinogenic effectiveness of derivatives of nitrosodiethylamine in rats, *Cancer Res.,* 38, 2391, 1978.
12. **Lijinsky, W. and Taylor, H. W.,** The change in carcinogenic effectiveness of some cyclic nitrosamines at different doses, *Z. Krebsforsch,* 92, 221, 1978.
13. **Hecht, S. S., Chen, C. B., Ohmorij, T., and Hoffman, D.,** Comparative carcinogenicity in F344 rats of the tobacco-specific nitrosamines, *N*-nitrosonornicotine and 4-(*N*-methyl-*N*-nitrosamino)-*1*-(3-pyridyl)-*1*-butanone, *Cancer Res.,* 40, 298, 1980.
14. **Singer, G. M. and Taylor, H. W.,** Carcinogenicity of *N*-nitrosonornicotine in Sprague-Dawley rats, *J. Natl. Cancer Inst.,* 57, 1275, 1976.
15. **Mirvish, S. S., Bulay, O., Runge, R. G., and Patil, K.,** Study of the carcinogenicity of large doses of dimethylnitramine, *N*-nitroso-L-proline, and sodium nitrite administered in drinking water to rats, *J. Natl. Cancer Inst.,* 64, 1435, 1980.
16. **Pelfrene, A. and Garcia, H.,** Chemically induced esthesioneuroblastomas in rats, *Z. Krebsforsch.,* 86, 113, 1976.
17. **Taylor, H. W. and Lijinsky, W.,** Tumor induction in rats by feeding heptamethyleneimine and nitrite in water, *Cancer Res.,* 35, 812, 1975.
18. **Goodall, C. M., Lijinsky, W., and Tomatis, L.,** Tumorigenicity of *N*-nitrosohexamethyleneimine, *Cancer Res.,* 28, 1217, 1968.
19. **Lijinsky, W. and Taylor, H. W.,** The effect of substituents on the carcinogenicity of *n*-nitrosopyrrolidine in Sprague-Dawley rats, *Cancer Res.,* 36, 1988, 1976.
20. **Zeller, W. J.,** Investigation of the influence of copper and cobalt ions on carcinogenesis due to diethylnitrosamine, *Arch. Geschwulstforsch.,* 45, 634, 1975.
21. **Mohr, U., Reznik, G., and Pour, P.,** Carcinogenic effects of Di-iso-propanol-nitrosamine in Sprague-Dawley rats, *J. Natl. Cancer Inst.,* 58, 361, 1977.
22. **Wiessler, M. and Schmähl, D.,** The carcinogenic action of *N*-nitroso compounds fourth communication: *N*-nitroso-*O,N*-diethyl-hydroxylamine, *Z. Krebsforsch.,* 83, 205, 1975.
23. **Druckrey, H., Ivankovic, S., Mennel, H. D., and Preussmann, R.,** Selective induction of nasal cavity tumors in rats by *N,N'*-Dinitrosopiperazine, nitrosopiperidine, nitrosomorpholine, methylallyl-, dimethyl- and methylvinylnitrosamine, *Z. Krebsforsch.,* 66, 138, 1964.
24. **Garcia, H. and Lijinsky, W.,** Tumorigenicity of five cyclic nitrosamines in MRC rats, *Z. Krebsforsch.,* 77, 257, 1972.

25. **Henderson, B. E. and Louie, E.,** Discussion of risk factors for nasopharyngeal carcinoma, *IARC Sci. Publ.,* 20, 251, 1978.
26. **Reznik, G., Mohr, U., and Krüger, F. W.,** Carcinogenic effects of D-*n*-propylnitrosamine, β-hydroxypropyl-*n*-propylnitrosamine, and methyl-*n*-propylnitrosamine on Sprague-Dawley rats, *J. Natl. Cancer Inst.,* 54, 937, 1975.
27. **Taylor, H. W. and Nettesheim, P.,** Influence of administration route and dosage schedule on tumor response to nitrosoheptamethyleneimine in rats, *Int. J. Cancer,* 15, 301, 1975.
28. **Pour, P., Salmasi, S., Runge, R., Gingell, R., Wallcave, L., Nagel, D., and Stepan, K.,** Carcinogenicity of *N*-nitrosobis(2-hydroxypropyl)amine and *N*-nitrosobis(2-oxopropyl)amine in MRC rats, *J. Natl. Cancer Inst.,* 63, 181, 1979.
29. **Lijinsky, W. and Taylor, H. W.,** Increased carcinogenicity of 2,6-dimethylnitrosomorpholine compared with nitrosomorpholine in rats, *Cancer Res.,* 35, 23, 1973.
30. **Reznik-Schüller, H. M.,** Nasal cavity carcinogenesis induced by nitrosomethylpiperazine in F344 rats, in preparation.
31. **Bottema, T.,** Experimentelle Gezwellen in het Neusslijmvlies van de Rat, Ph.D. thesis, University of Amsterdam, The Netherlands, 1971.
32. **Azzopardi, A. and Thurlbeck, W. M.,** Oxidative enzyme pattern of the bronchial mucous glands, *Am. Rev. Resp. Dis.,* 97, 1038, 1968.
33. **Kraft, P. L. and Tannenbaum, S. R.,** Distribution of *N*-nitrosomethylbenzylamine evaluated by whole body radioautography and densitometry, *Cancer Res.,* 40, 1921, 1980.
34. **Herrold, K. M.,** Induction of olfactory neuroepithelium tumors in Syrian hamsters by diethylnitrosamines, *Cancer,* 17, 114, 1964.
35. **Reznik-Schüller, H. M.,** Ultrastructure of *N*-diethylnitrosamine-induced tumors in the nasal olfactory region of the Syrian golden hamster, *J. Pathol.,* 124, 161, 1978.
36. **Montesano, R. and Saffiotti, U.,** Carcinogenic response of the respiratory tract of Syrian golden hamsters to different doses of diethylnitrosamine, *Cancer Res.,* 28, 2197, 1968.
37. **Stenback, F.,** Glandular tumors of the nasal cavity induced by diethylnitrosamine in Syrian golden hamsters, *J. Natl. Cancer Inst.,* 50, 895, 1973.
38. **Herrold, K. M.,** Epithelial papillomas of the nasal cavity. Experimental induction in Syrian hamsters, *Arch. Pathol.,* 78, 189, 1964.
39. **Reznik-Schüller, H. M. and Mohr, U.,** Ultrastructure of *N*-nitrosodibutylamine-induced tumors of the nasal cavity in the European hamster, *J. Natl. Cancer Inst.,* 57, 401, 1976.
40. **Pour, P., Cardesa, A., Althoff, J., and Mohr, U.,** Tumorigenesis in the nasal olfactory region of Syrian golden hamsters as a result of Di-*n*-propylnitrosamine and related compounds, *Cancer Res.,* 34, 16, 1974
41. **Althoff, J., Eagan, M., and Grandjean, C.,** Carcinogenic effect of 2,2'-dimethyldipropylnitrosamine in Syrian hamsters, *J. Natl. Cancer Inst.,* 55, 1209, 1975.
42. **Pour, P., Krueger, F. W., Althoff, J., and Mohr, U.,** Effect of beta oxidized nitrosamines on Syrian hamsters. III. 2,2'-Dihydroxy di-*n*-propylnitrosamine, *J. Natl. Cancer Inst.,* 54, 141, 1975.
43. **Pour, P., Wallcave, L., Gingell, R., and Mohr, U.,** Carcinogenic effect of *N*-nitroso (2-hydroxypropyl) (2-oxopropyl)amine, a postulated proximate pancreatic carcinogen in Syrian hamsters, *Cancer Res.,* 39, 3828, 1979.
44. **Pour, P., Krüger, F. W., Cardesa, A., Althoff, J., and Mohr, U.,** Tumorigenicity of methyl-*N*-propylnitrosamine in Syrian golden hamsters, *J. Natl. Cancer Inst.,* 52, 456, 1974.
45. **Althoff, J., Grandjean, C., and Gold, B.,** Carcinogenic effect of subcutaneously administered *N*-nitroso-2,6-dimethylmorpholine in Syrian golden hamsters, *J. Natl. Cancer Inst.,* 60, 197, 1978.
46. **Reznik, G., Mohr, U., and Lijinsky, W.,** Carcinogenic effect of *N*-nitroso-2,6-dimethylmorpholine in Syrian golden hamsters, *J. Natl. Cancer Inst.,* 60, 371, 1978.
47. **MacKay, B., Luna, M., and Butler, G. J.,** Adult neuroblastoma. Electron microscopic observations in nine cases, *Cancer,* 37, 1334, 1971.
48. **Schade, A. R.,** Sinneszellen und Nervenzellen, in *Grundlagen der Cytologie,* Hirsch, K. G., Ruska, H., and Sitte, P., Eds., Gustav Fischer Verlag, Stuttgart, 1973, 579.
49. **Greenblatt, M. and Rijhsinghani, K.,** Comparative cytopathologic alterations induced by alkylnitrosamines in nasal epithelium of the Syrian hamster, *J. Natl. Cancer Inst.,* 42, 421, 1969.
50. **Seifert, K. and Ule, D.,** Die Ultrastruktur der Riechschleimhaut der neugeborenen und jugendlichen weissen Maus, *Z. Zellforsch.,* 76, 147, 1967.
51. **Yamamoto, M.,** An electron microscopic study of the olfactory mucosa in the bat and rabbit, *Arch. Histol. Jpn.,* 38, 359, 1976.
52. **Frisch, D.,** Ultrastructure of mouse olfactory mucosa, *J. Anat.,* 121, 87, 1967.
53. **Althoff, J., Grandjean, C., Gold, B., and Runge, P.,** Carcinogenicity of *1*-oxopropylpropylnitrosamine in Syrian hamsters, *Z. Krebsforsch. Klin. Oncol.,* 90, 221, 1977.

54. **Althoff, J., Cardesa, A., Pour, P., and Mohr, U.**, Carcinogenic effect of *N*-nitrosohexamethyleneimine in Syrian golden hamsters, *J. Natl. Cancer Inst.*, 73, 323, 1973.

55. **Herrold, K. M.**, Histogenesis of malignant liver tumors induced by dimethylnitrosamine. An experimental study with Syrian hamsters, *J. Natl. Cancer Inst.*, 39, 1099, 1967.

56. **Hilfrich, J., Schmeltz, T., and Hoffmann, D.**, Effects of *N*-nitrosodiethanolamine and *1,1*-diethanol-hydrazine in Syrian golden hamsters, *Cancer Lett.*, 4, 55, 1978.

57. **Haas, H., Mohr, U., and Krüger, F. W.**, Comparative studies with different doses of *N*-nitrosomorpholine, *N*-nitrosopiperidine, *N*-nitrosomethylurea, and dimethylnitrosamine in Syrian golden hamsters, *J. Natl. Cancer Inst.*, 51, 1295, 1973.

58. **McCoy, G. D., Hecht, S. S., Chen, C. B., Katayama, S., Rivenson, A., Hoffman, D., and Wynder, E. L.**, Influence of chronic ethanol consumption on the metabolism and carcinogenicity of *N*-nitrosopyr-rolidine and *N'*-nitrosonornicotine in Syrian golden hamsters, *Proc. Am. Assoc. Cancer Res.*, 21, 100, 1980.

59. **Lijinsky, W., Ferrero, A., Montesano, R., and Wenyon, C. E.**, Tumorigenicity of cyclic nitrosamines in Syrian golden hamsters, *Z. Krebsforsch.*, 74, 185, 1970.

60. **Rivenson, A., Ohmori, T., Hecht, S. S., and Hoffman, D.**, Organotropic carcinogenicity of tobacco specific *N*-nitrosamines, *Proc. 5th Meet. Eur. Assoc. Cancer Res., Vienna*, Abstr., Kugler Publications, Vienna, 1980, 51.

61. **Hilfrich, J., Hecht, S. S., and Hoffman, D.**, A study of tobacco carcinogenesis. XV. Effects of *N*-nitrosonornicotine and *N*-nitrosoanabasine in Syrian golden hamsters, *Cancer Lett.*, 2, 169, 1977.

62. **Reznik, G.**, Experimentelle Karzinogenese im Respirationstrakt am Modell des Europäischen Feldhamsters (*Cricetus cricetus* L.), *Fortschr. Med.*, 95, 2627, 1977.

63. **Mohr, U., Althoff, J., Speilhoff, R., and Bresch, H.**, The influence of hibernation upon the carcinogenic effect of *N*-diethylnitrosamine in European hamsters, *Z. Krebsforsch.*, 80, 285, 1973.

64. **Reznik, G., Reznik-Schüller, H., and Mohr, U.**, Carcinogenicity of *N*-nitrosodiethylamine in hibernating and non-hibernating European hamsters, *J. Natl. Cancer Inst.*, 58, 673, 1977.

65. **Reznik-Schüller, H. and Mohr, U.**, Ultrastructure of *N*-nitrosodibutylamine-induced tumors of the nasal cavity in the European hamster, *J. Natl. Cancer Inst.*, 57, 401, 1976.

66. **Althoff, J., Mohr, U., Page, N., and Reznik, G.**, Carcinogenic effect of dibutylnitrosamine in European hamsters (*Cricetus cricetus*), *J. Natl. Cancer Inst.*, 53, 795, 1976.

67. **Reznik, G. and Mohr, U.**, Effect of Di-isopropanolnitrosamine in European hamsters, *Br. J. Cancer*, 36, 479, 1977.

68. **Mohr, U., Reznik, G., and Reznik-Schüller, H. M.**, Carcinogenic effect of *N*-nitrosomorpholine and *N*-nitrosopiperidine on European hamsters (*Cricetus cricetus*), *J. Natl. Cancer Inst.*, 53, 231, 1974.

69. **Reznik, G., Mohr, U., and Lijinsky, W.**, Carcinogenicity of subcutaneously injected nitrosoheptame-thyleneimine in European hamsters, *J. Natl. Cancer Inst.*, 61, 239, 1978.

70. **Reznik, G., Mohr, U., and Kmoch, N.**, Carcinogenic effect of different nitroso-compounds in Chinese hamsters. I. Dimethylnitrosamine and *N*-diethylnitrosamine, *Br. J. Cancer*, 33, 411, 1976.

71. **Reznik, G., Mohr, U., and Kmoch, N.**, Carcinogenic effects of different nitroso-compounds in Chinese hamsters: *N*-dibutylnitrosamine and *N*-nitrosomethylurea, *Cancer Lett.*, 1, 183, 1976.

72. **Reznik, G., Mohr, U., and Kmoch, N.**, Carcinogenic effects of different nitroso-compounds in Chinese hamsters. II. *N*-nitrosomorpholine and *N*-nitrosopiperidine, *Z. Krebsforsch.*, 86, 95, 1971.

73. **Cardesa, A., Pour, P., Haas, H., and Mohr, U.**, Histogenesis of tumors from the nasal cavities induced by diethylnitrosamine, *Cancer*, 37, 346, 1976.

74. **Green, U. and Ketkar, M.**, The influence of diazepam upon the carcinogenic effect of diethylnitrosamine in gerbils, *Z. Krebsforsch.*, 92, 55, 1978.

75. **Haas, H., Kmoch, N., Mohr, U., and Cardesa, A.**, Susceptibility of gerbils (meriones unguiculatus) to weekly subcutaneous and single intravenous injections of *n*-diethylnitrosamine, *Z. Krebsforsch*, 83, 233, 1975.

76. **Hoffmann, F. and Graffi, A.**, Carcinoma of the nasal cavity in mice, following topical application of diethylnitrosamine to the skin of the back, *Acta Biol. Med. Ger.*, 12, 623, 1964.

77. **Hoffmann, F. and Graffi, A.**, Nasal cavity tumors in mice after percutaneous diethylnitrosamine appli-cation, *Arch. Geschwulstforsch.*, 23, 274, 1964.

78. **Hilfrich, J., Althoff, J., and Mohr, U.**, Stimulation of the rate of induction of lung tumors by diethyl-nitrosamine in 0-20-mice, *Z. Krebsforsch.*, 75, 240, 1970.

79. **Dickhaus, S., Reznik, G., Green, U., and Ketkar, M.**, The carcinogenic effect of beta-oxidized dipro-pylnitrosamine in mice, *Z. Krebsforsch*, 90, 253, 1977.

80. **Green, U., Konishi, Y., Ketkar, M. B., and Althoff, J.**, Comparative study of the carcinogenic effect of *N*-Bis-2-hydroxypropyl-nitrosamine and N-Bis-2-acetoxypropyl-nitrosamine on NMR1 mice, *Cancer Lett.*, 9, 257, 1980.

81. **Adamson, R. H. and Sieber, S. M.,** The use of nonhuman primates for chemical carcinogenesis studies, in *Regulatory Aspects of Carcinogenesis and Food Additives: The Delaney Clause,* Academic Press, New York, 1979, 275.
82. **Smith, R. L. and Caldwell, J.,** Drug metabolism in nonhuman primates, in *Drug Metabolism From Microbe to Man,* Parke, D. V. and Smith, R. L., Eds., Taylor & Francis, London, 1977, 331.
83. **Dalgard, D. W., Correa, P., Waalkes, T. P., and Adamson, R. H.,** Induction of mucoepidermoid carcinoma in prosimians with *N*-nitrosodiethylamine, *Proc. Am. Assoc. Cancer Res.,* 16, 87, 1975.
84. **Hirao, K., Matsumura, K., Imagawa, A., Enomoto, Y., Hosogi, Y., Kani, T., Fujikawa, K., and Ito, N.,** Primary neoplasms in dog liver induced by diethylnitrosamine, *Cancer Res.,* 34, 1870, 1974.
85. **Hosugi, Y.,** The development of experimental nasal and paranasal cavity tumors in dogs and their radiologic study, *J. Nara. Med. Assoc.,* 24, 712, 1974.

Chapter 4

EXPERIMENTAL NASAL CAVITY TUMORS INDUCED BY TOBACCO-SPECIFIC NITROSAMINES (TSNA)*

A. Rivenson, K. Furuya, S. S. Hecht, and D. Hoffmann

TABLE OF CONTENTS

I.   Introduction 80

II.   Formation and Occurrence of TSNA 80

III.   Bioassays of TSNA 80

IV.   Microscopic Anatomy and Histogenesis of Nasal Cavity Tumors Induced by
        TSNA 82

Acknowledgments 85

References 112

---

*   Figures for this chapter appear at the end of the text.

I. INTRODUCTION

Cigarette smoking is one of the most unphysiologic habits acquired by man. In order to voluntarily inhale smoke one must suppress powerful natural reflexes designed to protect the respiratory apparatus against noxious factors. In addition, the cigarette smoke induces or promotes cancers. Of course, one can argue that "like the definition of sin, the definition of a carcinogen which has significance to the environmental cancer problem is not an easy one ."[1]

Yet, if a product clearly qualifies as "a carcinogen which has significance", that one is undoubtedly cigarette smoke. Not only the most thorough epidemiological studies but also an enormous amount of experimental data point to the conclusion that cigarette smoking is closely related to the development of a variety of cancers. The demonstration of the tumorigenic potential of tobacco-specific nitrosamines (TSNA) represents one step with important implications for the experimental approach of tobacco-related cancers. Theoretically, the existence of TSNA has been long suspected because the carcinogenic activity of the cigarette smoke could not be fully explained by the presence of various other compounds.[2]

II. FORMATION AND OCCURRENCE OF TSNA

The structures of some tobacco alkaloids and the nitrosamines derived from them (TSNA) are illustrated in Figure 1. The major alkaloid in most tobacco varieties is nicotine. Minor alkaloids include nornicotine, anabasine, and anatabine. The possible presence in tobacco smoke of alkaloid-derived nitrosamines was suggested by Boyland and co-workers[3,4] who carried out the first bioassays of N'-nitrosonornicotine (NNN) and N'-nitrosoanabasine (NAB) as described below.[4] However, the presence of NNN in tobacco smoke was first reported in 1974.[5] Surprisingly high levels of NNN were also detected in unburned tobacco.[6,7] Studies on the origin of NNN in tobacco and tobacco smoke indicated that the tertiary amine nicotine was a more important precursor than the secondary amine nornicotine, in contrast to expectations based solely on chemical reactivity.[5,7,8] This led to the hypothesis that nitrosamines other than NNN could be derived from nicotine.[10]

This hypothesis was verified experimentally in 1978 by studies which showed that the nitrosaminoketone NNK and the nitrosaminoaldehyde NNA were formed in the nitrosation of nicotine and that the former was present in tobacco.[9,11] The advent of the thermal energy analyzer (TEA) for nitrosamine analysis led to thorough studies on the occurrence of tobacco-specific nitrosamines in tobacco, in main- and sidestream tobacco smoke, and in the saliva of snuff dippers.[12,13] The levels of NNN, NNK, and NATB in tobacco are generally between 1 to 50 ppm; concentrations in main- and sidestream tobacco smoke vary from 0.1 to 6 µg per cigarette.[12] Trace amounts of NAB have been detected in tobacco smoke but NNA has not been detected. The relatively high levels of TSNA in tobacco, tobacco smoke, and saliva of snuff dippers make it likely that these compounds are involved in the tobacco-related cancers which include cancers of the lung, larynx, oral cavity, esophagus, pancreas, and bladder in smokers and of the oral cavity in snuff dippers.[13-15]

III. BIOASSAYS OF TSNA

In the first carcinogenicity assays, conducted by Boyland and co-workers,[3] NNN in arachis oil was injected intraperitoneally in 20 male and 20 female Chester Beatty mice (total dose, 0.5 mmol per mouse), and 7 of 40 mice developed multiple pulmonary adenomas compared to 1 of 30 mice in the control groups. High doses (7.9 to 11.5 mmol per rat) of NAB induced esophageal tumors in 25 out of 32 rats which were given the nitrosamine in the drinking water. The tumors appeared after 50 to 70 weeks of treatment.[4]

The carcinogenicity of NNN in rats was first reported in 1975.[16] In this comparative study of NNN and NAB, each nitrosamine was administered in the drinking water for 30 weeks to groups of 20 male Fischer 344 rats. The total doses per rat were 3.3 mmol of NAB and 3.6 mmol of NNN. The experiment was terminated after 48 weeks. In the NNN group, 14 of 20 animals developed tumors, mainly esophageal papillomas and carcinomas. One pharyngeal tumor and 3 nasal cavity tumors were also observed. In contrast, NAB induced tumors in only 2 of the 20 animals. This experiment demonstrated that NNN was a more potent carcinogen than NAB. The lower tumor yield from NAB compared to Boyland's experiment was probably due to the lower dose and the shorter lifetime of the animals.

When NNN was administered in the drinking water to a group of 15 female Sprague-Dawley rats (total dose, 8.8 mmol per rat) tumors of the esophagus were not observed; all 15 animals developed what was called "adenocarcinomas of the olfactory epithelium". This experiment demonstrates a difference in the organospecificity of NNN in Sprague-Dawley and Fischer 344 rats.[17]

The mode of administration is also an important factor in determining the organospecificity of NNN in the rat. When a total dose of 3.4 mmol of NNN was administered by subcutaneous injection in trioctanoin over a 20-week period to a group of 12 male and 12 female Fischer 344 rats, nasal cavity tumors were observed in 92% of the males and in 75% of the females. Esophageal tumors were not detected.[18] The difference in target organ between this assay and the experiment in which NNN was given in the drinking water was not due to the vehicle because a similar yield of nasal cavity tumors was obtained when NNN was injected subcutaneously in saline.[19] The induction of esophageal tumors by NNN administered in the drinking water is particularly relevant to the situation in tobacco chewers who are exposed to NNN orally and have an excess risk for esophageal cancer.[14]

When NNK was assayed in Fischer 344 rats by subcutaneous injection in trioctanoin, with a regimen and dose identical to that used for NNN, nasal cavity tumors were induced in 83% of the males and 83% of the females.[18] In addition, NNK induced liver tumors in 83% of the males and 100% of the females and lung tumors in 67% of the males and 67% of the females. These results demonstrate that NNK is a more powerful carcinogen than NNN in the Fischer 344 rat, an observation that may be related to its activity as a methylating agent, as discussed in Chapter 10.

Comparative tumorigenicity experiments in strain A/J female mice also showed that NNK was a more powerful tumorigen than either NNN or NNA.[9] Each compound (0.1 mmol) was administered by intraperitoneal injection over a period of 7 weeks; the experiment was terminated 30 weeks later. NNK induced more lung adenomas per mouse than did NNN, while the incidence of lung adenomas in mice treated with NNA was not greater than in control mice. Two salivary gland tumors were also observed in animals treated with NNN.

The carcinogenic activity of NNN in the Syrian Golden hamster was first reported in 1977.[20] NNN or NAB (total dose, 2 mmol per hamster) were each administered by subcutaneous injection in saline over a period of 25 weeks. Within 83 weeks, 12 of 19 hamsters given NNN developed tracheal tumors and 1 had a tumor of the nasal cavity. None of the animals treated with NAB developed tumors. Thus, the relative carcinogenic activities of NNN and NAB were the same with Fischer 344 rats and Syrian Golden hamsters. NNK proved to be a powerful carcinogen in the Syrian Golden hamster, as demonstrated in comparative bioassays with NNN.[21] In one assay, 30 hamsters were each given 19 subcutaneous injections of 0.048 mmol of NNN or NNK in trioctanoin (total dose, 0.9 mmol per hamster). This regimen of NNK was toxic and only 8 of the original 30 hamsters survived the first 10 weeks of the experiment. Nevertheless, 19 animals developed nasal cavity tumors. Among the NNN group, 1 animal developed a lung adenoma and 5 had tracheal papillomas. In a second assay, 20 hamsters received each 75 subcutaneous injections of 0.012 mmol of NNN or NNK over a 25-week period (total dose, 0.9 mmol per hamster). Eleven of the

NNK-treated animals developed carcinomas of the nasal cavity, 16 had lung adenomas and/ or adenocarcinomas, and 7 developed tracheal papillomas. Among the animals treated with this dose of NNN, only 1 developed a lung adenoma and one had a tracheal papilloma. Thus NNK is clearly a more potent carcinogen than NNN in Syrian Golden hamsters, as well as in strain A/J mice and Fischer-344 rats.

The organospecificity of NNK and NNN in the Syrian Golden hamster was demonstrated in an experiment in which these nitrosamines were dissolved in olive oil and applied to the lips and the oral cavity.[22] NNN and NNK each were applied twice weekly for 30 weeks (total dose, approximately 1.5 mmol) to groups of 12 male and 12 female hamsters. Among the NNK-treated animals 5 of 12 males and 6 of 12 females had nasal cavity tumors and 9 of 12 males and 9 of 12 females developed tumors of the lung. Papillomas of the oral cavity were observed in only 1 male and 1 female. NNN induced nasal cavity tumors in 2/12 males and 1/ 12 females and tracheal tumors in 1/12 males and 1/12 females. One oral cavity papilloma was observed. Thus, the results were similar to those obtained upon subcutaneous injection indicating a lack of sensitivity of the Syrian Golden hamster oral cavity to these nitrosamines.

Because of the known synergism between chronic alcohol consumption and cigarette smoking as risk factors for cancers of the head and neck, the effect of chronic alcohol consumption on the carcinogenicity of NNN and a structurally related nitrosamine which occurs in tobacco smoke, N-nitrosopyrrolidine (NPYR), was examined in male Syrian Golden hamsters.[23] Groups of male Syrian Golden hamsters were maintained on ethanol-containing or control liquid diets for 4 weeks prior to and during carcinogen treatment. NNN or NPYR were administered by intraperitoneal injection, in saline, over a period of 25 weeks (total dose, 1 or 2 mmol). The incidence of tracheal and nasal cavity tumors in the NNN-treated animals was similar to that described above and was not affected by ethanol treatment. In contrast, ethanol treatment increased the sensitivity of the hamster trachea and nasal cavity to the effects of NPYR, particularly at the lower dose. At this dose, in animals on a control diet, 1 of 20 hamsters had a nasal cavity tumor and 4 of 20 hamsters had tracheal tumors, whereas in the ethanol-treated groups 8 of 18 hamsters has nasal cavity tumors and 9 of 18 had tracheal tumors. This is believed to relate to ethanol-induced increases in the rates of metabolic activation of NPYR, but not NNN, in the tissues of the Syrian Golden hamster nasal cavity and trachea.

The above-mentioned bioassays in rats, mice, and hamsters demonstrate the carcinogenic activities of the tobacco-specific nitrosamines NNN and NNK. NNK is a powerful carcinogen; NNN is a moderately active carcinogen. NAB appears to have only weak activity. The carcinogenicity of NATB is currently being assayed in Fischer-344 rats in a dose response study which also includes NNN and NNK. The emergence of NNK as a highly active carcinogen points to the role of the nitrosamines in the tobacco-induced cancers in man.

Due to their frequency, aggressiveness, and particular histologic structure, the experimental nasal cavity tumors provide an interesting material to study.

In our tests, the parameter "time" was invariable; autopsies of treated animals were performed at the time of death or at the termination of the experiment when all animals were sacrificed in a short interval of time. Hence, the only variable was the quantity of TSNA administered.

When the survival was adequate, most tumors (80%) were large, occupying the nasal cavity and/or invading the brain. Yet some were small or incipient, indicating a certain degree of individual sensitivity (or lack of it) for TSNA.

IV. MICROSCOPIC ANATOMY AND HISTOGENESIS OF NASAL CAVITY TUMORS INDUCED BY TSNA

With oscillations towards one predominant type or another, the experimental nasal cavity tumors (ENCT) induced by TSNA have a comparable histogenesis and analogous morphology with ENCT induced by other *n*-nitrosocompounds.

Basically, both olfactory and respiratory parts of the nasal mucosa participate in tumorigenesis.

The histologic structure of the early ENCT may or may not resemble the histologic appearance of the late, invasive ENCT. Frequently, the "early" aspects remain as small enclaves in the fully developed tumor or may completely disappear submerged by the more aggressive component which becomes the predominant tissue of the tumorous mass.

Examined in the "early stages", the TSNA nasal cavity tumors always show a multicentric development. In the respiratory part of the nasal mucosa, all phases from nonspecific inflammation to tumorous lesions can be observed. Chronic and acute inflammation, loss of cilia, and squamous metaplasia are precursors of squamous papillomas (Figures 2 to 5).

In the olfactory part, the images are more complex due to the more elaborated structure of this mucosa. As in the respiratory area, the process starts with the same nonspecific inflammatory reaction. The nerve-bundles may show degenerative changes even at this stage. Foci of disorderly dysplasia and atypia replace the sharp, architectural regularity of the olfactory epithelium (Figure 6). Intraepithelial and/or intramucosal nodules follow the hyperplastic stage (Figure 7). Most of the intraepithelial neurons degenerate due to the destruction of their axons by the inflammatory and tumorous process as well as the toxic activity of the product (Figure 6).

Among the factors contributing to the initial pleomorphic aspect of the nasal cavity tumors we may recall :

1. The presence of a large number of cell types (columnar ciliated, goblet, acinar glandular, bipolar-neuronal, sustentacular, Schwann, basal "stem") in a relatively limited space
2. The facile metaplastic conversion
3. The presence of an unyielding rigid, osseous cavity

This last mechanical factor plays an important role in the natural selection of the most vigorous and fastest growing tissue designed to survive the collision course. Less malignant and benign tumors, which initially have an important contribution to the makeup of the experimentally induced nasal cavity tumors, either disappear or remain as islands of quiescent or necrotic tissue. The hamsters seem to preserve more of these various types of metaplastic (mostly squamous) tissues than the rats, which in turn tend to have a more uniform pattern of the end-stage tumors.

All these data must be considered before deciding the diagnosis of nasal tumors induced by nitrosamines. As is well known, the human spontaneous cases of olfactory tumors provide a wide panel of suggested diagnoses from adenocarcinoma or transitional cell carcinoma to reticulum-cell-sarcoma and from esthesioneuroepithelioma to plain "carcinoma".[24,25]

In our cases, if we eliminate what can be easier eliminated (e.g., "lymphoma" or "sarcoma") and try to rationalize other possible diagnoses, we may end up with a more orderly evaluation.

Most of the metaplastic epidermoid tissues (including transitional) grow slowly and tend to be "differentiated". The number of mitoses in these tissues at any given time is very low. To the contrary, the supporting and basal cells of the olfactory area, after losing most of their neuronal partners to the toxicity of the product and to the prolonged inflammatory reaction, start proliferating (Figure 6). As long as the space is available, squamous papilloma (inverted or outgrowing) and olfactory epitheliomas grow independently without reciprocal interference. In the olfactory area, bizarrely shaped cells with uni- or multipolar extensions fill portions of the lamina propria previously occupied by nerve bundles and glands (Figure 8A and B). If the animal dies or is sacrificed at this stage, the multiplicity of tumorous foci and the variable histology may keep the pathologists arguing forever on the "real" label for a given histology section. Yet the important fact is that the plurality of tumor types represents just a transitional stage in what will be *the* nasal cavity tumor of the respective animal. With the exception of mice — which show a great resistance to nasal tumors induced by TSNA — (Figures 9 and 10) — all rodents used in our experiments continued to develop their "initial" or "early" tumors up to a critical point; that point was reached when the narrow, osseous cavity was filled with tumor. At that time, the competition for space and nutrition becomes a major factor in the future evolution of the tumorous process. It is only at that point that the neuroepithelial tumor of basal and supporting cells emerges as the malignant tumor of the area. Its high aggressiveness is due, presumably, to the return of component cells to their primitive, neuroepithelial stage of development.

Electron microscopic studies have repeatedly confirmed the olfactory sustentacular and basal-cell nature of various chemically induced experimental nasal cavity tumors.[26,27]

The light microscopy of the florid TSNA-induced tumors shows typically neurogenic characters: piriform, dendritic, or carrot-like elongated cells; numerous ependymal-type, organoid, rosettes (Figures 11 to 16). In some instances, the elongated cells may have their tapered foot process attached to a blood vessel or connective septum forming perivascular rosettes (Figure 14). The Homer-Wright pseudorosettes are also visible (Figure 15). As described by Ishikawa et al.,[28] we consider that the lumen-forming ependymal-like structures represent a differentiation beyond the so-called "true rosette" and correspond to an abortive primitive neural-tube development.

Yet, for some authors[26,27,29,30] the neuroepithelial character of the experimentally induced nasal cavity tumors is doubtful becuase of lack of neurofibrils (see Chapter 3.) It is not clearly explained why the presumed absence of neurofibrils (hence neuroblasts) would deprive these tumors of their neuroepithelial origin and make them less "neurogenic".* Embryologically, neurons, supporting cells, and basal cells derive together from the same neuroepithelial stem cell.[25,31] That is unanimously accepted. Perhaps it is not superfluous to recall that the primitive neuroepithelial cells of placodes differentiate into esthesioneuroblasts, which, as stem cells, further differentiate into olfactory neurons and sustentacular cells. A reserve of stem cells still exists in adults, as "basal" cells of the olfactory epithelium.[32,33]

Thorough and complex studies using light microscopy, ultramicroscopy, autoradiography, biochemical markers, and electrophysiology have proven the constant renewal of the olfactory neurons by the basal "stem" cells, which divide and differentiate in new perikarya.[32-43] "This would constitute a very exceptional case to the general rule that neurons are not formed in postnatal life."[44] It is not unreasonable to call the olfactory stem cells "undifferentiated neuroblasts".[45]

As a target for the carcinogen, the basal cells proliferate without control forming various types of olfactory neuroepithelial tumors. Theoretically, as a working hypothesis, we may assume that the accumulation of carcinogen at the level of olfactory mucosa can spark the derepression of old ontogenetic growth stereotypes of the basal and supporting cells. They regain the highly proliferative rate and the morphogenetic potential of the embryonic subependymal layer of the original neuroepithelial (neuroectodermal) tube. That gives them the appearance of elongated ependymal-like cells (forming true rosettes) or uni- or multipolar spongioblasts (Figure 17A, B, and C). Recently, it was shown that a similar conversion (to multipolar cells) occurs when olfactory basal cells are cultivated in vitro.[34]

Once the growing capacity of the olfactory cells surpasses the slow growth of other

---

*   The term neurogenic means (with respect to tumors) originating in the nervous system. The neuroepithelium is the epithelium of the ectoderm which generates the cerebrospinal axis. Calling the sustentacular and basal cells "nonneurogenic" would implicitly remove all gliomas (including Schwannomas) from the group of neurogenic tumors.

metaplastic (epidermoid or glandular) structures, these later tumors, if not necrotic, remain as benign or well-differentiated islands of tissue (Figure 18) or become necrotic in the body of the main tumor which is an esthesioneuroepithelioma. Due to a variety of causes, including mechanical factors (compression before and during the bone erosion), the fibrilar extensions of glio or neuroblastic type are less visible than in early development of the tumors. Nevertheless, numerous fibrils and dendritic cells can be seen by careful staining of sections with Mallory phosphotungstic hematoxilin (Figures 22 to 24). These cells are incrusted in the compact lobular mass of the tumor body, usually away from the rosettes. The cells composing the tumor lobules have little cytoplasm but prominent nuclei ("bare nuclei"). The morphology and colorability of these nuclei (clear, gray, or densely dark) (Figure 19) are reminiscent of the types of nuclei present in the normal cells of the olfactory epithelium.

The dynamics of the rosette formation is another element which deserve attention. Apparently, the true rosettes arise by the same mechanism seen in embryonic development: cytolysis of a central group of cells and radial organization of long "peg cells" around the newly created lumen (Figures 12B to 13B). The rosette-forming activity seems more accentuated in the rat than hamster. The latter animal also has a tendency to maintain larger and more numerous islands of epidermoid tissue, though usually without an obvious malignant potential.

As of this time, considering the facts accumulated — the location of the tumor, the shape and structure of the cells, and the morphogenetic capability to form typical rosettes and pseudorosettes — we diagnose the TSNA-induced neoplasmas (as well as most other nitrosamine-induced nasal cavity tumors) as "neuroepitheliomas of the olfactory area" according to the Herrold initial opinion.[35] Calling them "adenocarcinomas" or vaguely "carcinomas" would mean to use a misnomer and ignore the objective embryologic, histogenetic, morphogenetic, and cytologic data.

ACKNOWLEDGMENTS

This study was supported by PHS Grant Number CA29580 and CA21393, both awarded by the National Cancer Institute, DHHS.

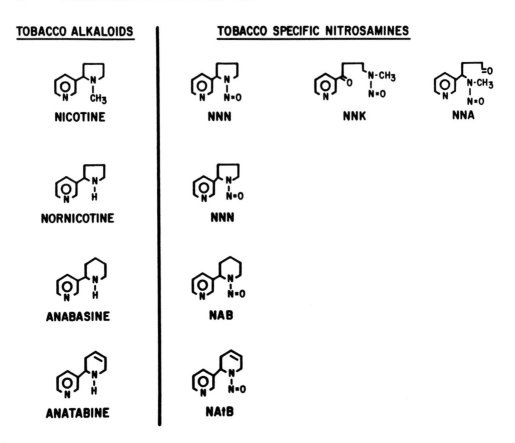

FIGURE 1.   The structure of some tobacco alkaloids and the nitrosamines derived from them (tobacco-specific nitrosamines).

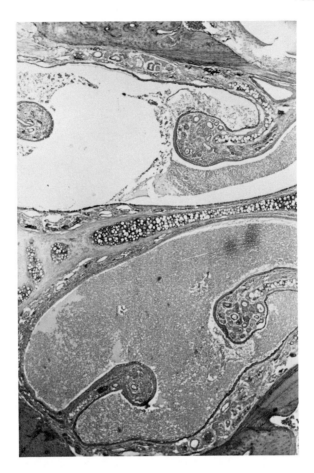

FIGURE 2. Rat, NNN treatment: extensive acute inflammatory reaction and pus formation. No epithelial proliferation in this case. (H
and E; ×10)

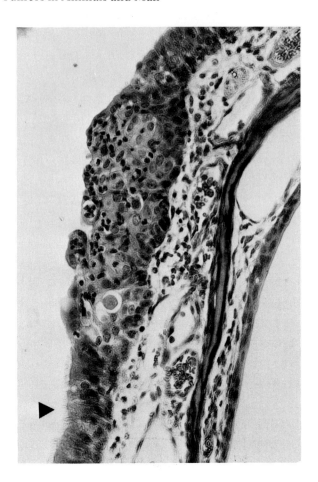

FIGURE 3.   Rat, NNN treatment: early lesions of the respiratory nasal cavity. Squamous metaplasia with dysplastic proliferation. Normal respiratory epithelium (arrowhead). (H and E; ×134)

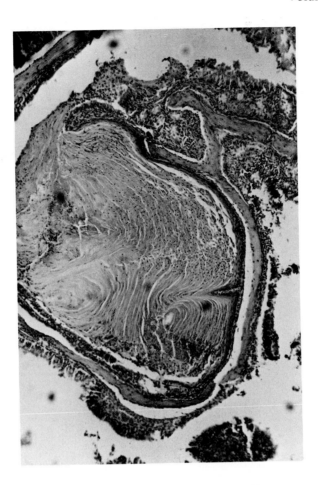

FIGURE 4. Hamster, NNK treatment: early tumor with squamous metaplastic conversion of nasal respiratory epithelium and massive accumulation of keratinized material in a choanal fold. The rest of respiratory mucosa is ravaged by inflammation. (H and E; ×29)

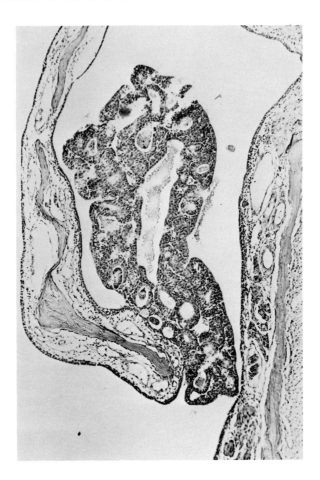

FIGURE 5.   Rat, NNK treatment: early proliferation of nasal respiratory epithelium. Squamous papilloma with cilindromatous and
pseudoglandular appearance. The inflammation is mild, which is
uncommon at this stage of tumor development. (H and E; ×29)

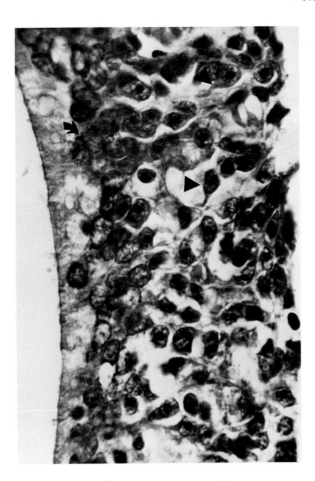

FIGURE 6. Rat, NNN treatment: early modifications in the olfactory epithelium. The polarization of neurons (arrowheads) and supporting cells is greatly disturbed and the entire epithelium is disorganized. Proliferation of supporting cells is suggested by the clustering of their nuclei (arrow). (H and E; ×670)

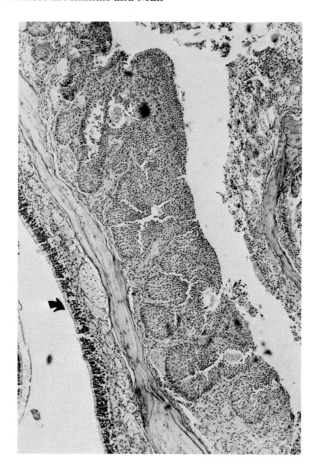

FIGURE 7.   Rat, NNK treatment: early tumor at the junction of the
respiratory-olfactory mucosa. Wide area of papillary (metaplastic)
proliferation, with transitional features. This is a common occurrence
in both rats and hamsters. Rarely seen in mice. Extensive acute and
chronic inflammation destroys the mucosa in the upper right side of
the photograph. The other parts of the olfactory epithelium (arrow)
seem unaffected at this level. (H and E; ×25)

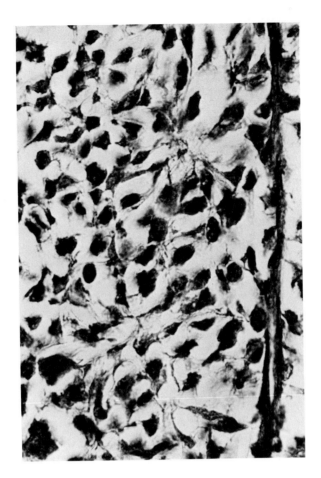

A

FIGURE 8.   (A, B) Rat, NNK treatment: early olfactory tumor. Dendritic cells. The extensions are avid for phosphotungstic hematoxylin stain and the similarity to uni- or bipolar spongioblasts is evident. One of the factors which greatly hinders the study of such tumors is the necessity to submit the tissue to decalcifying agents and the heat during paraffin embedding. That contributes to change in the usual silver and other reagents' specifity. The silver techniques for neurofibrils in the peripheral nervous system, applied on paraffin sections, are notoriously unreliable, especially after decalcification; this is well-known by those studying the nervous apparatus of bones or teeth.[48] Plastic embedding and sliding microtome sectioning without decalcification may bypass this impediment. It is also possible that frozen or celloidin sections (after decalcification) may be more adequate for the use of silver techniques unavailable on paraffin sections. (Bielschowsky, Cajal, Hortega, etc.) (PTAH; ×250)

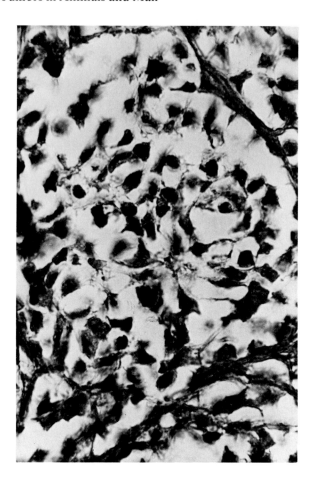

FIGURE 8B

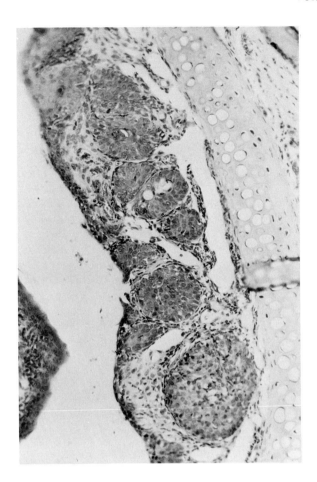

FIGURE 9.   Mouse, NNK treatment: squamous metaplastic endo-
phytic papillary nodules in respiratory mucosa. No malignant tumors
have been seen in our mice treated with TSNA. (H and E; ×29)

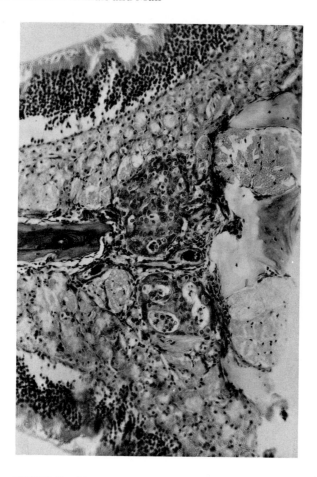

FIGURE 10.   Mouse, NNK treatment: early proliferative nodules
in the lamina propria of the olfactory mucosa. Uncertain histogenesis.
(H and E; × 50)

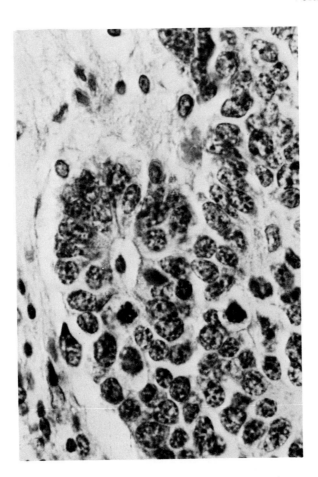

FIGURE 11.   Rat, NNK treatment: brain invasion by olfactory tumor. Various aspects of true (ependymal-like) rosettes. Note the
"sun-like" appearance, the usual presence of cellular debris in the
lumen, the "pseudocuticular membrane limiting the lumen",[47] and
mitoses in the rosette cells. (H and E; ×268)

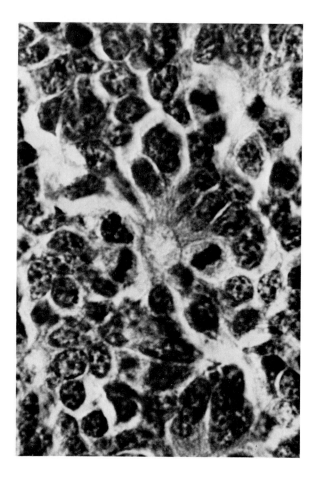

A

FIGURE 12.   (A, B, C, D) Rat, NNK treatment: fully developed
olfactory neuroepithelioma showing "ependymal-like rosette" for-
mations with very long piriform or carrot-shaped cells and numerous
mitoses, a character similar to Flexner rosettes in retinal neuroepithelioma. These rosettes are actually abortive tubular structures formed
continuously by the tumor cells reverted to their embryonic (neuroectodermal) morphogenetic program. Very often, cellular clumps
or debris can be found in the lumen of the rosettes. (H and E; ×670)

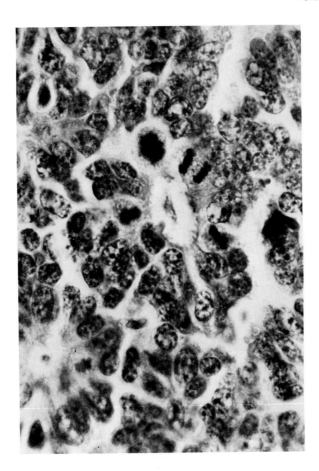

FIGURE 12B

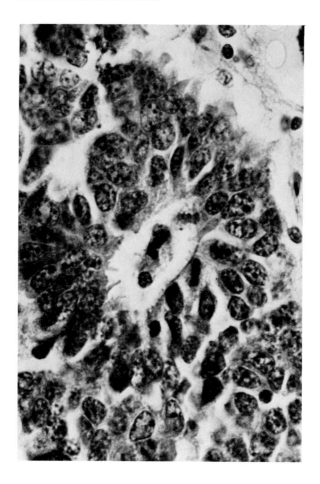

FIGURE 12C

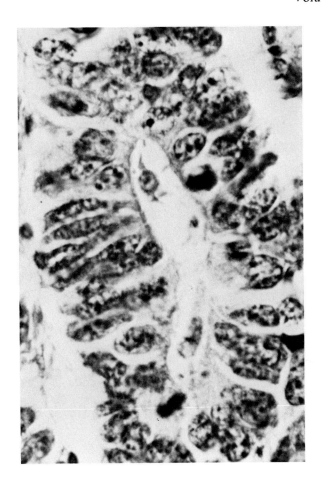

FIGURE 12D

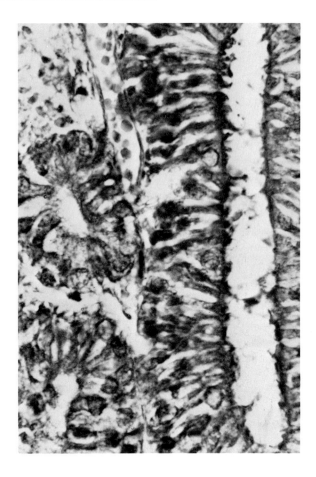

A

FIGURE 13.   (A, B) NNN treatment: ependymal-like rosettes with elongated cells. Some of these cells are inserted with one end to the rosette lumen membrane and the other end to a blood vessel. (H and E; ×670)

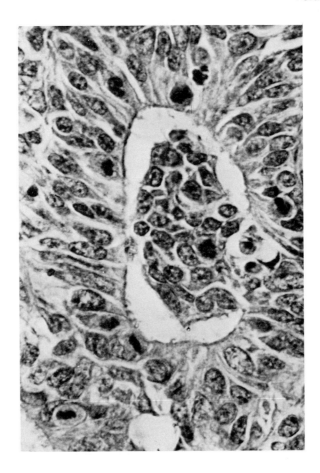

FIGURE 13B

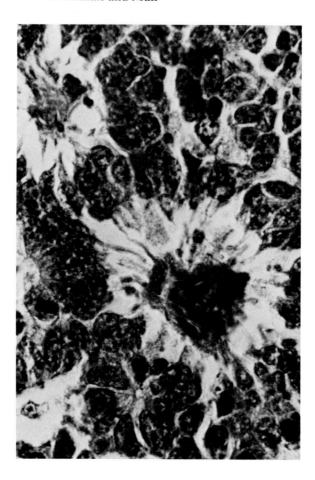

FIGURE 14.   Rat, NNN treatment: long piriform or racket-like cells attached by their foot process to vasculo-connective trabecules (pseudorosetting). (H and E; ×670)

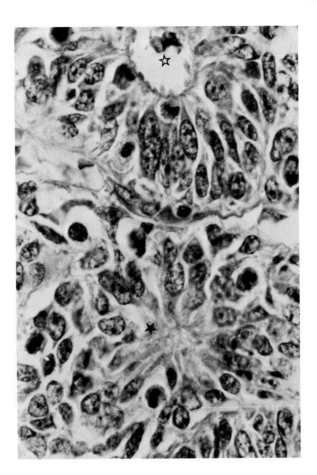

FIGURE 15.   Rat, NNK treatment: ependymal-like rosette (white star) and Homer Wright-like pseudorosette (black star) in a fully developed olfactory neuroepithelioma. Elongated cells, "carrot" or "peg" shaped, are arranged in a circular-radial mode, typical for this type of structure. The lumen of the true rosette contains cellular debris, attesting the morphogenesis by cytolysis of central core and radial rearrangement of the surrounding cells. (H and E; ×670)

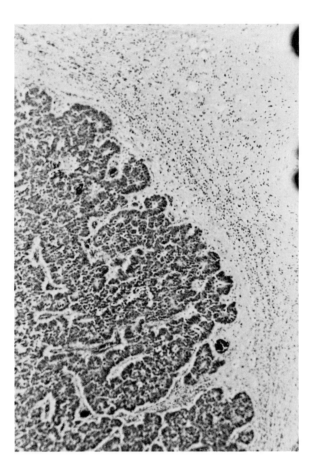

FIGURE 16.   Rat, NNN treatment: brain invasion by an olfactory
neuroepithelioma. Many true rosettes are seen. (H and E; ×25)

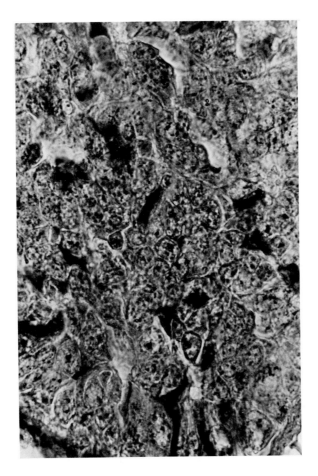

A

FIGURE 17. (A, B, C) Hamster, NNK treatment: advanced olfactory neuroepithelioma. Bi- and unipolar spongioblast-like cells in the tumor mass. (PTAH stain; ×250, ×670, ×670)

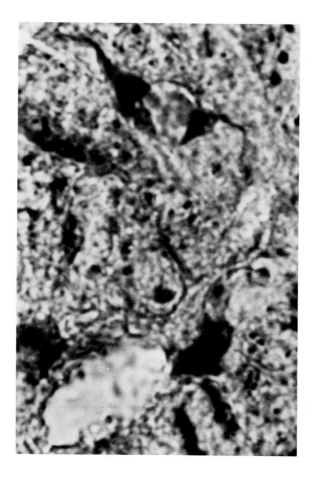

FIGURE 17B

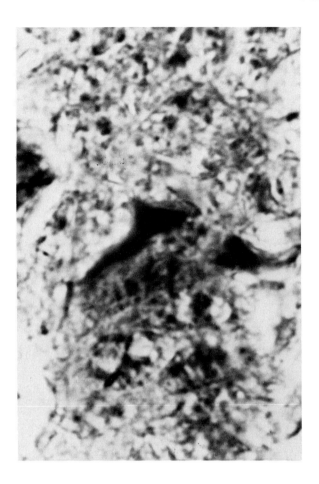

FIGURE 17C

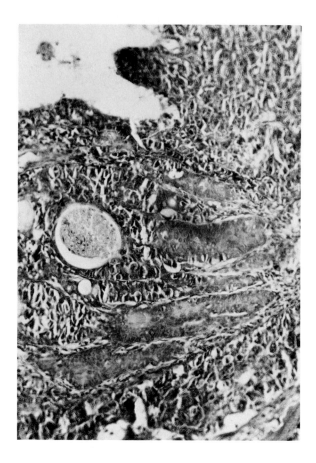

FIGURE 18.   Hamster, NNK treatment: neuroepithelial tumor with
areas of epidermoid tissue as remaining enclaves. (H and E; ×67)

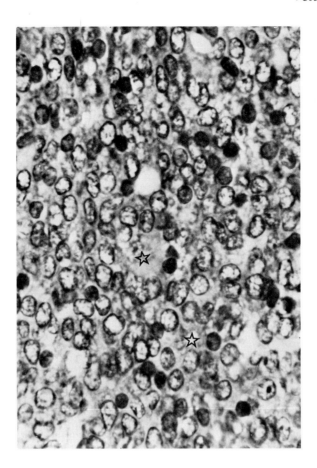

FIGURE 19.   Hamster, NNK treatment: in the "undifferentiated" parts of neuroepithelial tumors, the compactness of tissue and crowding of nuclei suggest a "medullary" aspect. "Dark", "gray", and "clear" nuclei can be seen as well as abortive sketches of pseudo-rosettes (stars). (H and E; ×250)

REFERENCES

1. **Eckardt, R. E.,** Environmental carcinogenesis: guest editorial *Cancer Res.,* 22, 395, 1962.
2. **Roe, F. J. C., Salaman, M. H., Cohen, J., and Burgan, J. G.,** Incomplete carcinogens in cigarette smoke condensate: tumor promotion by a phenolic fraction, *Br. J. Cancer,* 13, 623, 1959.
3. **Boyland, E., Roe, F. J. C., and Gorrod, J. W.,** Induction of pulmonary tumors in mice by nitrosonornicotine, a possible constituent of tobacco smoke, *Nature (London),* 202, 1126, 1964.
4. **Boyland, E., Roe, F. J. C., Gorrod, J. W., and Mitchley, B. C. V.,** The carcinogenicity of nitrosoanabasine, a possible constituent of tobacco smoke, *Br. J. Cancer,* 23, 265, 1964.
5. **Hoffmann, D., Rathkamp, G., and Liu, Y. Y.,** On the isolation and identification of volatile and nonvolatile *N*-nitrosamines and hydrazines in cigarette smoke, in *N-Nitroso Compounds in the Environment,* IARC Scientific Publ. No. 9, Bogovski, P., Walker, E. A., and Davis, W., Eds., International Agency for Research on Cancer, Lyon, 1974, 159.
6. **Hoffmann, D., Hecht, S. S., Ornaf, R. M., and Wynder, E. L.,** *N'*-nitrosonornicotine in tobacco, *Science,* 186, 265, 1974.
7. **Hecht, S. S., Ornaf, R. M., and Hoffmann, D.,** *N'*-nitrosonornicotine in tobacco; analysis of possible contributing factors and biologic implications, *J. Natl. Cancer Inst.,* 54, 1237, 1974.
8. **Mirvish, S. S., Sams, J., and Hecht, S. S.,** Kinetics of nornicotine and anabasine nitrosation in relation to *N'*-nitrosonornicotine occurrence in tobacco and to tobacco-induced cancer, *J. Natl. Cancer Inst.,* 59, 1211, 1977.
9. **Hecht, S. S., Chen, C. B., Hirota, N., Ornaf, R. M., Tso, T. C., and Hoffmann, D.,** Tobacco-specific nitrosamines: formation from nicotine in vitro and during tobacco curing and carcinogenicity in strain A mice, *J. Natl. Cancer Inst.,* 60, 819, 1978.
10. **Klus, H. and Kuhn, H.,** Untersuchungen über die nichtflüchtigen *N*-Nitrosamine der Tabakalkaloide, *Fachliche Mitt. Oesterr. Tabakregie,* 14, 251, 1973.
11. **Hecht, S. S., Chen, C. B., Ornaf, R. M., Jacobs, E., Adams, J. D., and Hoffmann, D.,** Reaction of nicotine and sodium nitrite; formation of nitrosamines and fragmentation of the pyrrolidine ring, *J. Org. Chem.,* 43, 72, 1978.
12. **Hoffmann, D., Adams, J. D., Brunnemann, K. D., and Hecht, S. S.,** Assessment of tobacco-specific *N*-nitrosamines in tobacco products, *Cancer Res.,* 39, 2505, 1979.
13. **Hoffmann, D. and Adams, J. D.,** Carcinogenic tobacco-specific *N*-nitrosamines in snuff and in the saliva of snuff dippers, *Cancer Res.,* 41, 4305, 1981.
14. U.S. Department of Health, Education and Welfare, Smoking and Health, A Report of the Surgeon General, 284-109/6619, U.S. Government Printing Office, Washington, D.C., 1979.
15. **Winn, D. M., Blot, W. J., Shy, C. M., Pickle, L. W., Toledo, A., and Fraumeni, J. F., Jr.,** Snuff dipping and oral cancer among women in the southern United States, *N. Engl. J. Med.,* 304, 745, 1981.
16. **Hoffmann, D., Raineri, R., Hecht, S. S., Maronpot, R., and Wynder, E. L.,** Effects of *N'*-nitrosonornicotine and *N'*-nitrosoanabasine in rats, *J. Natl. Cancer Inst .,* 55, 977, 1975.
17. **Singer, G. M. and Taylor, H. W.,** Carcinogenicity of *N'*-nitrosonornicotine in Sprague-Dawley rats, *J. Natl. Cancer Inst.,* 57, 1275, 1976.
18. **Hecht, S. S., Chen, C. B., Ohmori, T., and Hoffmann, D.,** Comparative carcinogenicity in F-344 rats of the tobacco-specific nitrosamines, *N'*-nitrosonornicotine and 4-(*N*-methyl-*N*-nitrosamino)-*l*-(3-pyridyl)-*l*-butanone.
19. **Hecht, S. S., Young, R., Rivenson, A., and Hoffmann, D.,** On the metabolic activation of *N*-nitrosomorpholine and *N'*-nitrosonornicotine: effects of deuterium substitution, in *N-Nitroso Compounds: Occurrence and Biological Effects,* IARC Scientific Publ., No. 41, Bartsch, H., O'Neill, I. K., Castegnaro, M. and Okada, M., Eds., Lyon, 1982, 499.
20. **Hilfrich, J., Hecht, S. S., and Hoffmann, D.,** Effects of *N'*-nitrosonornicotine in Syrian Golden hamsters, *Cancer Lett.,* 2, 169, 1977.
21. **Hoffmann, D., Castonguay, A., Rivenson, A., and Hecht, S. S.,** Comparative carcinogenicity and metabolism of 4-(methylnitrosamino)-1-(3-pyridyl)-1-butanone and *N'*-nitrosonornicotine in Syrian golden hamsters, *Cancer Res.,* 41, 2386, 1981.
22. **Rivenson, A., Hecht, S. S., McCoy, G. D., and Hoffmann, D.,** unpublished data, 1980.
23. **McCoy, G. D., Hecht, S. S., Katayama, S., and Wynder, E. L.,** Differential effects of chronic ethanol consumption on the carcinogenicity of *N*-nitrosopyrrolidine and *N'*-nitrosonornicotine in male Syrian Golden hamsters, *Cancer Res.,* 41, 2849, 1981.
24. **Elkon, D., Hightower, S. I., Lim, M. L., Cantrell, R. W., and Constable, S. C.,** Esthesioneuroblastoma, *Cancer,* 44, 1087, 1979.
25. **Chaudhry, A. P., Haar, J. G., Koul, S., and Nickerson, P. A.,** Olfactory neuroblastoma; a light and ultrastructural study of two cases, *Cancer,* 44, 564, 1979.

26. **Reznik-Schüller, H.,** Ultrastructure of *N*-diethylnitrosamine induced tumours in the nasal olfactory region of the Syrian Golden hamster, *J. Pathol.,* 124, 161, 1978.

27. **Reznik, G., Reznik-Schüller, H., Ward, J. M., and Stinson, S. F.,** Morphology of nasal-cavity tumours in rats after chronic inhalation of 1,2-dibromo-3-chloropropane, *Br. J. Cancer,* 42, 772, 1980.

28. **Ishikawa, T., Masahito, P., and Takayama, S.,** Olfactory neuroepithelioma in a domestic carp *(Cyprinus carpio), Cancer Res.,* 38, 3954, 1978.

29. **Pour, P., Cardesa, A., Althoff, J., and Mohr, U.,** Tumorigenesis in the nasal olfactory region of Syrian Golden hamsters as a result of Di-*n*-propylnitrosamine and related compounds, *Cancer Res.,* 34, 16, 1974.

30. **Cardesa, A., Pour, P., Haas, H., Althoff, J., and Mohr, U.,** Histogenesis of tumors from the nasal cavities induced by diethylnitrosamine, *Cancer,* 37, 346, 1976.

31. **Hamilton, W. J., Boyd, J. D., and Mossman, H. W.,** *Human Embryology,* Williams & Wilkins, Baltimore, 1952, 314.

32. **Yamamoto, M.,** An electron microscopic study of the olfactory mucosa in the bat and rabbit, *Arch. Histol. Jpn.,* 38, 359, 1976.

33. **Takagi, S. F. and Yajima, T.,** Electrical activity and histological changes in the degenerating olfactory epithelium, *J. Gen. Physiol.,* 48, 559, 1965.

34. **Takagi, S. F.,** Degeneration and regeneration of the olfactory epithelium, in *Handbook of Sensory Physiology,* Vol. 6, Beidle, L. M., Ed., Springer-Verlag, Berlin, 1971, 76.

35. **Nagaharay, Y.,** Experimentelle Studien über die Histologischen Veränderungen des Geruchsorgans nach der Olfactoriesdurchschneidung, Beiträge zur Kenntnis des feineren Baus des Geruchsorgans, *Jpn. J. Med. Sci.,* 5, 165, 1940.

36. **Andres, K. H.,** Der Feinbau der regio Olfactoria von Makrosmatikern, *Z. Zellforsch.,* 69, 140, 1966.

37. **Andres, K. H.,** Differenzierung und Regeneration von Sinneszellen in der regio Olfactoria, *Naturwissenschaften,* 17, 500, 1965.

38. **Moulton, D. J.,** Cell renewal in the olfactory epithelium of the mouse, in *Conference on Odor: Evaluation, Utilization and Control,* Caier, W. S., Ed., New York Academy of Sciences, New York, 1967, 52.

39. **Graziadei, P. P. C.,** Cell dynamics in the olfactory mucosa, *Tissue and Cell,* 5, 113, 1971.

40. **Graziadei, P. P. C. and Metcalf, J. F.,** Neuronal dynamics in the olfactory mucosa of the adult vertebrates, *Am. Anat.,* 10, 11, 1971.

41. **Harding, J., Graziadei, P. P. C., and Margolis, F. L.,** Olfactory chemoreceptor cell: heretical neurons?, *Trans. Am. Soc. Neurochem.,* 7, 162, 1976.

42. **Harding, J. and Margolis, F. L.,** Denervation in the primary olfactory pathway of mice. III. Effect on enzyme of carnosine metabolism, *Brain Res.,* 110, 351, 1976.

43. **Harding, J., Graziadei, P. P. C., Montigraziadei, G. A., and Margolis, F. L.,** Denervation in the primary olfactory pathway of mice. IV. Biochemical and morphological evidence for neuronal replacement following nerve section, *Brain Res.,* 132, 11, 1977.

44. **Ham, A. W. and Cormack, D. H.,** *Histology,* 8th ed., J. B. Lippincott, Philadelphia, 1979, 728.

45. **Goldstein, N. I. and Quinn M. R.,** A novel cell line isolated from the murine olfactory mucosa, *In Vitro,* 17, 593, 1981.

46. **Herrold, K.,** Induction of olfactory neuroepithelial tumors in Syrian hamsters by diethylnitrosamine, *Cancer,* 17, 114, 1964.

47. **Gerard-Marchant, R. and Micheau, C.,** Microscopical diagnosis of olfactory esthesioneuromas: general review and report of five cases, *J. Natl. Cancer Inst.,* 35, 75, 1965.

48. **Linder, J. E.,** A simple and reliable method for the silver impregnation of nerves in paraffin sections of soft and mineralized tissues, *J. Anat.,* 127, 542, 1978.

Chapter 5

HISTOPATHOLOGY OF THE NASAL CAVITY IN LABORATORY ANIMALS EXPOSED TO CIGARETTE SMOKE AND OTHER IRRITANTS

David Walker

TABLE OF CONTENTS

I.   Introduction 116

II.   The Animal Model... 116
        A.   Structure and Function.. 116
        B.   Particulate Deposition 117
        C.   Microbiological Status... 117

III.   Microanatomy of the Rat Nasal Cavity...................................... 118
        A.   General 118
        B.   Specific Transverse Level 119

IV.   Nasal Histopathology after Cigarette Smoke Exposure 122
        A.   Methodology 122
        B.   Author's Results.. 123
                1.   Nasal Septum 123
                2.   Turbinates... 125
                3.   Nasolacrimal Duct 125
                4.   Maxillary Sinus 125
                5.   Other Epithelia.. 125
        C.   Others' Results 126
                1.   Short-Term Studies....................................... 126
                2.   Long-Term Studies....................................... 126
        D.   Comment 126

V.   The Distribution of Lesions Caused by Other Inhaled Irritants 127
        A.   Examples 127
                1.   Cigarette Smoke Constituents 127
                2.   Sulfur Dioxide 129
                3.   Carcinogens 129
                4.   Pyrolysis Products....................................... 129
                5.   Formulated Industrial Products 130
        B.   Comment 130

Acknowledgments 132

References... 133

I. INTRODUCTION

As the normal entrance to the respiratory tract, the nasal cavity is the first target for air-borne irritants and the first physical barrier impeding their progress to the lower conducting airways. It thus has a protective function for which it is well-designed, not only to provide but also to maintain by preserving its own integrity. Primarily, its intricate structure and large surface area encourage the inertial impaction of coarse particles, those with mass median aerodynamic diameter of about 10 μm or more. Secondly, its mucosa rich in goblet and ciliated cells promotes their mucociliary clearance, at the same time humidifying the air. Finally, its extensive vasculature facilitates absorption to reduce pulmonary insult and, if necessary, expedites inflammatory response. If these defensive mechanisms are impaired, the risk of damage to the lower respiratory system increases. It is therefore important, in the experimental evaluation of inhaled irritants, to examine the nasal cavity not only for induced damage but also for preexisting coincidental or spontaneous disease. Also, histo-pathological examination of this region is essential for data on pharmaceutical preparations to be administered by the nasal route.[1] Surprisingly, because of its obvious significance, the nasal cavity has been ignored in many inhalation studies. Omissions have been attributed to dearth of anatomical knowledge, technical difficulties, and, paradoxically, to the possibility of infection complicating the results.[2,3]

II. THE ANIMAL MODEL

The choice of an animal model for investigating potential toxicity in man is always a compromise between the ideal and the available. Ideally the model should imitate human structure and function but usually choice is determined more by practicality and economics. For studies on nasal irritancy, the important considerations on structure and function include anatomy, breathing pattern, mucociliary clearance, and distribution of particulate impaction. Much of this information, well-documented for man, is incomplete for laboratory animals. Nevertheless some interspecies differences are known and should be contemplated before selecting a model. Also it is important to choose animals free from respiratory disease.

A. Structure and Function

The human nose comprises two nasal cavities separated by a median septum. Each cavity possesses three turbinate bones (dorsal, middle, and ventral), which project as curving lamellae from its lateral wall, and communicates with four paranasal sinuses (frontal, maxillary, ethmoidal, and sphenoidal). The sinuses, like the cavities, secrete mucus which, as it joins the nasal stream en route for the pharynx, continually bathes those turbinate areas most likely to be injured by inspired materials.[4] The anterior part of the middle turbinate is one impact site of wood dust and consequently a predilection area for squamous metaplasia.[5] Normally most people breathe preferentially through their noses even though this resists airflow. Oral respiration is usual only during exercise or following nasal occlusion.

Although animals other than some primates do not have a "nose" demarcated from the rest of the head their nasal cavities resemble, in very general terms, that of man. An obvious difference which has impressed many investigators is the presence of intricate scroll-like turbinates unlike the simpler human lamellae. Their comparative anatomy has been summarized by Proctor and Chang (Chapter 1, Volume I) and Wynder and Hoffman.[6] Such complexity does not apply to the chicken which, for this reason, has been preferred for studies on mucociliary transport.[7] The paranasal air sinuses, on the other hand, are seemingly less developed. In the rat, the pocket-like maxillary recess is described as the only developed paranasal sinus, and flow of mucus from it into the nasal cavity is questioned.[8] In the mouse, actual communication between these two chambers is doubted.[2] The ethmoid area is excluded from the functional volume of the guinea pig's respiratory system because it receives very little or no tidal air.[9] Similarly, this region is protected in the mouse by the airflow trajectory unless it voluntarily sniffs.[2,10]

The guinea pig is unable to breathe through its mouth even after heavy exercise,[11] and it is commonly stated that nose breathing is obligatory in other laboratory rodents.[2,12,13] This has been challenged by the observation of oral breathing in rats exposed to cigarette smoke and the subsequent demonstration of considerable particulate matter in their lower jaws.[14] However, of all the common laboratory animals, it is only the dog which readily by-passes its nasal defense by mouth breathing like man.

B. Particulate Deposition

Most of the data on particulate deposition in laboratory animals has been generated from dosimetry studies on cigarette smoke. Undiluted mainstream smoke contains up to 5×10^9 heterogeneous particles per milliliter with round and spherical forms ranging in diameter from 0.2 to 1.0 μm with a median particle diameter of about 0.4 μm.[15] One might therefore expect a large proportion of smoke total particulate matter (TPM) to percolate the nasal filter on its way to the lung. However there are implications that nasal filtration is a major obstacle in laboratory animals to the development of inhalation toxicity studies.[6,12] These were disputed by Binns and co-workers (see Beven, Reference 16) in a comprehensive series of experiments using a versatile purpose-built smoking machine[16] and decachlorobiphenyl as particulate phase marker. Their preliminary communication on rats stated that the largest proportion of TPM retained was in the lungs.[17] Then they produced comparative figures, expressed as percentage TPM throughout the respiratory system, for head (predominantly nasal) deposition in the rat, guinea pig, golden hamster, and mouse of 10.0, 11.3, 14.4, and 27.2%, respectively.[14] Their subsequent values for TPM in the rat's head, following either continuous or intermittent exposure, were almost consistently below 10% of the whole,[18,19] in agreement with other workers using a completely different exposure system.[20] They also noticed that relative deposition in the rat's head was increased both by nonacclimatization and by higher smoke concentration which encourages rapid growth of particle size.[21] Other investigators also related higher nasal deposition to more concentrated smoke by comparing results on Syrian Golden hamsters used in "closed" and "open" exposure systems.[22] There are less data on smoke dosimetry for nonrodent species, although one value of 32% has been published for nasal absorption of organic matter in the rabbit.[23] It can be inferred, from a review of these and earlier papers, that the number of cigarette smoke particles impacted in the nasal cavities of laboratory animals is a relatively small proportion of the whole.

C. Microbiological Status

The complicating effects of respiratory infection on the interpretation of experimental pulmonary pathology have been stressed repeatedly. This is no less true for the conducting airways, especially the nasal cavity, since rhinitis is an extremely common manifestation of respiratory disease. Assuming availability, specific pathogen free (SPF) animals should be preferred. Goblet cells, for example, are considerably more prevalent in the bronchi of conventional rats than in those which are Caesarean-derived.[24]

Since animals of known microbiological status are not always available, it is prudent of the experimental pathologist to be aware of the various infections which might affect the nasal cavity. In the domestic species, most viruses and bacteria implicated in respiratory infections attack the nasal epithelium. As diseases of veterinary significance, they have been well-documented and reviewed for the dog.[25] In the smaller laboratory species, the nasal cavity may be infected by bacteria (e.g., pasteurellosis in rabbits),[26] mycoplasmas (e.g., chronic respiratory disease in rats),[27] viruses (e.g., Sendai disease in mice),[28] or mites (e.g., symptomless infestation in hamsters).[29] Also the pathologist should recognize those infections which cause rhinitis but are better known for their effects in other organs, e.g., sialoda-cryoadenitis in rats.[30] Finally he should not disregard the possibility of artifacts from su-boptimal environmental conditions since it has been shown that high levels of ammonia in animal cages may alter the epithelial lining of the conducting airways.[31]

III. MICROANATOMY OF THE RAT NASAL CAVITY

A. General

Interpretation of reactive, particularly subtle, changes in the nasal cavity of an experimental animal requires, as in all investigative histopathology, a thorough knowledge of the normal tissues. Unfortunately, such information is not readily available in comprehensive detail. Probably this is because nasal complexity has deterred investigators or prompted them to study the simpler airways. Certainly the trachea has attracted more attention from the his-tologists and electron microscopists. Anatomical texts[32] and histological atlases,[33] although helpful, provide insufficient detail for the experimental pathologist. However, there have been several useful papers written about the rat, albeit focused on specific areas. For that reason and because the rat is a common model for inhalation studies this species alone is considered here.

The disposition of the various organs, tissues, and adnexa of the nasal cavity, especially its lining epithelia, is such that — whatever the plane of section — parallel cuts more than 1 mm apart will inevitably display altered distributions, often markedly so. This is a vital concept for the experimental pathologist to grasp if he is to compare like with like without bias between different groups of animals. It is therefore the author's habit to become familiar with a minimal number of levels and orientations. This is more rewarding and far more economic than serial sectioning to discover focal lesions. The importance of standard-level sectioning has also been emphasized for the larynx.[34]

The most important tissues in inhalation studies on nasal irritants are the epithelial linings of the cavities and sinuses. The three main types — squamous, respiratory, and olfactory —have been used in the rat to designate zones of the cavity.[32] The anterior zone or vestibule is lined by stratified squamous epithelium which extends posteriorly along the bottom of the ventral meatus to the exit of the incisive duct. Most of the middle zone, including the maxillary sinus and the nasal and maxillary turbinates, is invested with respiratory-type epithelium. The posterior zone and the ethmoturbinates are covered by olfactory mucosa. Katz and Merzel[35] mapped the distribution of these epithelia on the septum in a sagittal plane from measurements on photographs of semiserial transverse sections and then pro-ceeded to derive their areas with a planimeter. The smallest area, stratified squamous epi-thelium, is 15% of the whole and unique in the first 2.5 mm of the vestibule. Respiratory-type epithelium occupies the largest area, nearly 44% of the whole, extending as an oblique band from anterodorsal to posteroventral. The remainder of the septum is olfactory, a triangular area with its base at the posterior extremity of the cavity and its apex anteriorly in the roof.

Ten types of cell have been identified in the epithelium lining the respiratory airways of the rat between the upper trachea and the distal bronchioli.[36] The ultrastructure of nasal epithelium has not been so thoroughly investigated although microvillous cells have been identified in the respiratory zone.[37] They extend for a variable distance into the anterior nasal cavity from the squamous vestibular cells to the ciliated cells with which they are also interpersed. Olfactory epithelium is composed of three types of cells: deep basal, middle sensory, and superficial sustacular. Their zonal arrangements[38] and ultrastructure[39] have been described in the context of studies on selective olfactory toxicity.

The lamina propria of the nasal cavity is highly vascular especially around the turbinate bones. It is infiltrated lightly and diffusely by mononuclear inflammatory cells and there are focal accumulations of lymphocytes, frequently near the nasolacrimal ducts. Globule leucocytes have been described among the epithelial cells of both respiratory and olfactory regions, particularly in females.[35] Serous glands and their ducts are numerous in the propria of the septum and lateral walls and Bowman's glands occur in the olfactory mucosa. In the septum, between the olfactory mucosa and the vomeronasal organ, the more dorsal glands are PAS-negative and the more ventral are PAS-positive.[35] (See also Chapters 1 and 2, Volume I.)

The histology and histochemistry of the maxillary sinus and its associated glands have been described comprehensively by Vidic and Greditzer.[8] The epithelium lining of the sinus is a mixture of pseudostratified and simple ciliated columnar virtually lacking goblet cells. The sinus is completely surrounded by two glands, the lateral (nasal of Steno) ventroanteriorly and the maxillary dorsoposteriorly. The former is predominantly mucus and secretes via a duct into the nasal cavity. The latter is predominantly serous and its ducts open directly into the sinus.

B. Specific Transverse Level

One transverse level of section favored by the author for light microscopy is illustrated in Figure 1. This discloses all three types of lining epithelia, numerous glands and their ducts, both nasal and maxillary turbinates, the nasolacrimal ducts, and the paired vomeronasal organ (of Jacobson). It is also advantageous in presenting on the septal surfaces a well-ciliated epithelium which includes many goblet cells but not, in the SPF rat, too numerous to make counting tedious.

Olfactory epithelium lines each dorsal meatus and the medial surfaces of the vomeronasal tubes. Stratified squamous epithelium, around the bottom of the ventral meatus, is keratinized infrequently and then only slightly. The rest of the cavity is invested by respiratory-type epithelium. This has a connotation of morphological continuity but in reality there are wide variations in cell types and their relative distributions throughout the lining of the conducting airways. This has become evident with the increasing use of transmission and scanning electron microscopy, particularly in relation to the trachea and intrapulmonary airways.[36,40] Some of this variation can be discerned in the nasal cavity, at the level illustrated, even by light microscopy.

The respiratory-type epithelium lining the septum includes both goblet cells and tall pseudostratified columnar cells with prominent cilia. Similar cells also invest the medial and ventral surfaces of the nasal turbinates. Thus the dorsal meatus, with its tall olfactory cells in the roof of the cavity, is lined by a thick layer of epithelium. Elsewhere the respiratory epithelium is considerably lower, sometimes almost cuboidal, less luxuriantly or even sparsely ciliated, and lacks goblet cells. Although there are individual exceptions, this lower type of epithelium covers both surfaces of the maxillary turbinates, the lateral aspect of the nasal turbinate, and the lateral wall of the cavity around the middle meatus. Ventrally, below the maxillary turbinate, the lateral lining of the cavity becomes more ciliated and populated densely with goblet cells. Epithelium lining the lateral surfaces of the vomeronasal tubes is also nonciliated and devoid of goblet cells but is frequently infiltrated by neutrophils. The lining of the nasolacrimal ducts is similarly nonciliated and frequently includes squamous foci in the normal animal.

There are more goblet cells per unit surface area in the nasal cavity of the rat than in any other region of its conducting airways. However their population density varies not only with level and site within level but also between apparently normal individuals, sometimes considerably. At the level illustrated in Figure 1, they are invariably present and highly concentrated in the septal epithelium from a point opposite the ventral edge of the median cartilage around the vomeronasal bulge to the junction with vestibular squamous cells. The

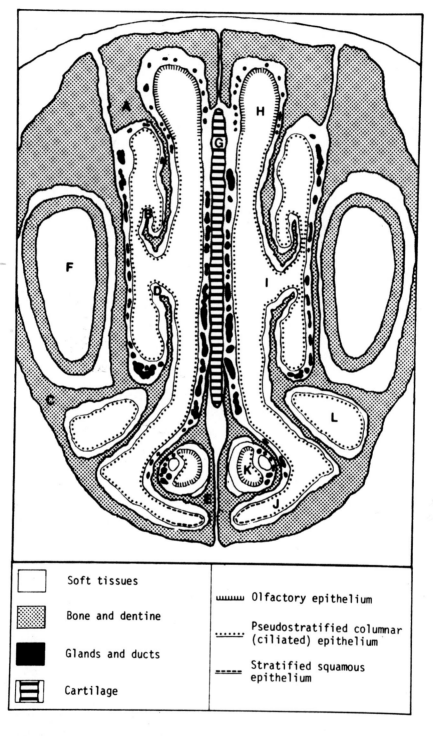

FIGURE 1.   Transverse section of the rat nasal cavity: line drawing from a normal specimen with schematic representation of tissue types. (A) Nasal bone; (B) nasal (dorsal) turbinate; (C) maxillary bone; (D) maxillary (ventral) turbinate; (E) vomer bone; (F) incisor tooth root pulp; (G) septal cartilage; (H) olfactory region (dorsal meatus); (I) respiratory region (middle meatus); (J) vestibular region (ventral meatus); (K) vomeronasal organ; and (L) nasolacrimal duct.

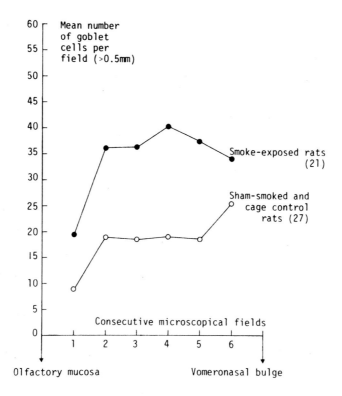

FIGURE 2.   Goblet cell hyperplasia induced by smoke (diluted 1 in 8 and 1 in 12) from cigarettes composed entirely of tobacco: distribution of effect on the straight part of the nasal septum.

opposing ventrolateral wall of the cavity is similarly constantly and densely populated so that the ventral meatus must be supplied with copious acid mucosubstance. Usually there are fewer goblet cells in the straight part of the septum but the population density here is more variable, ranging from sparse to moderate. Variability probably reflects microbiological status. Characteristically at this level goblet cells are infrequent in the dorsal parts of the septal surface below the olfactory junction and on the opposing medial aspects of the nasal turbinates. This septal distribution is depicted graphically in Figure 2. Normally, there are no goblet cells in the epithelia lining the lateral aspects of the nasal turbinates, both surfaces of the maxillary turbinates, the lateral walls of the cavity, the nasolacrimal ducts, and the vomeronasal tubes. A quantitative difference in goblet cells between male and female, as reported for the trachea,[41] has not been observed.

The morphology of nasal goblet cells varies, like their density, with site. In the dorsal, sparsely populated sites of the septal surface they are usually slender, poorly differentiated, and stain faintly by the Mowry technique.[42] In more ventral sites, they are characteristically goblet-like with apical accumulations of predominantly acid mucosubstance which stains a vivid blue or, less frequently, purple. In some cells subjacent stems of red PAS-positive granules may be demonstrated. In others, especially those sited on the vomeronasal bulge, the apical distension with blue secretory granules extends almost to the base of the cell.

The distribution of glands at this level is shown in Figure 1. Serous glands and their ducts are common in the septum and lateral walls of the cavity. They do not stain by the Mowry technique except for two groups: one in the septal propria around the ventral quarter of the median cartilage and the other within the bony case of the vomeronasal organ. These show a red reaction indicative of neutral mucosubstance. The smaller Bowman's glands confined to the olfactory propria stain a mixture of red and blue. Also, not illustrated, are occasional intraepithelial glands which secrete acid mucosubstance.

IV. NASAL HISTOPATHOLOGY AFTER CIGARETTE SMOKE EXPOSURE

It might be asked, quite reasonably, if there is any purpose in examining the nasal cavities of laboratory animals exposed to cigarette smoke since nasal disease does not contribute to the excess mortality associated with smoking.[15] Moreover, mainstream smoke is inhaled via the mouth not the nose. Many cigarette smokers, however, exhale through their nasal cavities and, perhaps more significantly, sidestream smoke passes this route. Thus the animal model is at least reasonably valid for studies on passive smoking. Also since animals will not usually inhale smoke by mouth, the nasal cavity is inevitably exposed and therefore provides an organ of potential pathological change, almost as an accident of experimental design. Even so, it has to be stated at the outset that many studies on cigarette smoke toxicity have excluded its examination and in most of the others the nasal changes reported are trivial by comparison with those in the larynx and lung.

A. Methodology

Numerous systems of exposure have been devised for inhalation studies. Their relative advantages and disadvantages have been presented.[43] The older whole-body chambers developed for industrial contaminants[44] have generally been superseded in studies on cigarette smoke by head-only systems.[45] The objectives of system design should include the prevention of undue aging of smoke and the limitation of particle growth by rapid aerosol dilution. Also an essential prerequisite for all techniques is validation by dosimetry prior to pathology. The author's results were all obtained on rats exposed by the head-only system devised and used by Binns and co-workers (see Beven, Reference 16). The method of examining the nasal cavity has been reported briefly[46] and will now be described in more detail.

After exposure the animal is anesthetized and exsanguinated. The lower jaw is removed and the head is fixed in 10% buffered formalin. The level of nasal cavity required may be identified externally by a dorsal point midway between the nostril and the inner canthus and a ventral point just in front of the first palatine ruga. After fixation, the head is sawed transversely in front and behind these points to provide a specimen of nasal cavity 3 to 4 mm thick which includes the required level. The skin and soft tissues are excised and the specimen is decalcified in 20% ethylenediamine tetra-acetic acid. It is then processed conventionally, embedded in paraffin wax, and sectioned from the narrower anterior surface. With a little experience the microtomist recognizes the correct level (Figure 1) in the block by naked eye identification of the incisor teeth roots and position of the nasolacrimal ducts, etc. Sections, 5-μm thick, are stained with hematoxylin and eosin and also by the alcian blue-periodic acid Schiff method omitting nuclear counter-stain.[42] The technique has to be modified if different levels are required, but a single standard section is adequate for most short-term bioassays on irritants.

Multiple levels were compared by Lucia and co-workers[2] in their assessment of nasal damage by pyrolysis products in the mouse.[2] They routinely prepared four transverse sections from each nasal cavity, 1.5 to 2 mm apart, from the vestibule to the ethmoid sinus region. They concluded that their two middle levels through the respiratory zone were the most informative because the others were protected — the vestibular by resistant squamous cells and the ethmoidal by an "air shunt".

Before evaluating induced changes, it is necessary to confirm suitability of the sections with respect to quality and level. Enumeration of goblet cells is impractical on thick sections and tedious on those with high population densitites. A dorsal increase in the septal concentration of goblet cells is usual in levels obtained too anteriorly. Morphological criteria of incorrect level, in relation to Figure 1, are summarized as follows:

1.   Too anterior: transverse concavity in dorsal edge of septal cartilage, nasal turbinate markedly scrolled, absence of olfactory mucosa, mid-septal goblet cell population high

2. Too posterior: presence of maxillary sinus, nasolacrimal duct lateral to incisor tooth root, transverse axis of vomeronasal tube horizontal, mid-septal goblet cell population sparse

All suitable sections from a study are shuffled and examined "blindly", i.e., without knowledge of the animal's grouping. Each area of tissue or type of change is assessed for all sections before the next one. Although time consuming, this avoids diagnostic drift. Goblet cell densities are estimated conveniently in the straight part of the septum. They may be counted in the epithelium on one side, commencing at the olfactory junction then progressing ventrally through, say, six medium power objective ($\times 25$) fields (Figure 2). Or, to avoid the difficulty of enumerating the dorsal poorly differentiated cells, count sites may be fixed to the third and fourth fields below the olfactory junctions on both sides. Alternatively, population densities may be estimated for both sides (2×3 mm) through a low power objective ($\times 2.5$) and accorded conventional scores or grades. Usually, but not invariably, the number of goblet cells is similar for both septal surfaces.

Reproducibility of counts on the same section is good, but more advantageous quantitative techniques for estimating goblet cell densities have been proposed by others. Greater reliability is claimed for small biopsies based on whole-mount preparations of human nasal septa[47] and results from the use of an image-analyzing computer have been compared favorably with manual counts.[48] Actual technique is perhaps less important than standard sampling, an allusion of preceding remarks. It is relevant, in this context, to note that goblet cell hyperplasia in the human bronchus tends to be linear, not diffuse.[49]

B. Author's Results

The author's results are based on the examination by light microscopy of approximately 700 nasal cavities, sectioned and stained as described above. The rats, all SPF Wistar-derived, were used in a series of five short-term experiments. For an initial period of a few days, they were gradually acclimatized to cigarette smoke and then exposed for two 10-min periods daily. The duration of all experiments was 6 weeks except in one study designed to investigate progressive changes between 2 and 12 weeks. All rats were killed within 24 hr of their final exposure except in another study designed to investigate regression between 1 and 42 days later. The cigarettes tested included those composed entirely of tobacco and others modified to provide lower TPM deliveries. Smoke was diluted with air in ratios varying from 1 in 5 to 1 in 20. Groups were segregated according to both cigarette type (TPM delivery) and smoke dilution. Both cage controls and sham-smoked animals were included and group size was 12, 18, or 24.

The nasal findings from one of these experiments have been published.[46,50] The following extranasal changes were attributed unequivocally and almost invariably in the five studies, to smoke exposure from cigarettes composed entirely of tobacco, if not from modified types: squamous metaplasia and keratinizing hyperplasia in the larynx, goblet cell hyperplasia in the trachea and intrapulmonary bronchus, hyperplasia and hypertrophy of pulmonary macrophages, and cuboidal cell metaplasia around the alveolar ducts. These also were reported for one of the five studies.[46,50,51]

1. Nasal Septum

The respiratory epithelium lining the nasal septum was never metaplastic nor even deciliated in any rat exposed to cigarette smoke. Also there were no changes, either in size or staining affinity, of the septal glands. Occasional ducts contained minimal cellular exudates in both smoke-exposed and control animals.

Goblet cell hyperplasia, after 6 weeks exposure, was demonstrated in some, but not all, experiments. In one study, cells were enumerated in four mid-septal fields, two on each

Table 1
GROUP MEAN COUNTS OF GOBLET CELLS PER FIELD (>0.5 MM) IN THE NASAL SEPTA OF RATS EXPOSED FOR 6 WEEKS TO CIGARETTE SMOKE DILUTED 1 IN 8 FROM FLUE-CURED TOBACCO

Cigarette code	Mean TPM delivery (milligrams per cigarette)	Number of rats[a]	Range	Mean	Standard deviation
—	Sham-smoked	18	0.3—42.8	18.0	15.4
D	9.4	10	12.3—45.0	28.4	10.0
C	12.0	16	24.5—55.5	40.0	10.2
B	16.4	20	11.0—55.3	40.4	10.5
A	18.1[b]	19	32.5—59.5	43.1	7.4

[a] Reduced from the original group size of 24 by the number of unsatisfactory sections.
[b] Maximum TPM delivery (cigarette composed entirely of tobacco).

Table 2
GROUP MEAN COUNTS OF GOBLET CELLS PER FIELD (> 0.5 MM) IN THE NASAL SEPTA OF RATS EXPOSED FOR 6 WEEKS, IN TWO EXPERIMENTS (1 AND 2), TO SMOKE FROM CIGARETTES COMPOSED ENTIRELY OF FLUE-CURED TOBACCO

Smoke concentration	Experiment	Number of rats[a]	Range	Mean	Standard deviation
Sham-	1	18	0.3—42.8	18.0	15.4
smoked	2	12	1.0—40.7	14.2	11.9
1 in 12	1	15	23.3—50.0	39.4	8.2
	2	12	8.7—48.4	30.2	11.5
1 in 8	1	19	32.5—59.5	43.1	7.4
	2	9	7.7—52.5	39.9	13.1
1 in 5	1	16	8.5—50.8	35.9	10.9

[a] Reduced from the original group sizes of 24 (1) and 18 (2) by the number of unsatisfactory sections.

side, and hyperplasia was positively related to TPM delivery of the cigarette (Table 1). Individual counts varied markedly, especially in the sham-smoked rats although this group alone possessed the lowest values. Counts on both sides of the nasal septum in the same individual were usually, but not invariably, similar and no consistent difference was detected between the sexes. In another similar study, goblet cells were counted in six consecutive fields on one side of the septum commencing at the olfactory junction. The hyperplasia, for cigarettes composed entirely of tobacco, was most evident in the middle part of the septum (Figure 2). The data from these two studies, albeit derived differently, were combined to illustrate the relation between response and concentration of smoke (Table 2). The number of goblet cells appeared to increase as concentration was raised from 1 in 12 to 1 in 8 but not from 1 in 8 to 1 in 5. In a third similar experiment, however, goblet cell hyperplasia was not demonstrated in the nasal cavities of any group of smoke-exposed rats, although it was conspicuous in both trachea and intrapulmonary bronchus.

Two further studies in this series were complementary and designed to investigate regression and progression of the histopathological changes observed at 6 weeks in the preceding experiments. In the regression study, rats were exposed as usual for a duration of 6 weeks but the holding period to killing was varied from 1 to 42 days. In the progression study rats were killed as usual within 24 hr of the last exposure but duration was varied from 2 to 12 weeks. The pathological findings, excluding the nasal cavity, in these studies have been reported for smoke diluted 1 in 12.[52] Goblet cell population densities were estimated in the nasal septa of rats exposed to smoke diluted 1 in 8. The estimates suggested that goblet cells increased within 2 weeks of exposure but this hyperplasia was neither marked nor progressive as the duration of inhalation was extended to 12 weeks. Moreover, it subsided rapidly — within 4 days — after cessation of exposure.

2. Turbinates

Slight hyperplasia of epithelium was observed occasionally in rats exposed to smoke around the ventral surfaces of the nasal turbinates. Focal squamous metaplasia was relatively rare. Overall frequencies for the five experiments follow.

Control (cage and sham-smoked)	0/224 (0.0%)
Smoke-exposed (all groups)	16/451 (3.5%)

The numbers recorded in each experiment were too small to relate with TPM delivery values, smoke dilutions, or exposure durations. The squamous foci developed in the nasal turbinates, most commonly on their lateral spurs or projections and around their free edges, but never on their medial surfaces. Less frequent sites were dorsal in the lateral walls of the cavity and dorsolateral aspects of the maxillary turbinates. Thus the lower, less profusely ciliated regions of respiratory epithelia were affected preferentially.

3. Nasolacrimal Duct

Goblet cells were never present in the linings of the nasolacrimal ducts but foci of squamous metaplasia were common, sometimes associated with underlying lymphoid nodules, in both control and smoke-exposed rats. They appeared to be more frequent at incorrect anterior levels but serial sectioning was not carried out to verify this. Their presence was neither attributed to the effects of cigarette smoke nor otherwise explained. Focal accumulations of lymphocytes were often revealed in the lamina propria around the ducts but, in all experiments, they were more numerous in control animals. Overall frequencies for the five experiments follow.

Control (cage and sham-smoked)	79/236 (33%)
Smoke-exposed (maximum TPM 6 weeks duration)	23/181 (13%)

4. Maxillary Sinus

In one study, the maxillary sinus was extirpated, together with its associated glands, by a mid-sagittal approach in the posterior nasal cavity. The epithelial lining of the sinus was normal in all rats exposed to smoke. There was no evidence of goblet cell hyperplasia, deciliation, metaplasia, or suppurative reaction. The blue reaction for acid mucosubstance in glandular tissue was questionably increased in animals exposed to smoke from cigarettes composed entirely of tobacco.

5. Other Epithelia

Significant changes in the olfactory mucosa were not observed in rats exposed to smoke. Also, the vestibular squamous epithelium was never hyperplastic nor extensive beyond its usual confines. Both epithelia lining the vomeronasal tubes were unaffected by smoke and the pharynx, examined in three studies, was always normal.

C. Others' Results

1. Short-Term Studies

Few investigators of cigarette smoke toxicity have focused their attention on the nasal region as a specific target organ. Two notable exceptions were Vidic and colleagues[53] working on the rat and Basrur and Harada[3] using the Syrian Golden hamster. Both groups demonstrated acute suppurative reaction, mucus hypersecretion, epithelial hyperplasia or metaplasia, and after removal of the insult, reversibility. Vidic and co-workers, confining their attention to the maxillary sinus, discovered — after only 6-min chamber exposure — desquamation of the ciliated lining cells and acute inflammatory reaction which was manifest 4 days later by frank pus in the lumen. Their findings in rats subjected to 6 days exposure (2 × 6 min/ day) were squamous metaplasia, microabscess formation and goblet cell hyperplasia in the lining epithelium together with maxillary adenitis. These changes had virtually resolved 2 weeks after the cessation of exposure. Basrur and Harada used an intermittent smoke delivery machine producing a nominal 10% aerosol. In hamsters killed after 4 weeks exposure (8 cigarettes per day, 5 days/week) they found vacuolar degeneration and basal cell hyperplasia of respiratory epithelium, neutrophil infiltration, and hyperactivity of goblet cells in the maxillary sinus. During a 1- or 2-week recovery period, the rhinitis subsided, although in animals exposed to smoke from their strongest cigarettes, atypical hyperplasia persisted in rosette and adenoid forms. Surface morphology, prior to recovery, revealed a decrease in the ciliated cell zone and an extension of the anterior squamous tissue. Also parakeratosis was observed in the vestibular mucosa but olfactory epithelium was spared. Matulionis,[39] on the other hand, described ultrastructural changes in the olfactory cells of mice after short-term exposure to 10% cigarette smoke. On the basis of effect in one strain of mouse but not in another, he postulated a genetically determined susceptibility.

2. Long-Term Studies

The chronic effects of cigarette smoke in the nasal cavities of laboratory animals are both unremarkable and similar for a wide range of species, experimental designs, exposure systems, and smoke concentrations or doses. The histopathological changes most commonly reported in long-term inhalation studies are hypertrophy, hyperplasia, and squamous metaplasia of the respiratory epithelium. Often these have been qualified as focal, recorded as infrequent, and merited little of the investigator's comment by comparison with concomitant, more conspicuous, findings in the larynx and lung. Hyper- or metaplastic nasal epithelia, particularly those investing the turbinates, have been described, following prolonged exposure, in the mouse (e.g., Wynder et al.),[12] rat (e.g., Dalbey et al.),[54] hamster (e.g., Bernfeld et al.),[55] and dog (e.g., Zwicker et al.).[56] In the last-mentioned example exposure was via tracheotomy and alteration to turbinate epithelium was apparently evoked by exhalation. According to the data of Coggins and co-workers[57] hypertrophy and hyperplasia of nasal epithelium in rats exposed for 12 weeks require for their occurrence not only the particulate but also the vapor phase of cigarette smoke.

D. Comment

The results of numerous inhalation studies on cigarette smoke obtained by different laboratories using a variety of species and exposure systems are not readily comparable. Consequently, generalized statements and conclusions on the experimental effects of smoke are not easily conceived. Although this applies to nasal histopathology, some inference and conjecture are permissible.

Pathogenesis identifies cigarette smoke as an irritant. Its target tissue in the nasal region is the lining respiratory epithelium. The peracute effect is a rapid degeneration of epithelium which provokes an acute inflammatory, usually suppurative, reaction. This is followed by epithelial regeneration which then progresses to hyperplasia or squamous metaplasia. This proliferative change usually resolves after removal of the insult. The two descriptions of this sequence in the nasal region, referred to above,[3,53] are entirely consistent with the observations of Lam[58] on the ventral epithelium of the rat larynx. The findings, after 60 min of exposure to cigarette smoke, were necrosis and inflammatory reaction followed by regeneration within 20 hr and hyperplasia between 30 and 70 hr before a return to the normal state.

The acute inflammatory reaction could be attributed to opportunist infection following enhanced susceptibility. This speculation is consistent with the concept of the host's normal bacterial flora influencing susceptibility to cigarette smoke.[59] Wynder and co-workers[12] suggested increased susceptibility to nasal infection in their smoke-exposed mice, but implied a viral agent because of the presence of giant cells in the exudate. They also stressed the pathogenesis of epithelial proliferation from rhinitis and the reversibility of these changes. Presumably the absence of acute rhinitis in other short-term studies reflects either the time of killing or the microbiological status of the animals used. The apparent reduction in nasal lymphatic tissue described above (Section IV.B) might merit — to further the growing evidence of smoke immunosuppression — more constructive investigation, as recently applied to the lung.[60]

The other acute effect of cigarette smoke in the nasal cavity is hypersecretion of mucus. Probably this occurs in epithelial sites more protected or less insulted than those reacting as described above but the evidence for this is more conjectural, even equivocal. Goblet cell hyperplasia has been demonstrated in the maxillary sinus of the rat[53] and the hamster.[3] However, this was not the author's experience when, in the same rats he found hyperplastic goblet cells elsewhere including the nasal cavity proper. Moreover this change, on the septal surface, has not been demonstrated consistently in similar experiments. These apparent discrepancies may serve to emphasize the necessity for careful technique to reveal what seems to be a subtle change (Figure 3).

If the insult persists, albeit intermittently as in a long-term inhalation study, the chronic nasal effect is focal hyperplasia or squamous metaplasia of the respiratory, especially turbinate, epithelia. This seems to occur irrespective of species or smoke-exposure systems. Often it is infrequent and, to the author's knowledge, has never been interpreted as precancerous. Such a mild reaction — even trivial by comparison with changes lower in the airways — is consistent with low TPM impaction in the nasal region, referred to above. Dontenwill[61] predicted the improbability of nasal neoplasia in smoke-exposed animals by comparing the low load of particles per unit surface area with that in the larynx. This expression of dose per unit area has been criticized on the basis that TPM distribution is not uniform within an organ system.[62] From this it is interesting to conjecture on the reason for squamous predilection sites described above (Section IV.B) — either higher TPM impaction or lower, more sensitive, epithelium.

V. THE DISTRIBUTION OF LESIONS CAUSED BY OTHER INHALED IRRITANTS

It is relevant to repeat here that the irritant effects of cigarette smoke in laboratory animals are less pronounced in the nasal cavity than elsewhere in the respiratory system. Moreover, in the nasal cavity they are confined to the respiratory epithelium and even within this tissue they appear only at certain sites. Other inhaled irritants and toxicants also exhibit specific, but different, patterns in their distributions of target organs, tissues, sites, and cell types. It is the intention in this final section to cite examples which collectively illustrate this significant variation.

A. Examples
1. Cigarette Smoke Constituents
The Dutch group of Feron, Kruysse, and others included, in their research program on

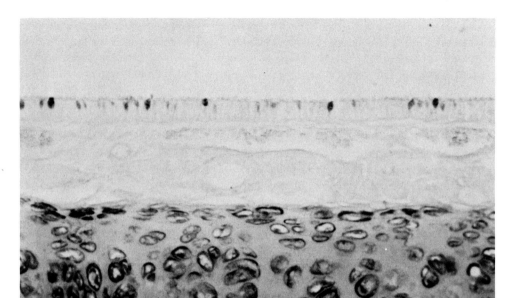

A

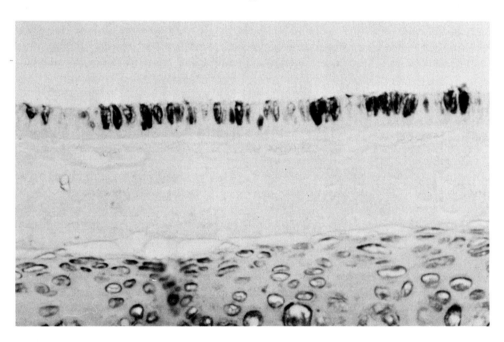

B

FIGURE 3.   Mid-septal goblet cell population in a control rat (A) and hyperplasia in another exposed to an irritant (B). It would be possible, in most experiments on cigarette smoke, to find examples which fit transposition of these captions, such is the variation in both response and the normal animal.

the biological effects of cigarette smoke components, the aldehydes acrolein and acetaldehyde and the unsaturated lactone butenolide. In different experiments, they exposed hamsters to acrolein,[63] acetaldehyde,[64] and butenolide[65] at maximum concentrations and durations of 5 ppm for 13 weeks, 4560 ppm for 90 days and 130 ppm for 13 weeks, respectively (all 6 hr/day, 5 days/week). Both aldehydes, in maximum concentration, caused necrotizing rhinitis and keratinizing squamous metaplasia of respiratory, if not olfactory, epithelia. The effects of butenolide did not exceed focal cuboidal or squamous metaplasia. Damage by the aldehydes was more severe in the nasal cavity or upper conducting airways than lower in the respiratory tract, in accordance with their differential uptake in the dog. Changes attributed to butenolide were confined entirely to the nasal cavity. The dorsomedial part of the nasomaxillary region was specified as a site of injury for all three smoke constituents.

2. Sulfur Dioxide

Giddens and Fairchild[10] exposed mice to 10 ppm of sulfur dioxide for periods of up to 72 hr. In reporting their findings, they implied an error of omission in previous studies on higher concentrations of the gas which revealed minimal lesions but neglected the nasal cavity. Nasal mucosal changes in their mice included deciliation, atrophy, metaplasia, necrosis, and suppurative rhinitis, but excluded goblet cell hyperplasia. Severity was positively related to exposure duration from 24 to 72 hr and changes were more conspicuous in conventional mice than in those of defined flora, another example of microbial contribution to inhalational toxicity. A lack of tracheobronchial injury was correlated with absorption of sulfur dioxide which is almost complete in the nasal mucosa. Distribution of effect was discussed in relation to airflow pattern and epithelial cell type. Respiratory epithelium, although deeper in the nasal cavity, was less resistant than anterior squamous tissue but olfactory cells incurred the most injury, in the dorsal nasomaxillary region. This suggested, to these investigators, an airflow arc which dipped to exit at the nasopharynx and so spare the ethmoid region.

3. Carcinogens

Nitrosamines show a remarkable selective toxicity for olfactory epithelium. This was demonstrated by Greenblatt and Rijhsinghani[38] in Syrian Golden hamsters 48 hr after single intraperitoneal injections of diethylnitrosamine and dimethylnitrosamine. Both compounds, at the same dose of 20 mg/kg, caused necrosis of olfactory tissue, especially the midzonal sensory cells, without altering either adjacent respiratory epithelium or the vomeronasal organ. Olfactory lesions, especially carcinomas, also surprised Feron and Kroes[66] in rats which they had exposed to an atmosphere of 5000 ppm vinyl chloride monomer for a year (7 hr/day, 5 days/week). The olfactory changes included both carcinomas and hyperplasias which were proliferations of atypical basal cells and Bowman's glands.

4. Pyrolysis Products

Lucia and co-workers were probably aware of variable distributions of reaction within the nasal cavity when they designed their experiment to compare pyrolysis products with hydrogen chloride. Their protocol included standard diagrams of nasal transverse sections for recording both location and extent of damage. They exposed different groups of mice for 10 min to various concentrations of gaseous hydrogen chloride (HCl) and the pyrolysis products of polyvinyl chloride (PVC), polyurethane foam (PUF), Douglas Fir (DF), etc. The nature of injury, 24 hr after exposure, was similar for all compounds but varied in severity from epithelial erosion and exudative rhinitis to submucosal ulceration, chondroid necrosis, and turbinate osteolysis. Low concentrations of HCl and PVC ulcerated the ventral respiratory epithelium near the squamous junction. As concentrations were raised, the ulcers increased in extent dorsally and contiguously, but vestibular squamous epithelium remained intact until high levels were generated. The pattern of injury to PUF differed markedly in that the ulcers were scattered at random throughout the mucosa and at high concentrations they increased in number but did not enlarge by contiguity. With DF there was less difference in vulnerability between squamous and respiratory epithelia. No explanation was offered for these variations in distribution but relatively mild damage in the ethmoid region was attributed to voluntary control of airflow into it.

5. Formulated Industrial Products

The author[67] also noticed a specific pattern in the distribution of nasal changes during studies on the acute inhalation toxicity of eight formulated oil products. Rats were exposed, in a head-only system, to mists generated in nominal concentrations of 1000 mg/m³ for 2 days (4 hr/day). The effects of this were minimal and the experiment was repeated with fumes of the oils at a lower nominal concentration of 450 mg/m³. Several of the fumes provoked squamous metaplasia in both the larynx and nasal cavity. In the more severely affected groups and individuals, the nasal respiratory epithelium (at the level of Figure 1) became squamous on the lateral and ventral surfaces of the nasal turbinate including its free edge, on all aspects of the maxillary turbinate, extensively along the lateral wall of the cavity and focally in the septum. The medial surface of the nasal turbinate always remained ciliated (Figure 4), and neither olfactory nor vestibular epithelia were changed. In less affected rats, the septum and the medial surface of the maxillary turbinate were spared and distribution on the lateral wall was focal. This recalled the effect of cigarette smoke (q.v.).

The epithelial change and its nasal distribution were completely different in another study to which the author contributed.[68] Rats were exposed, again in a head-only system, to an experimental organotin biocide for 3 days (4 hr/day), during which the concentration of the atmosphere was increased to an approximate maximum of 90 mg/m³. Extranasal lesions included necrotizing suppurative laryngotracheitis and focal impact necrosis at bronchial and bronchiolar bifurcations. The nasal changes were restricted almost entirely to the walls of the ventral meatus. Epithelia investing both turbinates, the lateral walls of the cavity, and the septum were completely unaffected, not even deciliated. Squamous epithelium lining the ventral meatus was necrotic and infiltrated by neutrophils which produced a purulent exudate in the lumen. This was not entirely an affinity of squamous cells for the biocide because, in the more severely affected rats, necrosis extended dorsally into respiratory epithelium around the vomeronasal bulge (Figure 5).

B. Comment

It should be evident from these examples that the anatomical distribution of injury varies considerably with the inhaled material. The variation applies not only to organ or tissue within organ but also to site within tissue. It may even apply to cell type within site since parenterally administered nitrosamines primarily alter the sensory cells of olfactory mucosa[38] and zinc sulfate introduced locally on nasal respiratory epithelium destroys preferentially the ciliated cells in one strain of mouse and the secretory cells in another.[69]

Specificity of effect-distribution also varies with the insult. At one end of the range there are materials which appear to attack nasal mucosa in a diffuse, random, or nonselective pattern. At the other end there are examples of specific affinity by each of the three nasal lining epithelia for different materials. However the evidence suggests that this specificity is not absolute and tends to disappear as atmospheric concentration or dose is increased.

Some determinants of target site are known, or at least reasonably postulated. For example, the rhinitis of sulfur dioxide correlates with its nasal solubility, and ethmoid sparing is explicable by consideration of airflow. Also the relation betwee particle size and deposition site has been known and stressed for years. However, it is not possible to provide, from current knowledge, a unifying hypothesis for the total variation in effect-distribution. Suffice it to say, dependence is multifactorial as follows:

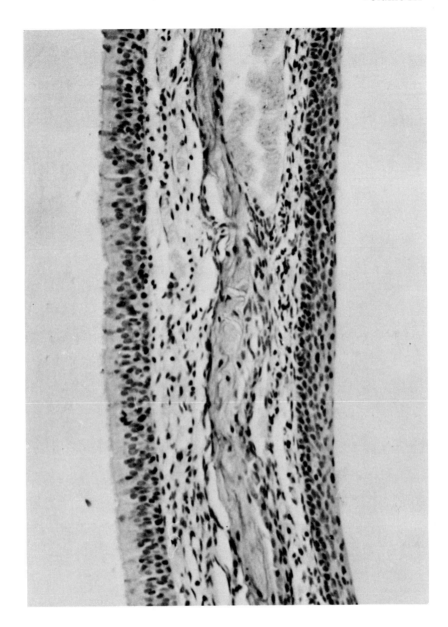

FIGURE 4. Nasal turbinate exposed to oil fumes: normal pseudostratified columnar ciliated epithelium on the medial (left) surface and metaplastic stratified squamous epithelium on the lateral (right) surface.

1. Particle size, concentration, shape, and hygroscopicity
2. Nasal aerodynamics and impact dose per unit surface area
3. Species anatomy, physiology, and genotype
4. Mucociliary flow rate and direction
5. Solubility of material or affinity of tissue
6. Cell metabolism, function, resistance, or susceptibility

If we are to further our knowledge of nasal toxicity and damage from aerial contaminants, these factors are areas for research in the experimental model. Even in the absence of such

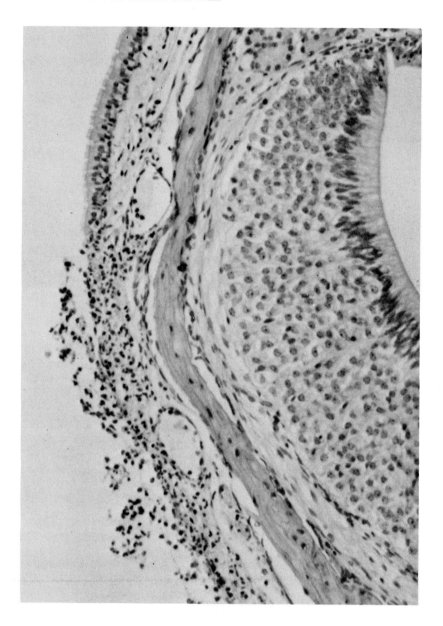

FIGURE 5.   Ventral meatus exposed to an experimental biocide: necrosis extending from ventral squamous vestibular tissue (below) into dorsal ciliated epithelium (above) around the vomeronasal bulge.

investigation the pathologist engaged in inhalation studies should be cognizant of variable effect-distribution and conduct his examination accordingly.

ACKNOWLEDGMENTS

The author thanks Mr. G. M. Barnes for the illustrations and Mrs. J. A. Clements for processing the manuscript.

REFERENCES

1. **Poynter, D.,** Inhalation toxicology: the questions which must be answered, in *Current Approaches In Toxicology,* Ballantyne, B., Ed., John Wright & Sons, Bristol, England, 1977, 101.
2. **Lucia, H. L., Barrow, C. S., Stock, M. F., and Alarie, Y.,** A semiquantitative method for assessing anatomic damage sustained by the upper respiratory tract of the laboratory mouse, *Mus musculis, J. Comb. Toxicol.,* 4, 472, 1977.
3. **Basrur, P. K. and Harada, T.,** Alterations in the nasal mucosa of Syrian Golden hamsters exposed to cigarette smoke, *Prog. Exp. Tumor Res.,* 24, 283, 1979.
4. **Proctor, D. F. and Swift, D. L.,** The nose — a defense against the atmospheric environment, in *Inhaled Particles III,* Vol. 1, Walton, W. H., Ed., Unwin Bros., Old Woking, England, 1971, 59.
5. **Hadfield, E. H.,** Damage to the human nasal mucosa by wood dust, in *Inhaled Particles III,* Vol. 2, Walton, W. H., Ed., Unwin Bros., Old Woking, England, 1971, 855.
6. **Wynder, E. L. and Hoffman, D.,** *Tobacco and Tobacco Smoke: Studies in Experimental Carcinogenesis,* Academic Press, New York, 1967, 202.
7. **Wakabayashi, M., Bang, B. G., and Bang, F. B.,** Mucociliary transport in chickens infected with Newcastle disease virus and exposed to sulfur dioxide, *Arch. Environ. Health,* 32, 101, 1977.
8. **Vidic, B. and Greditzer, H. G.,** The histochemical and microscopical differentiation of the respirator glands around the maxillary sinus of the rat, *Am. J. Anat.,* 132, 491, 1971.
9. **Schreider, J. P. and Hutchens, J. O.,** Morphology of the guinea pig respiratory tract, *Anat. Rec.,* 196, 313, 1980.
10. **Giddens, W. E. and Fairchild, G. A.,** Effects of sulfur dioxide on the nasal mucosa of mice, *Arch. Environ. Health,* 25, 166, 1972.
11. **Nixon, J. M.,** Breathing pattern in the guinea pig, *Lab. Anim.,* 8, 71 1974.
12. **Wynder, E. L., Taguchi, K. T., Baden, V., and Hoffman, D.,** Tobacco carcinogenesis. IX. Effect of cigarette smoke on respiratory tract of mice after passive inhalation, *Cancer,* 21, 134, 1968.
13. **Clark, D. G.,** The toxicology of new smoking materials, in *Proc. Eur. Soc. Toxicol.,* Vol. 18, Duncan, W. A. M. and Leonard, B. J., Eds., Excerpta Medica, Amsterdam, 1977, 128.
14. **Binns, R., Beven, J. L., Wilton, L. V., and Lugton, W. G. D.,** Inhalation toxicity studies on cigarette smoke. II. Tobacco smoke inhalation dosimetry studies on small laboratory animals, *Toxicology,* 6, 197, 1976.
15. Surgeon General, Smoking and Health, A Report of the Surgeon General, U.S. Department of Health, Education and Welfare, Washington, D.C., 1979, 2.
16. **Beven, J. L.,** Inhalation toxicity studies on cigarette smoke. I. A versatile exposure system for inhalation toxicity studies on cigarette smoke, *Toxicology,* 6, 189, 1976.
17. **Wilton, L. V. and Binns, R.,** Comparative inhalation toxicity of smoke from cigarettes during a six-week study, in *Proc. Eur. Soc. Toxicol.,* Vol. 18, Duncan, W. A. M. and Leonard, B. J., Eds., Excerpta Medica, Amsterdam, 1977, 270.
18. **Binns, R., Beven, J. L., Wilton, L. V., and Lugton, W. G. D.,** Inhalation toxicity studies on cigarette smoke. III. Tobacco smoke inhalation dosimetry study on rats, *Toxicology,* 6, 207, 1976.
19. **Binns, R., Lugton, W. G. D., Wilton, L. V., and Dyas, B. J.,** Inhalation toxicity studies on cigarette smoke. V. Deposition of smoke particles in the respiratory system of rats under various exposure conditions *Toxicology,* 9, 87, 1978.
20. **Kendrick, J., Nettesheim, P., Guerin, M., Caton, J., Dalbey, W., Griesemer, R., Rubin, I., and Maddox, W.,** Tobacco smoke inhalation studies in rats, *Toxicol. Appl. Pharmacol.,* 37, 557, 1976.
21. **Binns, R., Lugton, W. G. D., and Dyas, B. J.,** The effect of exposure conditions on cigarette smoke deposition in the respiratory system of male rats, in *Proc. Eur. Soc. Toxicol.,* Vol. 18, Duncan, W. A. M. and Leonard, B. J., Eds., Excerpta Medica, Amsterdam, 1977, 267.
22. **Kmoch, N., Reznik, G., and Mohr, U.,** Inhalation experiment with ^{14}C-labelled cigarette smoke. II. The distribution of cigarette smoke particles in the hamster respiratory tract after exposure in two different smoking systems, *Toxicology,* 4, 373, 1975.
23. **Dalhamn, T., Rosengren, A., and Rylander, R.,** Nasal absorption of organic matter in animal experiments, *Arch. Environ. Health,* 22, 554, 1971.
24. **Bell, D. P.,** Chronic respiratory disease in a caesarean-derived and a conventional rat colony, *Lab. Anim.,* 1, 159, 1967.
25. **Thompson, H., Wright, N. G., and Cornwell, H. J. C.,** Contagious respiratory disease in dogs, *Vet. Bull.,* 45, 479, 1975.
26. **Flatt, R. E.,** Bacterial diseases, in *The Biology of the Laboratory Rabbit,* Weisbroth, S. H., Flatt, R. E., and Kraus, A. L., Eds., Academic Press, London, 1974, chap. 9.
27. **Nelson, J. B.,** Respiratory infections of rats and mice with emphasis on indigenous mycoplasms, in *Pathology of Laboratory Rats and Mice,* Cotchin, E. and Roe, F. J. C., Eds., Blackwell Scientific, Oxford, 1967, chap. 10.

28. **Ward, J. M.,** Naturally occurring Sendai virus disease of mice, *Lab. Anim. Sci.,* 24, 938, 1974.
29. **Bornstein, S. and Iwarsson, K.,** Nasal mites in a colony of Syrian hamsters, *Lab. Anim.,* 14, 31, 1980.
30. **Jacoby, R. O., Bhatt, P. N., and Jonas, A. M.,** Pathogenesis of sialodacryoadenitis in gnotobiotic rats, *Vet. Pathol.,* 12, 196, 1975.
31. **Gamble, M. R. and Clough, G.,** Ammonia build-up in animal boxes and its effect on rat tracheal epithelium, *Lab. Anim.,* 10, 93, 1976.
32. **Hebel, R. and Stromberg, M. W.,** Respiratory system, in *Anatomy of the Laboratory Rat,* Williams & Wilkins, Baltimore, 1976, chap. D.
33. **Smith, E. M. and Calhoun, M. L.,** *The Microscopic Anatomy of the White Rat,* Iowa State University Press, Ames, 1968, 97.
34. **Smith, G.,** Structure of the normal rat larynx, *Lab. Anim.,* 11, 223, 1977.
35. **Katz, S. and Merzel, J.,** Distribution of epithelia and glands of the nasal septum mucosa in the rat, *Acta Anat.,* 99, 58, 1977.
36. **Jeffery, P. K. and Reid, L.,** New observations of rat airway epithelium: a quantitative and electron microscopic study, *J. Anat.,* 120, 295, 1975.
37. **Andrews, P. M.,** A scanning electron microscopic study of the extrapulmonary respiratory tract, *Am. J. Anat.,* 139, 399, 1974.
38. **Greenblatt, M. and Rijhsinghani, K.,** Comparative cytopathologic alterations induced by alkylnitrosamines in nasal epithelium of the Syrian hamster, *J. Natl. Cancer Inst.,* 42, 421, 1969.
39. **Matulionis, D. H.,** Ultrastructure of olfactory epithelia in mice after smoke exposure, *Ann. Otol.,* 83, 192, 1974.
40. **Breeze, R. G. and Wheeldon, E. B.,** The cells of the pulmonary airways, *Am. Rev. Resp. Dis.,* 116, 705, 1977.
41. **Hayashi, M. and Huber, G. L.,** Quantitative differences in goblet cells in the tracheal epithelium of male and female rats, *Am. Rev. Resp. Dis.,* 115, 595, 1977.
42. **Mowry, R. W.,** Alcian blue techniques for histochemical study of acidic carbohydrates, *J. Histochem. Cytochem.,* 4, 407, 1956.
43. **Phalen, R. F.,** Inhalation exposure of animals, *Environ. Health Persp.,* 16, 17, 1976.
44. **Gage, J. C.,** Experimental inhalation toxicity, in *Methods in Toxicology,* Paget, G. E., Ed., Blackwell Scientific, Oxford, 1970, chap. 9.
45. **Binns, R.,** Animal inhalation studies with tobacco smoke (a review), *Rev. Environ. Health,* 2, 81, 1975.
46. **Walker, D., Wilton, L. V., and Binns, R.,** Inhalation toxicity studies on cigarette smoke. VII. 6-week comparative experiments using modified flue-cured cigarettes: histopathology of the conducting airways, *Toxicology,* 10, 241, 1978.
47. **Mogensen, C. and Tos, M.,** Routine procedure for determining goblet cell density in the mucosa of the respiratory tract, *Acta Pathol. Microbiol. Scand. Sect. A,* 84, 435, 1976.
48. **Mawdesley-Thomas, L. E., Healey, P., and Barry, D. H.,** Experimental bronchitis in animals due to sulphur dioxide and cigarette smoke. An automated quantitative study, in *Inhaled Particles III,* Vol. 1, Walton, W. H., Ed., Unwin Bros., Old Woking, England, 1971, 509.
49. **Wang, N. S. and Ying, W. L.,** The pattern of goblet cell hyperplasia in human airways, *Hum. Pathol.,* 8, 301, 1977.
50. **Walker, D., Wilton, L. V., and Binns, R.,** The acute pathological effects of cigarette smoke inhaled by rats, in *Proc. Eur. Soc. Toxicol.,* Vol. 18, Duncan, W. A. M. and Leonard, B. J., Eds., Excerpta Medica, Amsterdam, 1977, 228.
51. **Walker, D., Wilton, L. V. and Binns, R.,** Inhalation toxicity studies on cigarette smoke. VI. 6-week comparative experiments using modified flue-cured cigarettes: histopathology of the lung, *Toxicology,* 10, 229, 1978.
52. **Smith, G., Wilton, L. V., and Binns, R.,** Sequential changes in the structure of the rat respiratory system during and after exposure to cigarette smoke, *Toxicol. Appl. Pharmacol.,* 46, 579, 1978.
53. **Vidic, B., Rana, M. W., and Bhagat, B. D.,** Reversible damage of rat upper respiratory tract caused by cigarette smoke, *Arch. Otolaryngol.,* 99, 110, 1974.
54. **Dalbey, W. E., Nettesheim, P., Griesemer, R., Caton, J. E., and Guerin, M. R.,** Chronic inhalation of cigarette smoke by F344 rats, *J. Natl. Cancer Inst.,* 64, 383, 1980.
55. **Bernfeld, P., Homburger, F., Soto, E., and Pai, K. J.,** Cigarette smoke inhalation studies in inbred Syrian Golden hamsters, *J. Natl. Cancer Inst.,* 63, 675, 1979.
56. **Zwicker, G. M., Filipy, R. E., Park, J. F., Loscutoff, S. M., Ragan, H. A., and Stevens, D. L.,** Clinical and pathological effects of cigarette smoke exposure in beagle dogs, *Arch. Pathol. Lab. Med.,* 102, 623, 1978.
57. **Coggins, C. R. E., Fouillet, X. L. M., Lam, R., and Morgan, K. T.,** Cigarette smoke induced pathology of the rat respiratory tract: a comparison of the effects of the particulate and vapour phases, *Toxicology,* 16, 83, 1980.

58. **Lam, R.,** Transient epithelial loss in rat larynx after acute exposure to tobacco smoke, *Toxicol. Lett.,* 6, 327, 1980.
59. **Holt, P. G. and Keast, D.,** Environmentally induced changes in immunological function: acute and chronic effects of inhalation of tobacco smoke and other atmospheric contaminants in man and experimental animals, *Bacteriol. Rev.,* 41, 205, 1977.
60. **Gregson, R. L. and Prentice, D. E.,** Aspects of the immunotoxicity of chronic tobacco smoke exposure of the rat, *Toxicology,* 22, 23, 1981.
61. **Dontenwill, W.,** Experimental investigations on the effect of cigarette smoke inhalation on small laboratory animals, in *Inhalation Carcinogenesis,* Hanna, M. G., Nettesheim, P., and Gilbert J. R., Eds., AEC Symp. Ser. 18, 1970, 389.
62. **Binns, R.,** Inhalation toxicity studies on cigarette smoke. IV. Expression of the dose of smoke particulate material applied to the lungs of experimental animals, *Toxicology,* 7, 189, 1977.
63. **Feron, V. J., Kruysse, A., Til, H. P., and Immel, H. R.,** Repeated exposure to acrolein vapor: subacute studies in hamsters, rats and rabbits, *Toxicology,* 9, 47, 1978.
64. **Kruysse, A., Feron, V. J., and Til, H. P.,** Repeated exposure to acetaldehyde vapor, *Arch. Environ. Health,* 31, 449, 1975.
65. **Feron, V. J., Kruysse, A., Immel, H. R., and Til, H. P.,** Repeated exposure to butenolide vapour: subacute study in Syrian Golden hamsters, *Toxicology,* 15, 65, 1979.
66. **Feron, V. J. and Kroes, R.,** One-year time-sequence inhalation toxicity study of vinyl chloride in rats. II. Morphological changes in the respiratory tract, ceruminous glands, brain, kidneys, heart and spleen, *Toxicology,* 13, 131, 1979.
67. **Collings, A. J., Walker, D., and Browne, N. A.,** unpublished data, 1979.
68. **Walker, D. and Collings, A. J.,** unpublished data, 1978.
69. **Matulionis, D. H.,** Light and electron microscopic study of the effects of $ZnSO_4$ on mouse nasal respiratory epithelium and subsequent responses, *Anat. Rec.,* 183, 63, 1975.

Chapter 6

RADIATION-INDUCED NASAL CAVITY TUMORS IN ANIMALS

Stephen A. Benjamin

TABLE OF CONTENTS

I.   General Aspects of Radiation Carcinogenesis 138
      A.   General Aspects 138
      B.   Dose, Dose Rate, and Distribution of Radiation 138
            1.   Dose... 138
            2.   Dose Rate 139
            3.   Dose Distribution.................................... 139
      C.   Terminology... 140
            1.   Types of Radiation 140
            2.   Radioactivity, Exposure, and Dose 140

II.   Cancer of the Nose and Paranasal Sinuses 140
      A.   Radiation-Induced Sinonasal Cancer in Humans 140
      B.   Radiation-Induced Cancer of the Nasal Passages and Paranasal Sinuses
            in Animals... 141
            1.   Studies in Rodents 141
            2.   Studies in Dogs..................................... 142
      C.   Pathogenesis of Radiation-Induced Sinonasal Cancer 150

III. Summary.. 152

References.. 152

I. GENERAL ASPECTS OF RADIATION CARCINOGENESIS

A. General Aspects

The carcinogenic potential of ionizing radiation has been recognized for many years and many comprehensive reviews of radiation carcinogenesis have been published.[1-4] While it is not the purpose of this chapter to review this field, the reader unfamiliar with this subject will undoubtedly benefit from a brief general discussion of the subject, as an understanding of the basic aspects of radiation effects is essential to understanding the information to follow.

The basic cellular events in neoplastic transformation of cells by radiation are not different from those caused by other physical, chemical, or viral agents in that all affect the cellular DNA causing some defect which may be transmitted from that cell to its daughter cells. Carcinogenesis appears to be a multistage process with the transformation or ''initiation'' step being followed by a ''promoting'' event which allows the potentially neoplastic cell to proliferate. Promoting factors may include local tissue damage or hormonal influences, which stimulate cells to divide. They may also include reduced immunologic function, in which case transformed cells, normally kept in check by the immune response, may proliferate unchecked. These events are as important for radiation carcinogenesis as they are for other carcinogens. It may be that radiation, through its ability to cause local tissue damage and immunologic suppression, can be both a tumor initiator and promotor. It is also clear that radiation-induced carcinogenic changes may be additive or synergistic with the action of other carcinogens.

Although ionizing radiation is capable of causing an absolute increase in cancers of many types in an exposed population, it may also be responsible for the earlier appearance of certain types of cancers, i.e., an age-related increase of neoplasms that may have appeared in the population at a later time. The identification or recognition of radiation-induced neoplasms often is not straightforward. When examined on a clinical and morphological basis, radiation-induced tumors are generally indistinguishable from ''spontaneous'' tumors of the same tissue origin. How, then, does one identify radiation-induced tumors in an exposed population? This is done by the use of statistical evaluation. Generally, two populations are identified and compared: one exposed to radiation and one unexposed. Radiation-induced cancers are considered to be those that appear in significant excess in the exposed group. Other factors may also help in recognizing radiation-induced cancer such as tumors appearing at known irradiated sites or in specific tissues receiving significant radiation dose.

B. Dose, Dose Rate, and Distribution of Radiation

1. Dose

The question of dose-response relationships is central to the entire field of radiation carcinogenesis and represents a subject of much debate and controversy. This is primarily related to uncertainty over low dose carcinogenesis.[5-7] There is less uncertainty concerning carcinogenesis at high radiation doses, but, even here, many questions concerning the pathogenesis of radiation-induced tumors remain.

Casarett,[3,58] in a review of the pathogenesis of radiation-induced cancer, addressed several important points. It is generally agreed that no ''threshold dose'' for radiation carcinogenesis exists and that the smallest dose of radiation has a finite probability of causing a genetic event which could ultimately result in a neoplastic cell. Obviously, measurement of such an event is impractical in terms of evaluating populations where so many other variables, such as genetic background, environment, age, sex, etc. are present. Most of what we know about cancers induced by radiation has been derived from populations exposed to relatively high levels of a variety of types of radiation. The discussion of nasal cavity tumors induced by radiation in this chapter is based primarily on studies of animals exposed to high radiation doses. The question of low dose radiation risk, while a highly important one, is not germane to the present subject, and the reader is referred to the National Academy of Sciences report, *The Effects on Populations of Exposure to Low Levels of Ionizing Radiation: 1980,*[7] for further information.

Recognizing that most pertinent data on carcinogenesis come from high level studies, it is important to understand the basic concepts of dose/effect relationships. With increasing radiation dose, the yield of cancers in an exposed group increases, to a point. At this point, the incidence of cancers plateaus after which it may even decrease as the dose increases further. This may be due to a number of factors, the most straightforward of which may deal with cell killing. If one delivers a high enough dose of radiation to a site, theoretically, the majority of, or all of, the cells that are capable of transforming and producing a tumor at that site may be killed. Taken one step further, if the individual dies because of acute radiation injury, there is obviously no individual at risk to develop tumors.

Assuming that the level of radiation dose to a cell is sublethal, what is the mechanism by which a carcinogenic event takes place? The number of damaging events or sublesions caused in the cell, or more accurately, the cell nucleus, is proportional to the absorbed dose of radiation. Theoretically, if two sublesions are spatially and temporally close they can interact causing a biological effect. Since radiation damage to DNA can be repaired, it is readily seen that at low doses, where the ionizing events are scattered, many sublesions may fail to interact and produce a permanent effect before repair takes place. It has been maintained that most somatic effects in higher organisms are produced by this mechanism.[5]

2. Dose Rate

Dose rate refers to the time span over which a specific dose of radiation is delivered to an exposed tissue. This parameter is important in view of the mechanisms just discussed. Radiation exposure at high dose rates causes a maximal response. A similar dose at lower rates produced by protracting or fractionating exposure over a longer period of time spreads out the ionizing events temporally, giving less chance for sublesion interaction and a greater chance for recovery of cells and tissues from the damage. Therefore, induction of cancer after irradiation at relatively low dose rates may require a higher total dose to achieve the same effect as irradiation of the same tissue at a high dose rate.

3. Dose Distribution

Radiation dose may be delivered from an external source such as an X-ray machine, or internally by radioactive isotopes incorporated into the body. In either case, whole body, partial body, or specific organ or tissue exposure may result. The latter is most common with internally deposited radionuclides. A variety of factors determine the specific radiation dose and effects in tissues from such radionuclides. These include the physical and chemical form of the compound, the amount given, the route of administration, the metabolism and excretion by the body, the type of radiation delivered, and the sensitivity of the tissue involved.[8]

These factors are of particular importance in the induction of neoplasms of the nasal cavity and associated structures. As will be seen, in order to deliver enough radiation dose to induce significant numbers of cancers, the radionuclide involved must localize in the nasal region and remain long enough to deliver the dose to the primary cells at risk. Because of their physical and chemical characteristics, specific radionuclides will have affinity for, and localize in, specific tissues and organs. For example, radiostrontium, a well-known component of fallout which enters the human food chain through milk, concentrates in bone when it is in its ionic form.[9] Thus, it is referred to as a bone seeker. It is not surprising that significant levels of ^{90}Sr in bone can give rise to bone cancers which are primarily osteosarcomas. Radiation dose may be delivered over very short to very long periods of time.

Doses from external exposures will be dependent, in part, on the dose rate and the length of exposure, as well as on the energy of the radiation. In the case of internally deposited radionuclides, the situation is more complex. A primary determinant of the tissue dose is the physical half-life of the radioactive element, which determines how rapidly the isotope decays. The biological half-life is how long the body takes to excrete 50% of the radionuclide. Taken together, these two factors determine the effective half-life of the radionuclide in the body, which is a critical factor in determining cumulative or total tissue doses. Most of the subsequent discussions of radiation-induced nasal tumors will involve studies with long-lived radionuclides which are retained in the body for long periods of time, resulting in chronic irradiation of pertinent tissues.

C. Terminology

A number of radiobiological terms will be used in this chapter. To ensure a full understanding they will be discussed here. The reader is referred to an excellent short review by Hobbs and McClellan[10] for further information.

1. Types of Radiation

The electromagnetic ionizing radiations include X- and gamma rays which are part of the electromagnetic spectrum and have extremely short wave lengths and high photon energies. Gamma rays tend to have shorter wave lengths and higher energies than X-rays. X-rays originate outside the nucleus of atoms, while gamma rays originate from unstable atomic nuclei which are releasing energy. Both are highly penetrating radiations.

Particulate radiations of interest here are also produced by radioactive decay of unstable elements. Alpha particles consist of two neutrons and two protons. They have a large mass and a double positive charge which result in poor penetrating power in tissues.

Beta particles are electrons which result from conversion of a neutron to a proton in the nucleus. They have greater range and penetration in tissues but much less ionizing power than alpha particles.

Neutrons are particles consisting of an electron and a proton. Their mass gives them considerable energy but the lack of charge allows them to penetrate tissues readily.

2. Radioactivity, Exposure, and Dose

The unit of expression of radioactivity is the curie (Ci) which is defined as 3.7×10^{10} nuclear disintegrations per second.

The roentgen (R) is a unit of exposure applied to gamma and X-radiations. It is a measure of ionizations in air, with 1 R equaling 2.58×10^{-4} C/kg of air.

The rad is the unit of radiation-absorbed dose; 1 rad equals 100 ergs/g in any medium.

Linear energy transfer (LET) refers to the rate at which ionizing radiations give up their energy in tissues. Heavy particles, such as alpha particles, are high LET as they give up their energy over a short path, causing closely spaced ionizations. X-rays, on the other hand, are low LET and cause scattered ionization events as they penetrate tissues.

The term relative biological effectiveness (RBE) is the ratio of the dose of one type of radiation to another required to produce an identical biologic effect. High LET radiations have a high RBE as they cause closely spaced ionizations which can interact more readily. Thus, for a given absorbed dose of radiation, high LET radiations will cause more cellular transformations which may lead to cancers.

II. CANCER OF THE NOSE AND PARANASAL SINUSES

A. Radiation-Induced Sinonasal Cancer in Humans

The first recognition of sinonasal cancer as being induced by radiation was in human beings.[11,12] Although sinonasal cancers account for less than 1% of all cancer deaths in the U.S., a variety of specific occupational and nonoccupational factors have been identified as playing a causal role.[13] Chemical agents which have been confirmed as causes of sinonasal cancer include the radioactive element radium. Exposure to most agents causing sinonasal cancer is by inhalation of airborne particulates and vapors. In the case of radium dial painters, radium salts were ingested and absorbed, depositing in bone. These individuals, and others who ingested, inhaled, or were given injections of radium salts, developed not only osteosarcomas, but also head and sinus carcinomas.[14] The head and sinus carcinomas are thought to be related to radiation of the epithelium from the radium in bone around the sinuses and from accumulation of the alpha-emitting radon and radon daughters in the sinuses themselves.[11] Such tumors of bone and surrounding tissues are often referred to as bone-related neoplasms. While the subject of radiation-induced sinonasal cancers in humans is addressed elsewhere in this volume, it is important to recognize that virtually all of the information relating to these effects in animals derives from experimental studies designed to further the understanding of the human conditions.

B. Radiation-Induced Cancer of the Nasal Passages and Paranasal Sinuses in Animals

Realization that various radioactive materials were potentially significant health hazards for an early nuclear energy industry led to the initiation of a number of experimental studies to evaluate the risks of these materials. Likely routes of exposure included ingestion and inhalation. Many radionuclides are absorbed and deposited in bone no matter what the exposure route. Inhaled radionuclides, depending of the chemical and physical form, either remain in the respiratory tract or translocate to other tissues, including bone.

Some of the earliest animal studies were designed to permit relating the effects of various radionuclides to one another and to provide a method for estimating toxicity in man. In these studies, radium has served as a standard for toxicity in animals and as a common denominator for extrapolation of effects from animals to man.[15,16] The formula for such extrapolations is

$$\frac{\text{Effect of X in animals}}{\text{Effect of }^{226}\text{Ra in animals}} = \frac{\text{Effect of X in humans}}{\text{Effect of }^{226}\text{Ra in humans}}$$

1. Studies in Rodents

Spontaneous neoplasms of the nasal cavity are apparently quite rare in rodents. Tumors of the jaws, usually of bony or dental tissue origin, and of the oral epithelium have been reported frequently in mice.[17] Two reports of spontaneous nasal cavity tumors in mice *(Mus musculus)* and Syrian hamsters *(Mesocricetus auratus)* were found. One neuroepithelioma and one angiosarcoma were found in 358 BALB/cf/Cd mice.[18] In two colonies of Syrian hamsters, five tumors of the nasal cavity, including two adenocarcinomas and three benign polyps,[19] were noted in 498 animals.

Finkel and Biskis[15] reviewed their studies of the effects of a variety of bone-seeking radionuclides on induction of cancers of bone and surrounding tissues. They gave CF1 female mice single intravenous injections of the alpha-emitters ^{226}Ra and ^{239}Pu and the beta-emitters ^{90}Sr and ^{45}Ca, all bone seeking radionuclides. Mice were injected with ^{226}Ra at levels of 0.6 to 4170 μCi/kg body weight. They developed significant numbers of osteosarcomas but only in animals which received between 1.2 and 100 μCi/kg. Animals receiving levels of 288 μCi/kg or above had no tumors and, when viewed histologically, it appeared that the bone, and therefore the cell population at risk, was dead. No specific tumors of the nasal epithelium were noted, however, some of the osteosarcomas arose in the maxillary bones and involved the nasal cavity. Similar findings were reported with animals injected with ^{239}Pu, except that fewer sarcomas of the head were seen.

Studies with ^{90}Sr- and ^{45}Ca-injected mice followed the same principles, with animals at the lowest and highest levels of injected activity showing no increase in tumors, but those in the intermediate levels having significant increases. The incidence of sarcomas of the head was more similar to that in the ^{239}Pu-injected mice than in the ^{226}Ra-injected mice. Finkel[20] did report the development of squamous cell (epidermoid) carcinomas of the oral cavity in these singly injected mice, but none of the nasal cavity.

Nilsson[21,22] also performed a series of studies of the pathologic effects of ^{90}Sr in mice. In his studies, CBA mice, 785 days old, were given ^{90}Sr nitrate intraperitoneally. Injected activities ranged from 0.2 to 1.6 µCi/g body weight. His findings differed from those of Finkel, in that while osteosarcomas remained the primary findings, carcinomas of the mucous membranes of the mouth and nose were common. In the 1.6 µCi/g group, carcinomas were almost as frequent as osteosarcomas and many animals had both.

In an elegant study of the pathology of these epithelial lesions, Nilsson[23] found that the earliest morphologic change in the ^{90}Sr-treated animals was focally increased mitotic activity in the stratum germinativum of the epidermis. Slight disarrangement, altered polarity, and increased size of basal cells were followed by disruption and atypia of the basal cell layer. These dysplastic changes progressed to involve all layers of the epidermis and included giant nuclei and premature keratinization. Finally, noninvasive squamous carcinoma *in situ* and invasive squamous carcinomas were seen. This pattern was true for the cutaneous membranes of the nose and the oral cavity.

Tumors were also seen in the olfactory membranes. The most important early change was a reduction, and later disappearance, of the nervous olfactory cells, swelling of the sustentacular cells, and the appearance of mitotic figures along the basal membrane. The tumor cells seemed to invade the mucosa from the basal membrane and appeared to be predominantly basal cells. These tumors of the olfactory mucous membrane appeared only in the highest dose group.

A total of 80 carcinomas or carcinomas *in situ* were found in 475 ^{90}Sr-exposed mice; none were seen in 95 controls and 70% were in the highest dose group (1.6 µCi/g). About 59% involved the hard palate and 16% involved the nose. Of the 13 tumors involving the nasal cavities, 3 were in the olfactory region and 10 were in the cutaneous part of the nose. The squamous cell carcinomas were generally well differentiated and keratin-producing. Interestingly, Nilsson also reported 20 carcinomas arising from the external ear canal in these mice, most originating from a sebaceous gland on the anterior outside wall of the external auditory meatus (so-called Zymbal gland).[22] Both the absolute incidence and the age-dependent incidence of head carcinomas were dose dependent. The latent period for both preneoplastic and frankly neoplastic changes was reduced at each increasing dose level.

Other experiments have been reported which involved the induction of tumors in the nasal region of rats by irradiation. Yokoro[24] studied young W/Fu rats given 800 R of X-rays to the head. The incidence of osteosarcomas that developed was low (5 out of 149 rats); however, three affected the maxilla, one the nasal bone, and one the frontal bone.

Jasmin et al.[25] injected radiocerium (^{144}Ce) in a colloidal suspension into the region of the maxillary sinus in Sprague-Dawley male rats. Eight of nine rats that lived past 200 days of age developed tumors of the paranasal sinus at the site of inoculation. Initial local activity in these animals ranged from 0.41 to 13.59 µCi. All the tumors were well-differentiated squamous cell carcinomas.

2. Studies in Dogs

Neoplasms of the nasal cavity and paranasal sinuses are not common in the dog and account for about 1% of all canine tumors.[26-30] These tumors tend to occur in older animals with peak incidences in the 8- to 12-year-old group. They are also more prevalent in long-nosed dogs. The great majority are malignant and involve the nasal cavity rather than the sinuses. Epithelial malignancies are more common than those of mesenchymal origin. Adenocarcinomas are most frequently reported and squamous cell carcinomas are next most common.

A number of studies have been performed with beagle dogs exposed to both alpha- and beta-emitting radionuclides administered by a variety of routes in a variety of physical and chemical forms. Since many of these studies were designed as a series of experiments administering several different radionuclides by a similar route, they will be discussed in this fashion.

At the University of Utah, studies have been performed in which beagle dogs 17 months of age were given single injections of graded activity levels of a number of radionuclides including ^{226}Ra, ^{239}Pu, and ^{90}Sr.[31-35] These studies were designed to evaluate the toxicity of single injected doses of various radionuclides as compared with radium, as discussed earlier. The studies involving ^{226}Ra and ^{239}Pu are still ongoing, while the ^{90}Sr study is complete.

Table 1 summarizes pertinent current findings. As in the mouse studies, osteosarcomas, chondrosarcomas, and hemangiosarcomas of the skeleton are the primary findings in dogs injected with these bone-seeking radionuclides. Several chondrosarcomas and an osteosarcoma involved the nasal cavity. Five dogs developed epidermoid carcinomas of the frontal sinus and one had a similar lesion of the tympanic bulla. Only one control dog had an osteosarcoma and none had nasal tumors. Since bone sarcomas and carcinomas of the head are rare in the beagle dog, the authors felt that most of the observed lesions could be related to radiation injury.[36]

Finkel et al.[37] reported studies of dogs injected with ^{90}Sr at Argonne National Laboratories. The occurrence of three epidermoid carcinomas of the nasal cavity in dogs given single or multiple injections of the radionuclide was reported. No dose relationship was reported to be evident for these tumors.

In another set of studies at the University of California, Davis, beagle dogs were administered ^{90}Sr in feed and by injection, and ^{226}Ra in a series of eight intravenous injections. Dogs were fed ^{90}Sr from the fetal stage (via the bitch) through 540 days of age. Radium injections also terminated at 540 days. The pattern of radiation dose delivered was more a continuous steady level through 1.5 years of age as compared with the singly injected dogs at Utah, where there was a steadily decreasing dose rate after injection of adults.

The single major difference in findings was a high incidence of myeloproliferative disorders in the ^{90}Sr-fed beagles. This was not seen in the multiple injection ^{226}Ra study. Table 2 summarizes selected pertinent findings in the California study. A chondrosarcoma of the nasal cavity, a frontal sinus carcinoma, 7 carcinomas of the nasal cavity, and 19 squamous carcinomas of the gingiva were seen in irradiated dogs, with no comparable lesions seen in the controls. Pool et al.[39] suggested that the high incidence of gingival carcinomas, many of which involved the maxillary bones and nasal cavity, was related to the high radionuclide burden in the bones of the head and in the teeth. He reported that cumulative skeletal doses at the time of first recognition of bone-related neoplasms were on the order of 3700 to 15,500 rads. The pathology of the neoplasms induced in the beagles which ingested ^{90}Sr was also discussed. A number of the osteosarcomas reported affected the maxillary region, including the nasal cavity and frontal sinuses. Many of the osteosarcomas were first recognized as lytic lesions, but usually they developed extracortical osteogenesis and a ''sunburst'' pattern radiographically. Metastatic lesions were common. Histologically, the osteosarcomas did not differ from such spontaneous lesions in dogs. The squamous cell carcinomas were also typical of such spontaneous lesions in the dog and did not tend to metastasize.

Of particular interest to induction of nasal cavity neoplasms are studies with radioactive materials delivered via inhalation. At the Lovelace Inhalation Toxicology Research Institute, a series of studies is underway to evaluate the dose-response relationships resulting from

Table 1

BONE-RELATED, AND NASAL CAVITY NEOPLASMS IN DOGS GIVEN SINGLE INJECTIONS OF
BONE-SEEKING RADIONUCLIDES

Radionuclides	Injected activity (μCi/ kg)	Total number of dogs	Type of neoplasm and site	Number of dogs affected	Earliest death with neoplasm (years since injection)	Radiation dose to skeleton (rads)
[226]Ra	0.006—11.9	194[a]	Osteosarcoma, skeleton	40	2.3	275—24095
			Chondrosarcoma, nasal cavity	1	11.7	324
			Squamous carcinoma, tympanic bulla	1	12.6	1685
[239]Pu	0.005—3.3	345[a]	Osteosarcoma or chondrosarcoma, skeleton	70	3.1	2—9292
			Osteosarcoma, nasal cavity	1	10.6	20
			Chondrosarcoma, nasal cavity	2	9.5	21, 33
			Squamous carcinoma, frontal sinus	2	5.7	2, 240
[90]Sr	0.517—105.0	156	Osteosarcoma, skeleton	15	2.6	6935—22079
			Hemangiosarcoma, skeleton	4	3.2	10837—13355
			Squamous carcinoma, frontal sinus	3	5.4	13480—18143
			Adenocarcinoma, nasal cavity	1	11.6	7053
Controls	0	133[a]	Osteosarcoma, skeleton	1	14.7	0

[a] Results of an ongoing study. As of 3/31/79, 107 dogs in the [226]Ra study and 230 dogs in the [239]Pu study remained alive.

Data from Wrenn, M. E., Research in Radiobiology, Annual Report, Radiobiology Division, University of Utah College of Medicine, Salt Lake City, 1979.

Table 2

SELECTED BONE-RELATED AND NASAL CAVITY NEOPLASMS IN DOGS AFTER CHRONIC INGESTION OF ^{90}Sr OR REPEATED INJECTIONS OF ^{226}Ra[40,41]

Radionuclide	Route of administration	Range of activities	Total number of dogs	Type of neoplasm and site	Number of dogs affected	Earliest death with neoplasm (years of age)	Lowest activity level affected
^{90}Sr	Ingestion	0.020—36.00 μCi/day	235[a]	Osteosarcoma and chondrosarcoma, skeleton	26	1.6	1.300 μCi/day
				Squamous carcinoma, gingiva	15	2.5	4.000 μCi/day
				Carcinoma, frontal sinus	1	9.2	12.000 μCi/day
				Carcinoma, nasal cavity	7	8.6	0.020 μCi/day
^{226}Ra	Multiple injections	0.003—1.25 μCi/kg	215[a]	Osteosarcoma and chondrosarcoma, skeleton	112	3.3	0.008 μCi/kg
				Chondrosarcoma, nasal cavity	1	9.3	0.003 μCi/kg
				Squamous carcinoma, gingiva	4	6.7	0.003 μCi/Kg
Controls	—	—	130[a]	No comparable neoplasms	—	—	—

[a] Results of ongoing study. As of 6/30/78, 189 dogs remained alive in the ^{90}Sr ingestion study and 124 in the ^{226}Ra study.

inhalation of beta-emitting radionuclides in various physical and chemical forms.[42] One-year-old beagle dogs inhaled a series of radionuclides of different half-lives in both soluble and relatively insoluble forms.

Some of the results of these studies involving the soluble radionuclides are outlined in Table 3. Dogs were given graded doses of ^{91}Y, ^{144}Ce, or ^{90}Sr in chloride forms. The effective half-lives of these radionuclides in the body were 59 days, 285 days, and 5 to 10 years, respectively.[43-48] After inhalation, the materials deposited in the upper and lower respiratory tract. The ^{90}Sr was absorbed rapidly from the lung and deposited in the skeleton. The ^{90}Sr cleared from the upper respiratory tract passed through the gastrointestinal tract and a portion of this was also absorbed. The ^{91}Y and ^{144}Ce were also absorbed from the lung and deposited in liver and skeleton, however, about 10% of the initial lung burden remained in the lung for a longer period. Therefore, the respiratory tract, liver, and skeleton received significant radiation doses. Besides the bone-related and nasal neoplasms listed in Table 3, one dog given ^{91}YCl$_3$ and two given ^{144}CeCl$_3$ developed pulmonary carcinomas and one ^{91}Y-exposed dog and seven ^{144}Ce-exposed dogs had hepatic hemangiosarcomas.

Companion studies were also performed in which dogs received the same radionuclides in a relatively insoluble form in fused aluminosilicate particles (FAP).[49-52] In this case, most of the radionuclide burden remained in the lung for long periods of time. The effective half-lives of ^{91}Y, ^{144}Ce, and ^{90}Sr FAP in the lung were 50, 180, and 400 days, respectively.[42] The lung and associated thoracic structures were, therefore, at greatest risk from radiation exposure. There was also translocation to sites such as liver and skeleton. These tissues received a lesser dose but were also at risk for late effects. Pulmonary neoplasia, as would be expected, was the primary finding in these dogs, however, some unexpected tumor types were noted. Among 65 dogs that died after being exposed to ^{91}Y FAP, 19 had pulmonary carcinomas of various cell types and 3 had hemangiosarcomas of structures closely associated with the lung, including the tracheobronchial lymph nodes, mediastinum, and heart. One dog had what grossly appeared to be a carcinoma of the nasal cavity at 9.3 years after exposure. The dose to the lung was 5600 rads. Among 65 dogs that died after inhalation of ^{144}Ce FAP, 9 had pulmonary carcinomas and 7 developed primary pulmonary hemangiosarcomas; 18 other dogs developed hemangiosarcomas of such irradiated tissues as tracheobronchial lymph nodes, mediastinum, heart, bone, and liver. In this group one dog developed a squamous cell carcinoma of the nasal cavity at 3.4 years after exposure. The dose to the lung in this dog was about 32,000 rads. Finally, among 81 dead dogs which inhaled ^{90}Sr FAP, 19 developed primary pulmonary hemangiosarcomas and only 3 had pulmonary carcinomas; 19 other dogs developed hemangiosarcomas of associated irradiated tissues. Two dogs developed nasal carcinomas at 2.8 and 6.8 years after exposure. Doses to lung in these dogs were 52,000 and 31,000 rads, respectively.

Several findings are of significance in this series of experiments. It is obvious that the localization of the radionuclide, hence the tissues irradiated rather than the specific radionuclide involved, is the prime determinant of the location of the late-occurring neoplasms. It is also evident that in dogs exposed to soluble or relatively insoluble beta-emitters, dose rate and cumulative dose play an important role in determining effects. Radionuclides with the shortest half-lives delivered the highest initial dose rates and delivered their radiation dose over a shorter period. Since very high dose rates and cumulative doses in short periods tended to result in acute injury many dogs died prior to developing cancers. The longer-lived radionuclides were considerably more effective in inducing cancer. Also, the more protracted radiation and the accumulation of high radiation doses favored the induction of hemangiosarcomas in ^{144}Ce- and ^{90}Sr-exposed dogs, as compared with epithelial tumor induction in ^{91}Y-exposed dogs. Benjamin et al.[53] have discussed the finding of large numbers of hemangiosarcomas in dogs exposed to both soluble and insoluble beta-emitting radionuclides.

With respect to nasal cavity and sinus tumors, it is interesting to note that in dogs exposed

Table 3

BONE-RELATED AND NASAL CAVITY NEOPLASMS IN DOGS THAT INHALED RELATIVELY SOLUBLE BETA-EMITTING RADIONUCLIDES[43,45,47]

Radionuclide and form	LTRB[a]	Major organs receiving radiation dose	Total number of dogs	Type of neoplasm and site	Numbers of dogs affected	Earliest death with neoplasm (years after exposure)	Radiation dose (rads)	
							Skeleton	Lung
$^{91}YCl_3$	14—540	Respiratory tract Skeleton Liver	46[b]	Squamous cell carcinoma, nasal cavity	3	5.5	860—2900	1000—3300
Controls	—		12[b]	No comparable neoplasms	—		—	—
$^{144}CeCl_3$	2.6—360	Respiratory tract Skeleton Liver	55[b]	Squamous cell carcinoma, nasal cavity	5	4.5	2800—6700	2100—5000
				Hemangiosarcoma, nasal cavity	1	7.2	2600	5500
				Osteosarcoma, skeleton	1	2.2	8100	—
Controls	—		15[b]	No comparable neoplasms	—		—	—
$^{90}SrCl_2$	0.97—120	Skeleton	72[b]	Osteosarcoma and chondrosarcoma, skeleton	20	2.4	2200—17000	—
				Hemangiosarcoma, skeleton	12	2.4	9900—18000	—
				Fibrosarcoma, skeleton	3	2.1	7600—19000	—
				Squamous carcinoma, nasal cavity	2	10.2	1200—13000	—
				Squamous carcinoma, frontal sinus	1	11.6	7300	—
				Basosquamous carcinoma, skull	1	7.2	7100	—
Controls	—		25[b]	No comparable neoplasms	—		—	—

a   LTRB = long-term retained burden in μCi/Kg body weight.

b   Results of ongoing study. As of 9/30/80, 15, 7, and 5 dogs remained alive in ^{91}Y, ^{144}Ce, and ^{90}Sr studies, respectively.

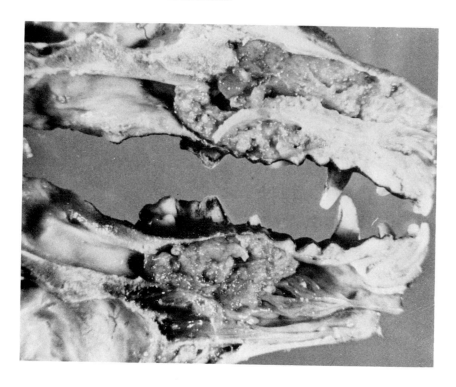

FIGURE 1.   Squamous cell carcinoma in a dog exposed by inhalation to ^{144}CeCl$_3$. The tumor filled the right nasal cavity and invaded the hard palate and internasal septum. (From Benjamin, S. A., Boecker, B. B., Cuddihy, R. G., and McClellan, R. O., *J. Natl. Cancer Inst.*, 63, 133, 1979. With permission.)

to ^{91}YCl$_3$ and ^{144}CeCl$_3$, nasal tumors outnumbered pulmonary tumors despite the fact that several thousand rads were delivered to the deep lung. Nasal cavity carcinomas were relatively more frequent and occurred at earlier ages in dogs which inhaled ^{91}YCl$_3$ and ^{144}CeCl$_3$, as compared with ^{90}SrCl$_2$. In contrast, little difference in nasal carcinoma occurrence was seen between dogs exposed to the three radionuclides in relatively insoluble form.

Histopathologic studies revealed that most of the nasal carcinomas in these studies were squamous cell carcinomas.[48] They were mostly well-differentiated tumors that were highly invasive and often progressed to bilateral turbinate involvement (see Figures 1 and 2). Metastases to lung and/or cervical lymph nodes were common. The nasal tumors were the cause of death or euthanasia in all cases reported, even if another malignancy, such as a lung carcinoma, was present concurrently. The only early lesion found was in a dog exposed to ^{144}CeCl$_3$, which died because of a mammary carcinoma. It had a lesion of the nasal turbinate epithelium characteristic of squamous carcinoma *in situ* (Figure 3). Of the two carcinomas in ^{90}SrCl$_2$-exposed dogs, one was a squamous carcinoma of the frontal sinus and the other was a basosquamous carcinoma of the skull in the region of the tympanic bulla. Presumably, both arose from epithelium lining these bony structures.

The high incidence of lung cancer in uranium miners, who also smoke, has led to studies of the separate and combined roles of radon daughters and cigarette smoking in respiratory tract carcinogenesis in dogs.[54] While neoplastic lesions were not observed, potentially preneoplastic pulmonary epithelial lesions, consisting of adenomatous and squamous hyperplasia, were frequent in dogs after 4 years of exposure. Of interest to this chapter, one dog exposed to radon daughters, uranium ore dust, and cigarette smoke had a pseudoepitheliomatous hyperplastic lesion with disorientation of basal cells in the nasal turbinate. This also could represent a preneoplastic change.

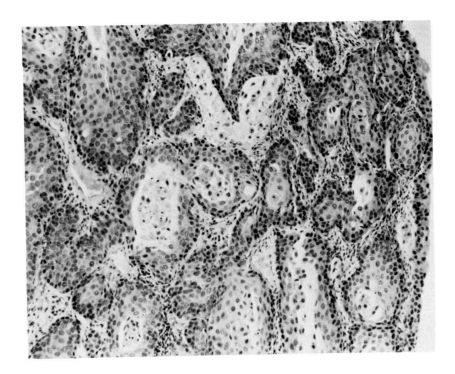

FIGURE 2. Squamous cell carcinoma involving the nasal passages of a dog exposed by inhalation to ^{144}CeCl$_3$. (H and E; × 100.) (Courtesy of Inhalation Toxicology Research Institute, Albuquerque, N.M.)

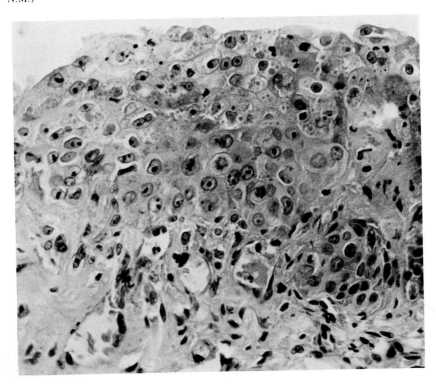

FIGURE 3. Squamous carcinoma *in situ* in the turbinate of a dog exposed to ^{144}CeCl$_3$ showing numerous mitoses and keratohyaline granule formation. (H and E; × 350.) (Courtesy of Inhalation Toxicology Research Institute, Albuquerque, N.M.)

The only study using external irradiation which has reported a nasal cavity tumor of potential significance is that being carried out at Colorado State University.[55] Beagle dogs were given single, acute, whole body exposures to 20 or 100 R of ^{60}Co gamma radiation at one of three prenatal or three postnatal ages up to 1 year of age to evaluate age-related radiation sensitivity. Out of 480 dogs irradiated in the perinatal period, 4 died with malignancies prior to 2 years of age. This is a very rare spontaneous event and to have four such deaths in a small irradiated population suggests a strong association with the radiation insult. One of these dogs, which received 20 R (approximately 16 rads) as a neonate, died at 1.9 years of age with a fibrosarcoma of the nasal cavity.

C. Pathogenesis of Radiation-Induced Sinonasal Cancer

As has been seen, tumors of the nasal cavity and paranasal sinuses can be induced in several species by radiation from a variety of sources, but primarily from internally deposited radionuclides. They can be differentiated from naturally occurring tumors of the same region only by the fact that they occur in much greater incidence in irradiated animals and because they are virtually all of a histologic type (squamous cell origin) that is not the primary type of nasal tumor (adenocarcinoma) seen spontaneously in animals. Although the pathogenesis of these tumors is complex, some speculations are possible. Much of our understanding actually derives from analysis of bone sarcomas induced by bone-seeking radionuclides.[15,21,32] In general, alpha-emitters are more oncogenic than beta-emitters and, the longer-lived isotopes, which deliver more chronic exposure, are more oncogenic than very short-lived ones. Furthermore, isotopes, such as plutonium and cerium, that deposit on bone surfaces tend to cause more tumors than do those, such as radium and strontium, which are distributed in the mineral volume of bone. The first two points have already been touched upon, i.e., alpha particles have a higher LET and RBE than beta particles and protracted radiation allows for less cell killing and a longer life span during which the individual remains at risk for cancer development. Localization of internally deposited radionuclides and the range in tissues of the radiation emitted also play an important role. It has been shown that the sensitive cells for osteosarcoma induction are the bone-forming endosteal cells. A radionuclide such as ^{239}Pu deposits on bone surfaces and delivers half its alpha radiation to the cell populations overlying the bone and half to the mineral below. In contrast, ^{226}Ra which distributes throughout the bone has more than 90% of its alpha radiation absorbed by the mineral because of the short path of the alpha particles. While ^{90}Sr also distributes throughout bone and while the beta emissions of ^{90}Sr have a lower RBE than do alphas, more beta radiation escapes the mineral (about 50%) to irradiate surrounding tissues because of the longer path in tissues.[32]

Applying this information to the induction of tumors of the nasal cavity, it is not surprising that such neoplasms are seen in animals exposed to bone-seekers. It is tempting to speculate that because of the greater range of beta radiation in tissues beta-emitters may be more efficient in causing tumors of epithelium overlying bone. This appears to be true with respect to findings in both mice and dogs, however, the numbers of tumors are relatively small and no absolute statement can be made.

Dogs injected with ^{226}Ra did not have any carcinomas of the paranasal sinuses[35,40,41] even though about one third of the bone-related cancers in humans exposed to ^{226}Ra were of this type.[11] Since sinus carcinomas were seen after ^{239}Pu and ^{90}Sr deposition in bone, one wonders whether the dog develops the same build-up of radon in the sinuses as occurs in humans.

The situation involving inhaled beta-emitting radionuclides has both similarities and differences when compared with studies of injected and ingested radionuclides. Where soluble radionuclide is deposited in bone the same principles hold true. This does not explain, however, the relatively high incidence and earlier appearance of nasal neoplasms in dogs which inhaled ^{91}YI$_3$ or ^{144}CeCl$_3$. Benjamin et al.[48] have discussed some of the other factors

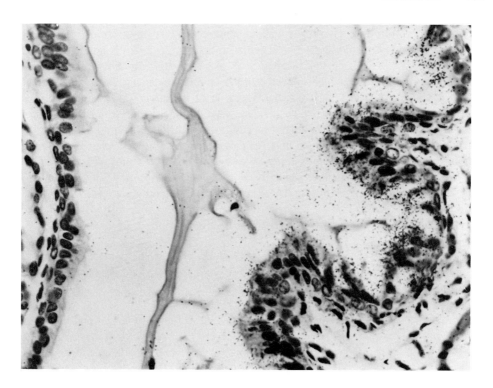

FIGURE 4. Autoradiograph of turbinate epithelium from dog killed 8 days after exposure to ^{144}CeCl$_3$, showing focally heavy concentration of radionuclide associated with the epithelial lining. (H and E; × 300.) (From Benjamin, S. A., Boecker, B. B., Cuddihy, R. G., and McClellan, R. O., *J. Natl. Cancer Inst.*, 63, 133, 1979. With permission.)

which may be involved. Doses to the skeleton of dogs which developed nasal tumors after inhalation of ^{91}Y or ^{144}Ce were generally lower than those of dogs exposed to ^{90}Sr which had bone-related sarcomas, nasal or head tumors. This suggests that other factors may have played a role.

One important factor is that yttrium and cerium both deposit on bone surfaces, which would lead to higher local dose rates to overlying epithelium. A second important factor relates to observed differences in concentrations of ^{91}Y, ^{144}Ce, or ^{90}Sr in the nasal turbinates relative to observed concentrations in the skeleton. Studies of ^{144}Ce concentrations in the nasal turbinates revealed that they were 10 to 100 times those of the average skeletal concentrations up to 32 days after inhalation exposure[56] and that they remained higher through 1.4 years after inhalation.[57] Autoradiographs of nasal turbinate tissue sections taken from dogs 8 days after inhalation suggested that the radionuclide was associated with focal areas of nasal epithelium (see Figure 4). This was thought to be related to precipitation and formation of insoluble compounds which were not readily cleared from the turbinate region. Similar findings were reported after ^{91}YCl$_3$ inhalation. Dogs which inhaled ^{90}SrCl$_2$ did not show this phenomenon. It is likely that doses to the nasal turbinate region in dogs that inhaled ^{144}Ce or ^{91}Y were considerably higher than the average skeletal or lung dose because of contributions from the radionuclides associated with both bone and respiratory epithelium.

Fewer nasal tumors were seen in dogs which inhaled relatively insoluble forms of beta-emitting radionuclides. This probably relates to the rapid and, apparently more complete, nasopharyngeal clearance observed for insoluble particles inhaled by dogs.[58]

There is good evidence that radiation-induced bone sarcomas seem to be induced by direct mechanisms involving localized tissue damage and repair.[21,22,39] Tumors tend to form in areas of bone with the highest radionuclide content, where there is focal bone damage and reparative changes, including increased cell proliferation.[39] Nilsson[23] showed that squamous carcinomas in ^{90}Sr-injected mice started at local sites in the stratum germinativum of the oral and nasal epithelium which showed probable irradiation damage and repair. The findings of local concentrations of ^{144}Ce associated with nasal epithelium and a carcinoma *in situ* of the nasal epithelium in dogs which inhaled ^{144}CeCl$_3$ and suggested that local injury may have been a factor in the development of nasal tumors in those studies.[48] Thus, it is likely that severe local injury and subsequent increased local cell turnover play an important role in the induction of radiation-induced nasal cavity neoplasms. It seems clear that factors such as local dose pattern, dose rate, cumulative dose, and local response to injury in this process are all important, however, their relative roles are still not fully defined.

III. SUMMARY

Neoplasms of the nasal cavity and paranasal sinuses have been induced in mice, rats, and dogs by radiation of different types and from varied sources. Most have been found in animals with internally deposited alpha- and beta-emitting radionuclides. Bone-seeking radionuclides, including ^{239}Pu, ^{226}Ra, and ^{90}Sr, deposit in the skeleton and deliver radiation to both bone and closely associated tissues such as epithelium of the oral and nasal cavities. Inhaled bone-seeking radionuclides such as ^{144}Ce and ^{91}Y in dogs result in a relatively higher occurrence of nasal tumors which is thought to be related to both irradiation from underlying bone and from radionuclide associated with the nasal epithelium. Bone sarcomas have been induced by irradiation of the turbinate and maxillary bones, however, the predominant type of tumor of the nasal passages and paranasal sinuses has been squamous cell carcinomas.

REFERENCES

1. **Casarett, G. W.,** Experimental radiation carcinogenesis, *Progr. Exp. Tumor Res.,* 7, 49, 1965.
2. **Upton, A. C.,** Radiation carcinogenesis, in *Methods in Cancer Research,* Vol. 4, Busch, H., Ed., Academic Press, New York, 1968, chap. 2.
3. **Storer, J. B.,** Radiation carcinogenesis, in *Cancer, A Comprehensive Treatise,* Vol. 1, Becker, F. F., Ed., Plenum Press, New York, 1975, chap. 16.
4. **Yuhas, J. M., Tennant, R. W., and Regan, J. D.,** *Biology of Radiation Carcinogenesis,* Raven Press, New York, 1976.
5. **Brown, J. M.,** The shape of the dose-response curve for radiation carcinogenesis. Extrapolation to low doses, *Radiat. Res.,* 71, 34, 1977.
6. **Upton, A. C.,** Radiobiological effects of low doses. Implications for radiobiological protection, *Radiat. Res.,* 71, 51, 1977.
7. **Radford, E. P.,** Chairman, Committee on the Biological Effects of Ionizing Radiations, *The Effects on Populations of Exposure to Low Levels of Ionizing Radiation: 1980,* National Academy Press, Washington, D.C., 1980.
8. **Casarett, G. W.,** Pathogenesis of radionuclide-induced tumors, in *Proc. Symp. Radionuclide Carcinogenesis,* Sanders, C. L., Busch, R. H., Ballou, J. E., and Mahlum, D. D., Eds., Natl. Tech. Inform. Serv., Springfield, Va., 1973, 1.
9. **Bennet, B. G.,** Global ^{90}Sr fallout and its occurrence in diet and man, in *Proc. Symp. Biomedical Implications of Radiostrontium Exposure,* Goldman, M. and Bustad, L. K., Eds., Natl. Tech. Inform. Serv., Springfield, Va., 1972, 17.
10. **Hobbs, C. H. and McClellan, R. O.,** Radiation and radioactive materials, in *Casarett and Doull's Toxicology. The Basic Science of Poisons,* 2nd ed., Doull, J., Klassen, C. D., and Amdur, M. O., Eds., Macmillan, New York, 1980, chap. 19.

11. **Evans, R. D., Keane, A. T., Kolenkow, R. J., Neal, W. R., and Shanahan, M. M.,** Radiogenic tumors in the radium and mesothorium cases studied at M.I.T., in *Proc. Symp. Delayed Effects of Bone-Seeking Radionuclides,* Mays, C. W., Jee, W. S. S., Lloyd, R. D., Stover, B. J., Dougherty, J. H., and Taylor, G. N., Eds., University of Utah Press, Salt Lake City, 1969, 157.

12. **Finkel, A. J., Miller, C. E., and Hasterlik, R. J.,** Radium-induced malignant tumors in man, in *Proc. Symp. Delayed Effects of Bone-Seeking Radionuclides,* Mays, C. W., Jee, W. S. S., Lloyd, R. D., Stover, B. J., Dougherty, J. H., and Taylor, G. N., Eds., University of Utah Press, Salt Lake City, 1969, 195.

13. **Roush, G. C.,** Epidemiology of cancer of the nose and paranasal sinuses: current concepts, *Head and Neck Surg.,* Sept./Oct., 3, 1979.

14. **Rubin, P.,** Comment: radionuclide carcinogenesis and sinus carcinoma, *JAMA,* 219, 354, 1972.

15. **Finkel, M. P. and Biskis, B. O.,** Experimental induction of osteosarcomas, *Progr. Exp. Tumor Res.,* 10, 72, 1968.

16. **Raabe, O. G., Book, S. A., and Parks, N. J.,** Bone cancer from radium: canine dose response explains data for mice and humans, *Science,* 208, 61, 1980.

17. **Gossner, W. and Luz, A.,** Tumors of the jaws, *Int. Agency Res. Cancer Sci. Publ.,* 23, 611, 1979.

18. **Rabstein, L. S. and Peters, R. L.,** Tumors of the kidneys, synovia, exocrine pancreas, and nasal cavity in BALB/cf/Cd mice, *J. Natl. Cancer Inst.,* 51, 999, 1973.

19. **Dour, P., Mohr, U., Cardesa, A., Althoff, J., and Kimoch, N.,** Spontaneous tumors and common diseases in two colonies of Syrian hamsters. II. Respiratory tract and digestive system, *J. Natl. Cancer Inst.,* 56, 937, 1976.

20. **Finkel, M. P.,** Late effects of internally deposited radioisotopes in laboratory animals, *Radiat. Res.,* 1, (Suppl.), 265, 1959.

21. **Nilsson, A.,** Pathologic effects of different doses of radiostrontium in mice. Dose effect relationship in ^{90}Sr-induced bone tumors, *Acta Radiol. Ther. Phys. Biol.,* 9, 155, 1970.

22. **Nilsson, A.,** Strontium-90-induced malignancies in mice, in *Proc. Symp. Biomedical Implications of Radiostrontium Exposure,* Goldman, M. and Bustad, L. K., Eds., Natl. Tech. Inform. Serv., Springfield, Va., 1972, 207.

23. **Nilsson, A.,** Pathologic effects of different doses of ^{90}Sr in mice. Development of carcinomas in the mucous membranes of the head, *Acta Radiol. Ther. Phys. Biol.,* 7, 27, 1968.

24. **Yokoro, K.,** Radiation carcinogenesis with special reference to the induction of osteogenic sarcomas by internal and external irradiations, *Acta Pathol. Jpn.,* 17, 348, 1967.

25. **Jasmin, J. R., Brocheriou, C., Klein, B., Morin, M., Smadja-Joffe, F., Cernmea, P., and Jasmin, C.,** Induction in rats of paranasal sinus carcinomas with radioactive cerium chloride, *J. Natl. Cancer Inst.,* 58, 423, 1977.

26. **Morgan, J. P., Suter, P. F., O'Brien, T. R., and Park, R. D.,** Tumors in the nasal cavity of the dog: a radiographic study, *J. Am. Vet. Radiol. Soc.,* 13, 18, 1972.

27. **Madewell, B. R., Priester, W. A., Gillette, E. L., and Snyder, S. P.,** Neoplasms of the nasal passages and paranasal sinuses in domesticated animals as reported by 13 veterinary colleges, *Am. J. Vet. Res.,* 37, 851, 1976.

28. **Confer, A. W. and DePaoli, A.,** Primary neoplasms of the nasal cavity, paranasal sinuses and nasopharynx in the dog. A report of 16 cases from the files of the AFIP, *Vet. Pathol.,* 15, 18, 1978.

29. **Norris, A. M.,** Intranasal neoplasms in the dog, *J. Am. Anim. Hosp. Assoc.,* 15, 231, 1979.

30. **Priester, W. A. and McKay, F. W.,** The occurrence of tumors in domestic animals, *Natl. Cancer Inst. Monogr.,* 54, 157, 1980.

31. **Taylor, G. N., Dougherty, T. F., Shabestari, L., and Dougherty, J. H.,** Soft-tissue tumors in internally irradiated beagles, in *Proc. Symp. Delayed Effects of Bone-Seeking Radionuclides,* Mays, C. W., Jee, W. S. S., Lloyd, R. D., Stover, B. J., Dougherty, J. H., and Taylor, G. N., Eds., University of Utah Press, Salt Lake City, 1969, 323.

32. **Mays, C. W., Dougherty, T. F., Taylor, G. N., Lloyd, R. D., Stover, B. J., Jee, W. S. S., Christensen, W. R., Dougherty, J. H., and Atherton, D. R.,** Radiation-induced bone cancer in beagles, in *Proc. Symp. Delayed Effects of Bone-Seeking Radionuclides,* Mays, C. W., Jee, W. S. S., Lloyd, R. D., Stover, B. J., Dougherty, J. H., and Taylor, G. N., Eds., University of Utah Press, Salt Lake City, 1969, 387.

33. **Dougherty, J. H., Taylor, G. N., and Mays, C. W.,** Strontium-90 toxicity in adult beagles after acute exposure, in, *Proc. Symp. Biomedical Implications of Radiostrontium Exposure,* Goldman, M. and Bustad, L. K., Eds., Natl. Tech. Inform. Serv., Springfield, Va., 1972, 259.

34. **Jee, W. S. S., Atherton, D. R., Bruenger, F., Dougherty, J. H., Lloyd, R. D., Mays, C. W., Nabors, J., Jr., Stevens, W., Stover, B. J., Taylor, G. N., and Woodbury, L. A.,** Current status of Utah long-term ^{239}Pu studies, in *Proc. Symp. Biological and Environmental Effects of Low-Level Radiation,* Vol. 2, International Atomic Energy Agency, Vienna, 1976, 79.

35. **Wrenn, M. E.,** *Research in Radiobiology, Annual Report, Radiobiology Division,* University of Utah College of Medicine, Salt Lake City, 1979.

36. **Mays, C. W., Jee, W. S. S., Taylor, G. N., and Stevens, W.,** Bone sarcoma induction in beagles by low doses from ^{239}Pu and ^{226}Ra, in *Research in Radiobiology, Annual Report, Radiobiology Laboratory,* University of Utah College of Medicine, Salt Lake City, 1978, 158.

37. **Finkel, M. P., Biskis, B. O., Greco, I., and Camden, R. W.,** Strontium-90 toxicity in dogs: status of Argonne study on influence of age and dosage pattern, in *Proc. Symp. Biomedical Implications Radiostrontium Exposure,* Goldman, M. and Bustad, L. K., Eds., Natl. Tech. Inform. Serv., Springfield, Va., 1972, 285.

38. **Pool, R. R., Williams, R. J. R., and Goldman, M.,** Strontium-90 toxicity in adult beagles after continuous ingestion, in *Proc. Symp. Biomedical Implications of Radiostrontium Exposure,* Goldman, M. and Bustad, L. K., Eds., Natl. Tech. Inform. Serv., Springfield, Va., 1972, 277.

39. **Pool, R. R., Williams, R. J. R., and Goldman, M.,** Induction of tumors involving bone in beagles fed toxic levels of strontium-90, *Am. J. Roentgenol. Radium Ther. Nucl. Med.,* 118, 900, 1973.

40. **Chrisp, C. E., Spangler, W. L., Pool, R. R., and Book, S. A.,** Cumulative causes of death in radionuclide-treated beagles, in *1978—1979 Annual Report, Radiobiology Laboratory, University of California, Davis,* Natl. Tech. Inform. Serv., Springfield, Va., 1979, 130.

41. **Book, S. A., Chrisp, C. E., Goldman, M., Parks, N. J., Philbrick, A. L., Pool, R. R., Raabe, O. G., Rosenblatt, L. S., Shifrine, M., Spangler, W. L., White, R. G., and Wilson, F. D.,** Comparative toxicity of strontium-90 and radium-226: experimental design and current status, in *1978—1979 Annual Report, Radiobiology Laboratory, University of California, Davis,* Natl. Tech. Inform. Serv., Springfield, Va., 1979, 200.

42. **McClellan, R. O., Benjamin, S. A., Boecker, B. B., Hahn, F. F., Hobbs, G. H., Jones, R. K., and Lundgren, D. L.,** Influence of variations in dose and dose rates on biological effects of inhaled beta-emitting radionuclides, in *Proc. Symp. Biological and Environmental Effects of Low-Level Radiation,* Vol. 2, International Atomic Energy Agency, Vienna, 1976, 3.

43. **Hahn, F. F., Muggenberg, B. A., Boecker, B. B., Jones, R. K., McClellan, R. O., and Pickrell, J. A.,** Toxicity of inhaled ^{91}YCl$_3$ in beagle dogs. XIV, in *Inhalation Toxicology Research Institute Annual Report 1979—1980,* Diel, J. H., Bice, D. E., and Martinez, B. S., Eds., Natl. Tech. Inform. Serv., Springfield, Va., 1980, 53.

44. **Benjamin, S. A., Boecker, B. B., Chiffelle, T. L., Hobbs, C. H., Jones, R. K., McClellan, R. O., Pickrell, J. A., and Redman, H. C.,** Neoplasia in beagle dogs after inhalation of ^{144}CeCl$_3$, in *Proc. Symp. Radionuclide Carcinogenesis,* Sanders, L L., Busch, R. H., Ballou, J. E., and Mahlum, D. D., Eds., Natl. Tech. Inform. Serv., Springfield, Va., 1973, 181.

45. **Muggenberg, B. A., Hahn, F. F., Boecker, B. B., McClellan, R. O., and Pickrell, J. A.,** Toxicity of inhaled ^{144}CeCl$_3$ in beagle dogs. XIV, in *Inhalation Toxicology Research Institute Annual Report 1979—1980,* Diel, J. H., Bice, D. E., and Martinez, B. S., Eds., Natl. Tech. Inform. Serv., Springfield, Va., 1980, 57.

46. **McClellan, R. O., Benjamin, S. A., Boecker, B. B., Chiffelle, T. L., Hobbs, C. H., Jones, R. K., Pickrell, J. A., and Redman, H. C.,** Neoplasms in dogs that inhaled ^{90}SrCl$_2$, in *Proc. Symp. Radionuclide Carcinogenesis,* Sanders, C. L., Busch, R. H., Ballou, J. E., and Mahlum, D. D., Eds., Natl. Tech. Inform. Serv., Springfield, Va., 1973, 215.

47. **Snipes, M. B., Muggenberg, B. A., Hahn, F. F., Boecker, B. B., Jones, R. K., McClellan, R. O., and Pickrell, J. A.,** Toxicity of inhaled ^{90}SrCl$_2$ in beagle dogs. XIV, in *Inhalation Toxicology Research Institute Annual Report 1979—1980,* Diel, J. H., Bice, D. E., and Martinez, B. S., Eds., Natl. Tech. Inform. Serv., Springfield, Va., 1980, 48.

48. **Benjamin, S. A., Boecker, B. B., Cuddihy, R. G., and McClellan, R. O.,** Nasal carcinomas in beagles after inhalation of relatively soluble forms of beta-emitting radionuclides, *J. Natl. Cancer Inst.,* 63, 133, 1979.

49. **Hahn, F. F., Muggenberg, B. A., Hobbs, C. H., McClellan, R. O., Mauderly, J. L., and Pickrell, J. A.,** Toxicity of ^{91}Y inhaled in a relatively insoluble form by beagle dogs. XI, in *Inhalation Toxicology Research Institute Annual Report 1979—1980,* Diel, J. H., Bice, D. E., and Martinez, B. S., Eds., Natl. Tech. Inform. Serv., Springfield, Va., 1980, 71.

50. **Boecker, B. B., Hahn, F. F., Muggenberg, B. A., Mauderly, J. L., McClellan, R. O., and Pickrell, J. A.,** Toxicity of ^{144}Ce inhaled in a relatively insoluble form by beagle dogs. XI, in *Inhalation Toxicology Research Institute Annual Report 1979—1980,* Diel, J. H., Bice, D. E., and Martinez, B. S., Eds., Natl. Tech. Inform. Serv., Springfield, Va., 1980, 76.

51. **Snipes, M. B., Hahn, F. F., Muggenberg, B. A., Mauderly, J. L., McClellan, R. O., and Pickrell, J. A.,** Toxicity of ^{90}Sr inhaled in a relatively insoluble form by beagle dogs. XI, in *Inhalation Toxicology Research Institute Annual Report 1979—1980,* Diel, J. H., Bice, D. E., and Martinez, B. S., Eds., Natl. Tech. Inform. Serv., Springfield, Va., 1980, 90.

52. **Hahn, F. F., Benjamin, S. A., Boecker, B. B., Chiffelle, T. L., Hobbs, C. H., Jones, R. K., McClellan, R. O., Pickrell, J. A., and Redman, H. C.,** Primary pulmonary neoplasms in beagle dogs exposed to aerosols of ^{144}Ce in fused-clay particles, *J. Natl. Cancer Inst.,* 50, 675, 1973.

53. **Benjamin, S. A., Hahn, F. F., Chiffelle, T. L., Boecker, B. B., Hobbs, C. H., Jones, R. K., McClellan, R. O., and Snipes, M. B.,** Occurrence of hemangiosarcomas in beagles with internally deposited radionuclides, *Cancer Res.,* 35, 1745, 1975.

54. **Filipy, R. E., Stuart, B. O., Palmer, R. F., Ragan, H. A., and Hackett, P. L.,** The effects of inhaled uranium mine air contaminants in beagle dogs, in *Experimental Lung Cancer. Carcinogenesis and Bioassays,* Karbe, E., and Park, J. F., Eds., Springer-Verlag, Berlin, 1974, 403.

55. **Thomassen, R. W., Angleton, G. M., Lee, A. C., Phemister, R. D., and Benjamin, S. A.,** Neoplasms in dogs receiving low-level gamma radiation during pre- and postnatal development, in *Proc. Symp. Late Biological Effects of Ionizing Radiation,* Vol. 2, International Atomic Energy Agency, Vienna, 1978, 181.

56. **Cuddihy, R. G., Boecker, B. B., McClellan, R. O., and Kanapilly, G. M.,** ^{144}Ce in tissues of beagle dogs after inhalation of CeCl$_3$ with special emphasis on endocrine glands and reproductive organs, *Health Phys.,* 30, 53, 1976.

57. **Boecker, B. B. and Cuddihy, R. G.,** Toxicity of ^{144}Ce inhaled as ^{144}CeCl$_3$ by the beagle: metabolism and dosimetry, *Radiat. Res.,* 60, 133, 1974.

58. **Cuddihy, R. G., Brownstein, D. G., Raabe, O. G., and Kanapilly, G. M.,** Respiratory tract deposition of inhaled polydisperse aerosols in beagle dogs, *Aerosol Sci.,* 4, 35, 1973.

Chapter 7

NASAL CAVITY CANCER IN LABORATORY ANIMAL BIOASSAYS OF ENVIRONMENTAL COMPOUNDS

Sherman F. Stinson

TABLE OF CONTENTS

I.   Introduction 158

II.   Experimental Techniques...158
    A.   Animal Model 158
    B.   Sampling Procedures 160
    C.   Sacrifice Times 161

III.   Pathogenesis and Pathology 161

IV.   Relevance of Animal Bioassays to Human Nasal Cancer.......................165

V.   Conclusions 166

References...167

I. INTRODUCTION

Until recently, the nasal epithelium of laboratory rodents has not been widely recognized as an important target site for carcinogenesis bioassays of environmental substances. This was probably due to a variety of factors, including the extremely low incidence of spontaneous nasal cavity neoplasms in rodents; the difficulty of examination and preparation of this intricate organ for histopathological assessment; the lack of familiarity of many pathologists with the normal histology and pathological lesions of this site; and the erroneous opinion that the nasal epithelium is of low sensitivity to carcinogens, especially those applied systemically. The induction of nasal carcinomas by systemic exposure to several different environmental agents and nitrosamines during the last decade has demonstrated the sensitivity of this site and has forced a reevaluation of the importance of the nasal cavity as an endpoint in carcinogenesis bioassays.

In 203 carcinogenesis bioassays reported by the Bioassay Program of the National Cancer Institute (NCI) as of November 1980, nasal carcinomas were induced in male and female rats in four studies.[1] All substances were given orally (feed, water, or gavage) or by injection. Of 25 positive target sites in these bioassays, the nasal cavities ranked twelfth in frequency in rats overall, but were the eighth most frequent site in males and seventh in females. In parallel studies run in mice, no nasal neoplasms were detected. These findings are more impressive when considered with the fact that in the bioassays, the nasal cavities were only examined grossly unless tumor masses were seen. Therefore early neoplasms, or tumors in concealed regions of the nasal cavities, could easily have been missed.[2] Since November 1980, three other compounds tested by the inhalation route of exposure have induced nasal carcinomas in rats and mice, making this the most frequent target site for inhalation studies.[2-6]

This report will present experimental techniques designed to optimize detection of proliferative lesions of the nasal cavities, including animal species, routes of exposure, and sampling methods. Environmental substances that have induced nasal neoplasms will be summarized and the lesions will be described. The relevance of animal carcinogenesis bioassays to human carcinogenesis, with respect to the nasal cavities, will also be discussed.

II. EXPERIMENTAL TECHNIQUES

A. Animal Model
Several factors must be considered when selecting a species for carcinogenesis bioassays where the nasal epithelium is a primary endpoint:

1. Practicability: availability, size, life span
2. Comparability to human nasal system: anatomy and physiology; distribution and type of neoplasms
3. Sensitivity of system: spontaneous occurrence of nasal lesion; susceptibility to carcinogenesis

If a bioassay is to be sensitive to the effects of weak carcinogens, large group sizes are essential. For this reason, the availability and size of the animal selected is important, especially for inhalation studies where the expense of equipment limits the usable exposure space. Likewise, a relatively short life span of the animal is important, not only due to the cost of maintaining large groups of animals for long periods of time, but also to expedite the time required to obtain useful information on suspect environmental carcinogens.

The nasal cavity is a complex organ consisting of several different epithelial types organized into varied anatomical structures and regions. For results obtained in an animal system to have relevance in man, some degree of anatomical and physiological comparability should exist. The anatomy and physiology of the nasal cavities in humans and experimental animals have been considered in detail in earlier chapters. Little information is available on the normal morphology and pathology of the nasal cavities of rodents except in rats, mice, and hamsters. Data on some primate species are also known, but these have not been used extensively for carcinogenesis studies due to limitations imposed by size and life span. Although the structural design of the nasal cavities differs between humans and the various laboratory animal species, the organization and epithelial types found are basically similar. Squamous epithelium lines the nares and parts of the extreme posterior regions. Modified respiratory epithelium covers the turbinals and surfaces of the air conducting passages and paranasal sinuses. Submucosal glands are abundant underlying the respiratory epithelium. Rodents lack the profuse submucosal lymphoid accumulations found in the human nasopharynx, although these are present in dogs and nonhuman primates. In the olfactory regions, the epithelium is of neuroepithelial origin. Sensory cells are found and, possibly, neuroendocrine cells are present.

The most common tumor of the upper respiratory tract in humans is nasopharyngeal carcinoma. It arises from the epithelium lining the nasopharynx and consists of poorly differentiated squamous cells intermixed with lymphoid elements. An analogus type of neoplasm has not been reported in rodents, possibly due to the lack of lymphoid deposits as well as other anatomical differences in these areas of rodent species. Other types of neoplasms have been found in the nasal cavities of rodents, however, and these and other nasal neoplasms can be indicative of risk for the development of human nasopharyngeal or other respiratory tract cancers as will be discussed later. Nasopharyngeal carcinomas, more similar to the human case, have been reported in dogs and other domestic species.[7] Although nasal cancer was found in two bioassays in nonhuman primates, nasopharyngeal carcinoma was not reported.[8]

In the respiratory regions of the human nasal cavities, squamous cell papillomas and carcinomas as well as adenocarcinomas are found, and olfactory neuroepithelial tumors occur in the olfactory areas.[9] All of these types of tumors have been reported in laboratory animals, and will be described in more detail later.

The sensitivity of a bioassay system for the detection of nasal cavity and nasopharyngeal carcinogens is determined by the relative innate susceptibility of the animal species to nasal carcinogenesis, but can be interfered with by a high spontaneous incidence of tumors. Rats, mice, and hamsters all have a very low spontaneous occurrence of nasal cancer. In a series of 2548 male and female rats and 5065 male and female mice, which were unexposed controls in noninhalation lifetime carcinogenesis bioassays of the NCI, no nasal neoplasms were detected.[10,11] Since the publication of these reports one benign and one malignant nasal tumors were found in a single female rat in a control group from an inhalation study.[6] No spontaneous nasal cancers were reported in series of 7200 or 531 male and female hamsters[12,13] or in a colony of 600 nonhuman primates.[8]

Nasal cavity neoplasms have been induced in several rodent species, predominantly by nitrosamines, but the lack of many comparative studies makes assessment of differential sensitivity to nasal epithelial carcinogenesis difficult. Male and female rats given p-cresidine, dioxane, procarbazine, or thio-TEPA orally developed nasal neoplasms while mice did not.[1] Further, rats inhaling vapors of dibromoethane, dibromochloropropane, or formaldehyde developed higher incidences of nasal tumors than did mice in parallel studies.[2,4,5,11] A wide variety of nitrosamines induce nasal tumors in rats.[15] Fewer have been tested in Syrian hamsters, with comparable tumor incidences to rats reported.[16,17] Sprague-Dawley rats exposed by inhalation to 0.1 ppm bis(chloromethyl)ether (BCME), however, developed a high incidence of nasal cancers, while Syrian hamsters under the same conditions developed none, indicating a lower susceptibility of the hamsters under these experimental conditions.[18] The

European hamster appears to be much more susceptible to nasal carcinogenesis with nitro-samines than either the Syrian hamster or the rat,[19] while the Chinese hamster is of lower sensitivity.[20,21] Gerbils have developed nasal carcinomas following injections with diethylnitrosamine.[22]

As nonhuman primates are not used extensively in carcinogenesis bioassays, information on the sensitivity of their nasal epithelium to carcinogenesis is sparse. Procarbazine did not induce nasal neoplasms in monkeys,[8] while nasal carcinomas were found in rats. Likewise, nitrosopiperidine, which produces nasal tumors in rodents, has not induced these neoplasms in monkeys, although studies were still in progress at the time of the report.[8] Aflatoxin B_1 did induce an olfactory neuroepithelioma, and diethylnitrosamine was highly carcinogenic to the nasal epithelium of monkeys in this series of bioassays.

In summary, several species of laboratory rodents as well as nonhuman primates and certain domestic species appear to provide acceptable animal models for carcinogenesis studies with the nasal cavities as a primary endpoint as an objective. The smaller rodents offer the advantages of high susceptibility (especially rats and hamsters) while requiring low maintenance costs and relatively short exposure and test periods. Larger species, such as nonhuman primates, are more expensive to purchase and maintain, but when expense and increased test times do not present an obstacle, they have the advantage that they are phylogenetically closer to man. The longer life spans allow experimental conditions to be designed which more closely approximate human exposure, which makes extrapolations to the human system easier in many cases.

B. Sampling Procedures

An optimal sampling procedure for the nasal cavities should provide detection, anatomical localization, and histopathological evaluation of all lesions that are present. In practice, these objectives have rarely been satisfied. Necropsy and pathological evaluation is one of the most expensive phases of a bioassay, and though the adequacy and usefulness of the study hinges on how thoroughly the examination is performed, compromises are invariably made. All too frequently, these compromises involve cursory and inadequate sampling of the nasal cavities.

The nasal cavity is a complex organ that is not easily examined grossly. Simple removal of the nasal bones and ''peering'' inside does not allow visualization of the paranasal sinuses, the nasopharyngeal duct, the nasolacrimal ducts, portions of the olfactory regions, and ethmoturbinals as well as other sites. Only relatively large lesions will be found by this technique. More thorough dismantling of the skull, while allowing some of these areas to be seen, results in tissue destruction that compromises histopathological evaluation.

One technique that has proven satisfactory for small laboratory rodents is to carefully remove the skin and, if desired, the calvarium and ventral structures such as the jaw and tongue, and fix the skull *in toto*. It is desirable to leave the brain with olfactory lobes intact as these are frequent sites of invasion and metastasis for nasal cancers. Often direct extension from a nasal tumor into the brain can be seen which may help to determine the primary site of a neoplasm of neural origin found in the brain. Following fixation, the skull is decalcified for the shortest effective period, and carefully sectioned with a sharp thin blade. After sectioning, the slices are meticulously examined grossly using a hand lens, and submitted for histologic processing.

Two factors must be considered when determining how to section the skull: the plane of sectioning and the number of sections to be taken. Longitudinal (sagittal) cuts facilitate gross observations and are excellent for examining the relationships and proximity of brain and nasal lesions. Tangential cuts through turbinates and paranasal structures, however, are often obtained which makes histologic assessment more difficult. In our experience, for routine sampling, cross (coronal) sections have been more satisfactory.

Maximizing the number of sections taken greatly increases the probability of detecting small lesions by gross and microscopic examination. Serial sections of 1- to 2-mm thickness are optimal, but the time and expense involved usually prohibits such thorough sampling. In any event, as different types of neoplasms develop in different regions of the nasal cavity, all major epithelial types must be sampled. If cross-sections are taken this will require a minimum of three sections. The first, through the anterior nasal cavity in the region of the incisors, will sample the predominantly squamous epithelial portion and the beginnings of the nasal turbinals and nasolacrimal ducts. The second, midway between the incisors and the first molar, will intersect the respiratory epithelium of the respiratory turbinals and the anterior portions of the maxillary sinuses. The third, in the area of the first molar, will transect the olfactory regions, paranasal sinuses, ethmoturbinals, and the anterior portions of the olfactory lobes. This section will also show portions of the lacrimal glands (organs often not examined histologically in bioassays) and the eyes. The exact plane of each section will vary from species to species, but experience will indicate the optimum position for the desired objectives. Further sections, as required, taken posteriorly will demonstrate the brain. Taken as described, these sections are thin enough to allow adequate gross examination of the nasal cavities prior to histologic processing.

If longitudinal sections are taken, a minimum of two is required. They should be taken approximately one third to one half of the distance from the midline to a plane perpendicular to the maxilla and incisive bones, on each side. The anterior-most part of the cuts should transect the nares. Gross visualization of most regions is good using this technique, but many important areas will not be seen histologically, such as the epithelium and glands of the nasal septum. If more detailed sectioning is done, however, care must be taken to avoid the risk of mutilating the intricate structures of nasal cavities.

C. Sacrifice Times

Most animal carcinogenesis bioassays are designed as lifetime studies. Lesions found in the nasal cavities at earlier times, however, can be important indicators of organ specificity and pathology found at termination.

In 13-week subchronic toxicity studies where rats and mice were exposed by inhalation to 0 to 25 ppm dibromochloropropane or 0 to 75 ppm dibromoethane, toxic lesions were found in the nasal cavities.[4] The lesions were dose related and consisted of necrosis, hyperplasia, and squamous metaplasia with dysplasia and cytomegaly. In the chronic study, rats and mice both developed nasal carcinomas in the same regions where toxic changes were found in the subchronic experiment. It was suggested that not only can subchronic toxicity indicate possible target sites, but that some early changes, such as cytomegaly, squamous metaplasia, and chronic inflammation may be predictive of a future carcinogenic response of the nasal epithelium. Further observations of early reactions associated with nasal carcinogenesis are needed.

III. PATHOGENESIS AND PATHOLOGY

Environmental substances that have induced nasal neoplasms in laboratory animals and the types of tumors found are listed in Table 1. As *N*-nitroso compounds are discussed in other sections of this series they are not included here.

Experimental exposure to a wide variety of environmental compounds has been associated with nasal cavity carcinogenesis in laboratory rodents. Hypotheses concerning structure-activity relationships are difficult to make at this point due to the relatively low number of positive agents and few chemicals tested in a given series of related substances. Some conclusions, however, can be drawn. Irritants, such as the chloromethyl ethers, formaldehyde, and formaldehyde with hydrochloric acid, had a strong potential as nasal carcinogens

Table 1
NASAL TUMORS INDUCED IN EXPERIMENTAL ANIMALS BY VARIOUS ENVIRONMENTAL SUBSTANCES

Substance	Experimental design				Animals with nasal neoplasms									Ref.
	Sp.[a]	Rt.[b]	No.[c]	Dose	Pap[d]	Ad[e]	SCCa[f]	AdCa[g]	NOSCa[h]	NECa[i]	Mes[j]	Metastasis	Other site	
Aflatoxin B1	NHP[k]	ip[l]	9	130 mg						1			Liver	8
^{14}Cerium chloride	Rat	in[m]	12	1—14 μCi										23
Cigarette smoke	Hamster	inh[n]	102	19.2%		1	8				1		Respiratory	24
Chloromethyl methyl ether	Rat	inh	40	1 ppm						1			Respiratory	25
Bis chloromethyl ether	Rat	inh	200	0.1 ppm						17			Respiratory	18
1,2-dibromo-3-chloropropane	Rat	inh	199	3—6 ppm	29	52	23	22	46				Respiratory	28
	Mouse	inh	190	0.6—3 ppm	3	10	13	10	31			Brain, l.n.	Respiratory	5,6
1,2-Dibromoethane	Rat	inh	200	10—40 ppm	1	65	12	97	46		4	Brain	Respiratory	29
	Mouse	inh	188	10—40 ppm	10	2	2	2	2		4		Respiratory	2
Dichlorobutene	Rat	?	?	?										30
Dimethyl sulfate	Rat	inh	27	3—10 ppm			4		+	1			Neurogenic	31
Dimethylcarbamoyl chloride	Rat	inh	93	1 ppm					+					32
1,4-Dioxane	Rat	Water	137	0.5—1%			46	5			1		Liver	33
	Rat	Water	120	0.8—1.8%			6						Liver	34
	Rat	Feed	360	0.001—1%			3						Liver	35
	Rat	inh	576	111 ppm	Negative									36
1,4-Dioxane + DMBA	Mouse	Skin	15	—		1	1							37
Epichlorohydrin	Rat	inh	340	10—100 ppm	1	15	15							38
Formaldehyde	Rat	inh	174	2—15 ppm	4	3	36		1					14
Formaldehyde + HCl	Rat	inh	?	15 + 10 ppm			25%							39
Hexamethylphosphoramide	Rat	inh	823	50—4000 ppb	39	1	340	6	65					40
Niridazole	Rat	Feed	27	250 ppm			1						Urinary	41
Phenylglycidil ether	Rat	inh	?	12 ppm					+					43
Procarbazine	Rat	ip	119	15—30 mg/kg				3		38		Brain	Ear canal	44
	Mouse	ip	105	15—30 mg/kg						22		Brain	Respiratory	44
Qunioxaline 1,4-dioxide	Rat	Feed	240	1—10 mg/kg		3	3	10	29	7	1	Lung, l.n.	Liver, urinary	45

Compound	Sp.[a]	Rt.[b]	No.[c]	Dose	Pap[d]	Ad[e]	SCCa[f]	AdCa[g]	NOSCa[h]	NECa[i]	Mes[j]	Site	Site	Ref
Substituted benzene compounds														
2-Methoxy analine	Rat	Feed	55	5000 ppm									Urinary	46
2-Methoxy-5-methyl analine	Rat	Feed	196	0.5—1%	1	1	2		2				Urinary, liver	26
2-Methoxy-5-methyl analine	Rat	Feed	186	0.5—1%	10	36	1			32		Brain	Urinary, liver	27
2,6-Dimethyl analine	Rat	Feed	?	?	10							(study incomplete)		47
1-Methoxy-4-nitro-2,3,5,6-tetrachlorobenzene	Rat	Feed	200	60—120 ppm	1	1	+		+					48
Phenacetin	Rat	Feed	101	1.25—2.5%	7	6	21	11					Urinary	42
Thio-TEPA	Rat	ip	130	0.7—2.8 mg/kg			2	2		6		Brain	Ear canal	49
Tetrachlorodibenzo dioxin	Rat	po[o]	50	0.01—0.1 μg/kg	5									50
Trimethoxycinnamaldehyde	Rat	ip,sc[p]	6	300 mg/kg	2	1								51
Cantonese salted fish	Rat	Feed	20	—	1	1	1						Liver	52

[a] Sp., species.
[b] Rt., route of exposure.
[c] No., number of animals.
[d] Pap, papilloma.
[e] Ad, adenoma.
[f] SCCa, squamous cell carcinoma.
[g] AdCa, adenocarcinoma.
[h] NOSCa, carcinoma of other type or type not specified.
[i] NECa, neuroepithelial carcinoma.
[j] Mes, mesenchymal neoplasm.
[k] NHP, nonhuman primate.
[l] ip, intraperitoneal.
[m] in, intranasal instillation.
[n] inh, inhalation.
[o] po, *per os*.
[p] sc, subcutaneous.

when given by inhalation, but only gastric carcinomas were induced by the oral route.[53,54] The opposite was true with dioxane, which induced nasal cancers when given in the water, feed, or on the skin, but not by inhalation.

Four structurally related substituted benzene comopunds tested by the NCI produced nasal cancers when fed to rats; amine and methoxy groups appeared to be important. 2-Methoxy aniline, 2-methoxy-5-methyl aniline, and 2,6-dimethylaniline were carcinogenic as was 1-methoxy-4-nitro-2,3,5,6-tetrachlorobenzene. Aniline, however, was not carcinogenic to the nasal epithelium,[55] nor was 4-methoxy-2-methylaniline.[56] It must be remembered that although reported incidences are low, these studies were done at a time when only gross examination of the nasal cavities was routinely done on NCI bioassays, making it very likely that early or small tumors were not detected. Two other methoxy- or ethoxy-substituted benzene compounds, phenacetin[42] and trimethoxycinnamaldehyde,[51] were also nasal carcinogens in rats.

Two of the positive compounds contain known nasal carcinogens. Cigarette smoke contains nitrosonornicotine, which induced 1 nasal carcinoma in 19 hamsters when injected subcutaneously.[57] Formaldehyde and hydrochloric acid react to form BCME, which was detected in the inhalation chamber in the test of this mixture.[36] Further, a third agent, Cantonese salted fish is suspected to contain diethylnitrosamine and possibly other nonvolatile nitrosamines.[52,58]

Species sensitivity was discussed previously and will not be covered further here. Three of the bioassays indicated a differential sex susceptibility. Female mice inhaling dibromochloropropane developed higher incidences of nasal neoplasms than did the males.[5] Nasal neoplasms were observed only in female rats eating Cantonese salted fish.[52] Contrary to these findings, male rats fed quinoxaline dioxide developed more nasal cancers than female rats.[45]

Systemic as well as direct routes of exposure were effective for inducing nasal carcinomas. This confirms results with nitrosamines demonstrating that the nasal epithelium is sensitive to systemic carcinogenesis. As mentioned previously, dibromochloropropane and debromoethane induced nasal neoplasms by inhalation but not by oral administration, while dioxane was ineffective when inhaled and carcinogenic when given systemically. These findings suggest differential absorption, distribution, retention, or metabolic properties which require further investigation. In the alkyl-bromide feeding studies, however, only gross examination of the nasal cavities was performed, so preneoplastic or early neoplastic lesions could have easily been missed.

A broad spectrum of neoplasms was observed in the experiments. The histopathological characteristics of these are adequately described in the cited references as well as other sections of this series. Papillomas and adenomas were found in most studies and were usually localized in the anterior portions of the nasal cavities. The origin of these was apparently from the squamous and respiratory epithelia, and from the submucosal mucus and serous glands.

Papillomas were squamous in nature. Lesions classified as adenomas included papillary adenomas, adenomatous polyps, benign adenocystic tumors, as well as other typical benign forms of mucinous or serous neoplasms. Squamous carcinomas were reported more frequently than adenocarcinomas. The location of these was variable, but the origin was believed to be from the respiratory regions of the anterior nasal cavities. They often grew quite large, eroding adjacent structures in the nasal cavities and skull and invading the brain. Other types of carcinomas reported included mixed adenosquamous, poorly differentiated, transitional cell (respiratory), basal cell, and not-specified classifications.

Neoplasms of neuroepithelial origin were frequently found. This can be a difficult diagnosis to confirm as these tumors (termed olfactory neuroblastomas or esthesioneuroepitheliomas) have most features in common with poorly differentiated adenocarcinomas at the light microscopic level. Adenocarcinomas also frequently invade the olfactory regions of the nasal cavities as well as the olfactory bulbs presenting further confusion as to origin unless careful sampling is done. Detailed reexamination of tissues from a bioassay of *p*-cresidine,[26] aided by electron microscopy, indicated that the tumors originally classified as neuroepithelial in origin, lacked neurogenic features (neurosecretory granules, neurotubules), but had features more consistent with a glandular origin.[27]

In addition to epithelial neoplasms, several types of mesenchymal tumors have been found in the nasal cavities. These include fibrosarcomas, hemangiosarcomas, undifferentiated sarcomas, an osteosarcoma, and a rhabdomyoma. The reported incidences are low.

In most of the studies, chronic sinusitis and rhinitis were associated with nasal carcinogenesis, in the early as well as in the later stages. This is important to note due to the association between chronic sinusitis and nasal cancer in humans (see chapter 6, Volume I).

Nasal carcinomas are frequently large and metastases are not uncommon, unlike most types of carcinomas in rodents. Metastatic sites that have been reported include the brain (including olfactory bulbs), cervical lymph nodes, and the lung.

The associated target sites in studies where nasal neoplasms were induced were the respiratory tract, liver, hematopoietic system, transitional epithelium of the urinary tract, ear canal, and prepucial gland. It is not unexpected that respiratory neoplasms were found in a high percentage of the studies due to the similarity of the respiratory epithelium to that found in the nasal cavities. The other organs are all common target sites for carcinogenesis bioassays and their relative frequency in these studies is similar to what has been observed in positive bioassays of the NCI. A related specificity of these sites to the nasal cavities, therefore, is not suggested.

IV. RELEVANCE OF ANIMAL BIOASSAYS TO HUMAN NASAL CANCER

A useful bioassay system must be sensitive and predictive. The development of nasal neoplasms in laboratory animals, and rodents in particular, as well as the characteristics of the system, have been presented in detail in this chapter. The sensitivity of these animals to the induction of nasal cancers is well-documented; further, the nasal epithelium appears to be one of the more sensitive organ sites in carcinogenesis bioassays. The question remains, however, concerning the significance of animal nasal tumors for predicting risk for the development of cancer in humans. Two types of evidence support the relevance of nasal carcinogenesis in animals to the induction of cancer in humans: morphologic and epidemiologic.

The histologic type, anatomical localization, and invasive and metastatic characteristics of laboratory animal nasal neoplasms are very similar to those found in humans. The most common site for tumor development in the animals was the nasoturbinals and nasal-septum in the respiratory (anterior) portions of the nasal cavities. The neoplasms arose from the respiratory epithelium and submucosal glands. The tumors extended posteriorly and laterally invading the olfactory regions, bones of the skull, olfactory bulbs and brain, and metastasizing to the brain and cervical lymph nodes. This is also the pattern for nasal cancer observed in humans. Early lesions found in animals, such as chronic inflammation, hyperplasia, and dysplasia are also associated with the development of nasal cancer in humans. Although nasopharyngeal neoplasms typical of the human case were not observed in laboratory animals, some substances that are associated epidemiologically with human nasopharyngeal cancer (such as nitrosamines) do induce nasal tumors in animals.

Several agents implicated in human carcinogenesis by epidemiological studies have induced nasal cancers in rodents. Workers exposed occupationally to chloromethyl and BCME have a much higher risk of developing oat cell cancers of the lung than the general population.[59,60] The suspected cell of origin of these neoplasms is the Kulschitsky cell, a neuroendocrine cell of neuroepithelial embryonic origin. Interestingly, the predominant nasal tumors induced in rodents by these chemicals were esthesioneuroblastomas, also tumors of neuroepithelial origin. As these cancers have "adenoid" features the possibility exists that they may also be of neuroendocrine origin. Detailed studies are needed to confirm the presence of neuroendocrine cells in the olfactory regions of the nasal cavities. These findings have particular importance in that no suitable animal model exists for the study of human oat cell carcinoma.

Other occupational or environmental groups with increased exposure to agents known to induce nasal neoplasms in laboratory animals are also predisposed to nasal epithelial carcinogenesis. Inhalation of cigarette smoke is associated with respiratory carcinogenesis in humans and some studies have also shown an increased risk of heavy smokers for the development of nasal cancers.[58] Wood workers have an unusually high incidence of nasal tumors.[61] Trimethoxycinnamaldehyde, a derivative of wood lignin constituents, was a nasal carcinogen in rats. Several occupational groups exposed to inorganic dusts (such as nickel workers) have increased incidences of nasal cavity cancer. Experimental exposure to several dusts has been associated with nasal epithelial carcinogenesis in animals (see Chapter 10, Volume II). Southern Chinese carry a high risk for nasopharyngeal cancer.[58] Consumption of large quantities of marine salted fish has been suggested as an etiologic agent. Cantonese salted fish was a nasal carcinogen in rats. Radiation has been implicated in the genesis of nasal cancers in man.[62] Radioactive cerrium induced nasal carcinomas in rats (also see Chapter 6).

Although much work is still necessary to firmly establish the predictive value of laboratory animal nasal carcinogenesis for human risk, the evidence already accumulated strongly suggests that compounds inducing these neoplasms in animals must be considered suspect nasal and/or respiratory carcinogens for man.

V. CONCLUSIONS

It cannot be disputed that the nasal epithelium is an important target site for carcinogenesis bioassays of environmental substances. Not only is it one of the more frequent positive endpoints, but evidence suggests that induction of nasal neoplasms in laboratory animals is indicative of carcinogenic risk for humans.

Techniques used in bioassays must provide for adequate gross and microscopic sampling of the nasal cavities to allow maximal localization and detection of lesions in this site. Further research is necessary to characterize the nasal epithelium and nasal tumors, especially in the olfactory regions. Also careful observations of early reactions associated with nasal carcinogenesis (such as chronic rhinitis and sinusitis) are needed. Additional carcinogenesis bioassays to confirm structure activity relationships for nasal carcinogenesis (such as with carboxy-alkyl and amine-substituted benzene analogs) must be conducted. Finally, additional detailed human epidemiologic studies should be done to analyze the relationship between induction of nasal cancer by environmental agents in animals and in humans.

REFERENCES

1. National Toxicology Program/Carcinogenesis Testing Program, Bioassay Results with Organ Sites Sequenced by Chemical Name, National Institutes of Environmental Health Sciences, Research Triangle Park, N. C., 1980.
2. **Stinson, S. F., Reznik, G., and Ward, J. M.,** Characteristics of proliferative lesions in the nasal cavities of mice following chronic inhalation of 1,2-dibromoethane, *Cancer Lett.,* 12, 121, 1981.
3. **Reznik, G., Stinson, S. F., and Ward, J. M.,** Lung tumors induced by chronic inhalation of 1,2-dibromo-3-chloropropane, *Cancer Lett.,* 10, 339, 1980.
4. **Reznik, G., Stinson, S. F., and Ward, J. M.,** Respiratory pathology in rats and mice after inhalation of 1,2-dibromo-3-chloropropane or 1,2 dibromoethane for 13 weeks, *Arch. Toxicol.,* 46, 223, 1980.
5. **Reznik, G., Ulland, B., Stinson, S. F., and Ward, J. M.,** Morphology and sex dependent manifestation of nasal tumors in B6C3F1 mice after chronic inhalation of 1,2-dibromo-3-chloropropane, *J. Cancer Res. Clin. Oncol.,* 98, 75, 1980.
6. **Reznik, G., Reznik-Schüller, H., Ward, J. M., and Stinson, S. F.,** Morphology of nasal-cavity tumors in rats after chronic inhalation of 1,2-dibromo-3-chloropropane, *Br. J. Cancer,* 42, 772, 1980.
7. **Ablashi, D. V. and Easton, J. M.,** *Animal Models for Nasopharyngeal Carcinoma,* IARC Scientific Publ. No. 20, International Agency for Research on Cancer, Lyon, 1978, 85.
8. **Adamson, R. H. and Sieber, S. M.,** The use of nonhuman primates for chemical carcinogenesis studies, in *Regulatory Aspects of Carcinogenesis and Food Additives: The Delaney Clause,* Academic Press, New York, 1979, 275.
9. **Willis, R. A.,** Epithelial tumors of the nasal and paranasal cavities, in *Pathology of Tumors,* Butterworths, London, 1967, 345.
10. **Goodman, D. G., Ward, J. M., Squire, R. A., Chu, K. C., and Linhart, M. S.,** Neoplastic and nonneoplastic lesions in aging F344 rats, *Toxicol. Appl. Pharmacol.,* 48, 237, 1979.
11. **Ward, J. M., Goodman, D. G., Squire, R. A., Chu, K. C., and Linhart, M. S.,** Neoplastic and nonneoplastic lesions in aging (C57BL/6N × C3H/HeN)F1 (B6C3F1) mice, *J. Natl. Cancer Inst.,* 63, 849, 1979.
12. **Kirkman, H.,** A preliminary report concerning tumors observed in Syrian hamsters, *Stanford Med. Bull.,* 20, 163, 1962.
13. **Pour, P., Mohr, U., Cardesa, A., Althoff, J., and Kmoch, N.,** Spontaneous tumors and common diseases in two colonies of Syrian hamsters. II. Respiratory tract and digestive system, *J. Natl. Cancer Inst.,* 56, 937, 1976.
14. **Swenberg, J. A., Kerns, W. D., Mitchel, R. I., Gralla, E. J., and Pavkov, K. L.,** Induction of squamous carcinomas of the rat nasal cavity by inhalation exposure to formaldehyde vapor, *Cancer Res.,* 40, 3398, 1980.
15. **Druckrey, H., Preussmann, R., Ivankovic, S., and Schmähl, D.,** Organotrope carcinogene Wirkungen bei 65 verschiedenen *N*-nitrosoverbindungen an BD-ratten, *Z. Krebsforsch.,* 69, 103, 1967.
16. **Pour, P., Cardesa, A., and Althoff, J.,** Tumorigenesis in the nasal olfactory region of Syrian golden hamsters as a result of di-*n*-propylnitrosamine and related compounds, *Cancer Res.,* 34, 16, 1974.
17. **Haas, H., Mohr, U., and Krüger, F. W.,** Comparative studies with different doses of *N*-nitrosomorpholine, *N*-nitrosopiperidine, *N*-nitrosomethylurea, and dimethylnitrosamine in Syrian golden hamsters, *J. Natl. Cancer Inst.,* 51, 1295, 1973.
18. **Kuschner, M., Laskin, S., Drew, R. T., Cappiello, V., and Nelson, N.,** Inhalation carcinogenicity of alpha halo ethers. III. Lifetime and limited period inhalation studies with bis(chloromethyl)ether at 0.1 ppm, *Arch. Environ. Health,* 30, 73, 1975.
19. **Mohr, U., Reznik, G., and Reznik-Schüller, H.,** Carcinogenic effects of *N*-nitrosomorpholine and *N*-nitrosopiperidine on European hamster *(Cricetus cricetus), J. Natl. Cancer Inst.,* 53, 231, 1974.
20. **Reznik, G., Mohr, U., and Kmoch, N.,** Carcinogenic effects of different nitroso-compounds in Chinese hamsters. I. Dimethylnitrosamine and *N*-diethylnitrosamine, *Br. J. Cancer,* 33, 411, 1976.
21. **Reznik, G., Mohr, U., and Kmoch, N.,** Carcinogenic effects of different *N*-nitroso-compounds in Chinese hamsters. II. *N*-nitrosomorpholine and *N*-nitrosopiperidine, *Z. Krebsforsch.,* 86, 95, 1976.
22. **Haas, H., Kmoch, N., Mohr, U., and Cardesa, A.,** Susceptibility of gerbils to weekly subcutaneous and single intravenous injections of *N*-diethylnitrosamine, *Z. Krebsforsch.,* 83, 223, 1975.
23. **Jasmin, J. R., Brocheriow, C., Klein, B., Morin, M., Smadja-Joffe, F., Cernea, P., and Jasmin, C.,** Induction in rats of paranasal sinus carcinomas with radioactive cerium, *J. Natl. Cancer Inst.,* 58, 423, 1977.
24. **Bernfeld, P., Homburger, F., and Russfield, A. B.,** Strain differences of inbred Syrian hamsters to cigarette smoke inhalation, *J. Natl. Cancer Inst.,* 53, 1141, 1974.
25. **Laskin, S., Drew, R. T., Capiello, V., Kuschner, M., and Nelson, N.,** Inhalation carcinogenicity of alpha halo ethers. II. Chronic inhalation studies with chloromethyl methyl ether, *Arch. Environ. Health,* 30, 70, 1975.

26. Bioassay of *p*-cresidine for possible carcinogenicity, NCI Carcinogenesis Tech. Rep. Ser. No. 142, DHEW Publ. No. (NIH) 79-1397, U.S. Government Printing Office, Washington, D.C., 1979.

27. **Reznik, G., Reznik-Schüller, H., Hayden, D. W., Russfield, A., and Murthy, A. S. K.,** Morphology of nasal cavity neoplasms in F344 rats after chronic feeding of *p*-cresidine, an intermediate of dyes and pigments, *Anticancer Res.,* 1, 279, 1981.

28. Bioassay of 1,2-dibromo-3-chloropropane for possible carcinogenicity, NCI Carcinogenesis Tech. Rep. Ser. No. 206, DHEW Publ. No. (NIH) 82-1762, U.S. Government Printing Office, Washington, D.C., 1982.

29. Bioassay of 1,2-dibromoethane for possible carcinogenicity, NCI Carcinogenesis Tech. Rep. Ser. No. 86, DHEW Publ. No. (NIH) 78-1336, U.S. Government Printing Office, Washington, D.C., 1978.

30. Dichlorobutene, *Chem. Regul. Rep.,* 3, 1324, 1979.

31. **Druckrey, H., Kruse, H., Preussmann, R., Ivankovic, S., and Landschultz, C.,** Cancerogenic alkylating substances. III. Alkylhalogenides, alkylsulfates, alkylsulfonates, and strained heterocyclic compounds, *Z. Krebsforsch.,* 4, 241, 1970.

32. Dimethylcarbamoyl chloride, NIOSH Current Intelligence Bull. No. 11, National Institute for Occupational Safety and Health, Washington, D.C., 1976.

33. Bioassay of 1,4-dioxane for possible carcinogenicity, NCI Carcinogenesis Tech. Rep. Ser. No. 80, DHEW Publ. No. (NIH) 78-1330, U.S. Government Printing Office, Washington, D.C., 1978.

34. **Hoch-Legeti, C., Argus, M., and Arcos, J.,** Induction of carcinomas in nasal cavity of rats by dioxane, *Br. J. Cancer,* 24, 164, 1970.

35. **Kociba, R. J., McCollister, S. B., Park, C., and Torkelson, T. R.,** 1,4-Dioxane. I. Results of a two-year ingestion study in rats, *Toxicol. Appl. Pharmacol.,* 30, 275, 1974.

36. **Torkelson, T. R., Leong, B. K. J., Kociba, R. J., Richter, W. A., and Gehring, P. J.,** 1,4-Dioxane. II. Results of a 2-year inhalation study in rats, *Toxicol. Appl. Pharmacol.,* 30, 287, 1974.

37. **King, M. E., Schefner, A. M., and Bates, R. R.,** Carcinogenesis bioassay of chlorinated dibenzodioxins and related chemicals, *Environ. Health Perspect.,* 5, 163, 1973.

38. **Laskin, S., Sellakumar, A. R., Kuschner, M., Nelson, N., LaMendola, S., Rusch, G. M., Katz, G. V., Dulak, N. C., and Albert, R. E.,** Inhalation carcinogenicity of epichlorohydrin in noninbred Sprague-Dawley rats, *J. Natl. Cancer Inst.,* 65, 751, 1980.

39. **Sellakumar, A. R., Albert, R. E., Rusch, G. M., Katz, G. V., Nelson, N., and Kuschner, M.,** Inhalation carcinogenicity of formaldehyde and hydrogen chloride in rats, *Proc. Am. Assoc. Cancer Res.,* 21, 106, 1980.

40. **Lee, K. P. and Trochimowicz, H. J.,** Induction of nasal tumors in rats exposed to hexamethylphosphoramide by inhalation, *J. Natl. Cancer Inst.,* 68, 157, 1982.

41. **Bulay, O., Clayson, D. B., and Shubik, P.,** Carcinogenic effects of niridazole in rats, *Cancer Lett.,* 4, 305, 1978.

42. **Isaka, H., Yoshi, H., Otsuji, A., Koike, M., Nagai, Y., Koura, M., Sufiyasu, K., and Kanabayashi, T.,** Tumors of Sprague-Dawley rats induced by long term feeding of phenacetin, *Gann,* 70, 29, 1979.

43. Phenylglycidil ether, *Chem. Regul. Rep.,* 31, 1336, 1979.

44. Bioassay of procarbazine for possible carcinogenicity, NCI Carcinogenesis Tech. Rep. Ser. No. 19, DHEW Publ. No. (NIH) 79-819, U.S. Government Printing Office, Washington, D.C., 1979.

45. **Tucker, M. J.,** Carcinogenic action of quinoxaline 1,4 dioxide in rats, *J. Natl. Cancer Inst.,* 55, 137, 1975.

46. Bioassay of *o*-anisidine hydrochloride for possible carcinogenicity, NCI Carcinogenesis Tech. Rep. Ser. No. 89, DHEW Publ. No. (NIH) 78-1339, U.S. Government Printing Office, Washington, D.C., 1978.

47. Bioassay of 2,6-xylidine for possible carcinogenicity, NCI Carcinogenesis Tech. Rep. Ser., U.S. Government Printing Office, Washington, D.C., in press.

48. Bioassay of 2,3,5,6-tetrachloro-4-nitroanisole for possible carcinogenicity, NCI Carcinogenesis Tech. Rep. Ser. No. 114, DHEW Publ. No. (NIH) 78-1369, U.S. Government Printing Office, Washington, D.C., 1978.

49. Bioassay of thio-TEPA for possible carcinogenicity, NCI Carcinogenesis Tech. Rep. Ser. No. 58, DHEW Publ. No. (NIH) 78-1308, U.S. Government Printing Office, Washington, D.C., 1978.

50. **Kociba, R. J., Keyes, D. G., Beyer, J. E., Carreon, R. M., Wade, C. E., Dittenber, D. A., Kalnins, R. P., Frauson, L. E., Park, C. N., Barnard, S. D., Hummel, R. A., and Humiston, C. G.,** Results of a two year chronic toxicity and oncogenicity study of 2,3,7,8-tetrachlorodibenzo-*p*-dioxin in rats, *Toxicol. Appl. Pharmacol.,* 46, 279, 1978.

51. **Schoental, R. and Gibbard, S.,** Nasal and other tumors in rats given 3,4,5-trimethoxycinnamaldehyde, a derivative of sinapaldehyde and of other x,b-unsaturated aldehydic wood lignin constituents, *Br. J. Cancer,* 26, 504, 1972.

52. **Huang, D. P. and Ho, J. H. C.,** Carcinoma of the nasal and paranasal regions in rats fed Cantonese salted marine fish, *IARC (Int. Agency Res. Cancer) Sci. Publ.,* 20, 315, 1978.

53. Bioassay of 1,2-dibromo-3-chloropropane for possible carcinogenicity, NCI Carcinogenesis Tech. Rep. Ser. No. 28, DHEW Publ. No. (NIH) 78-828, U.S. Government Printing Office, Washington, D.C., 1978.

54. Bioassay of 1,2-dibromoethane for possible carcinogenicity, NCI Carcinogenesis Tech. Rep. Ser. No. 86, DHEW Publ. No. (NIH) 78-1336, U.S. Government Printing Office, Washington, D.C., 1978.

55. Bioassay of aniline hydrochloride for possible carcinogenicity, NCI Carcinogenesis Tech. Rep. Ser. No. 130, DHEW Publ. No. (NIH) 78-1385, U.S. Government Printing Office, Washington, D.C., 1978.

56. Bioassay of *M*-cresidine for possible carcinogenicity, NCI Carcinogenesis Tech. Rep. Ser. No. 105, DHEW Publ. No. (NIH) 78-1355, U.S. Government Printing Office, Washington, D.C., 1978.

57. **Hilfrich, J., Hecht, S. S., and Hoffman, D.,** A study of tobacco carcinogenesis. XV. Effects of *N*-nitrosonornicotine and *N*-nitrosoanabasine in Syrian golden hamsters, *Cancer Lett.*, 2, 169, 1977.

58. **Henderson, B. E. and Louie, E.,** *Discussion of Risk Factors for Nasopharyngeal Carcinoma,* IARC Scientific Publ. No. 20, International Agency for Research on Cancer, Lyon, 1978, 251.

59. **Figueroa, G. W., Roszkowski, R., and Weiss, W.,** Lung cancer in chloromethyl methyl ether, *N. Engl. J. Med.*, 288, 1094, 1973.

60. **Sakabe, H.,** Lung cancer due to exposure to bis(chloromethyl)-ether, *Ind. Health,* 11, 145, 1973.

61. **Acheson, E. D., Cowdell, R. H., Hadfield, E., and Macbeth, R. G.,** Nasal cancer in wood workers in the furniture industry, *Br. Med. J.,* ii, 587, 1968.

62. **Finkel, A. J., Miller, C. E., and Hasterlik, R. J.,** Radium induced malignant tumors in man, in *Delayed Effects of Bone Seeking Radionuclides,* Mays, C. W., Jee, S. S., and Lloyd, R. D., Eds., University of Utah Press, Salt Lake City, 1969, 195.

Chapter 8

EPSTEIN-BARR VIRUS AND NASOPHARYNGEAL CARCINOMA

Lee S. Tuckwiller and Ronald Glaser

TABLE OF CONTENTS

I.   Introduction 172

II.   History of the Epstein-Barr Virus 172

III.   Biology of the Epstein-Barr Virus...172

IV.   The Association of EBV with Epithelial Cells 174

V.   An In Vitro Model for NPC..175

VI.   Histological Classification of Nasopharyngeal Carcinoma......................177

VII.   The Use of Antibody and Other Markers to Detect NPC in Patients 178

VIII.   Summary...180

References...182

I. INTRODUCTION

The ability of viruses to produce malignant disease in animals other than humans has been accepted for some time and has spurred the search for human tumor virus(es). The most likely candidate viruses, with direct association with human malignancy, have been the herpesviruses. Nonhuman herpesviruses have been clearly implicated in the induction of malignant disease in animals and include the etiologic agents of Marek's disease of fowl (the first disease of this kind to be controlled by a vaccine),[1] the Lucké adenocarcinoma of frogs,[2] and certain T-cell lymphomas of monkeys.[3] Of the human herpesviruses, Herpes simplex virus (HSV) type II has been associated with cervical carcinoma[4,5] and Epstein-Barr virus (EBV), the causative agent of infectious mononucleosis (IM),[6] with nasopharyngeal carcinoma (NPC)[7] and Burkitt's lymphoma (BL).[8] In this chapter, the biological properties of EBV and data which support the hypothesis that EBV is, at least in part, an important link in the chain of events leading to NPC, will be discussed.

One major difficulty in accepting EBV as a cancer-causing agent has been the ubiquity of the virus and the relatively rare instances of associated malignancy. While NPC is not a common form of cancer in most parts of the world including North America, there are geographic areas that are areas of high risk and incidence.[9-11] These areas include eastern China, primarily in the south (Canton), but also in the areas around Shanghai and the north (Peking) as well, but to a lesser degree. A native Alaskan population has been designated as a high risk group and an intermediate risk population in Tunisia has also been identified.[12] The geographic and population clustering of BL and NPC supports the theory of plural causality of these cancers and has led to a search for possible cofactors which might include other infectious agents, environmental carcinogens, and/or genetic predisposition (such as histocompatibility).

II. HISTORY OF THE EPSTEIN-BARR VIRUS

Based on epidemiological considerations, Burkitt[13] speculated that BL, a common tumor of African children, might be associated with an arthropod-borne vector, thus leading to the search for an infectious agent, viral or otherwise, which might be the cause of this malignant disease. EBV was first observed by Epstein et al.[14] by electron microscopic examination of cultured tumor cells from what is now known as African BL.[14] In 1970, EBV DNA was detected in both BL and NPC biopsies.[15] Since NPC tumors often have large numbers of infiltrating lymphocytes, and since EBV was known to be B-lymphocyte tropic, it was assumed that the EBV genome was in these lymphocytes. However, it has now been established that it is the epithelial cells of the tumor that are EBV genome positive and not the lymphocytes.[16] Thus, there existed a paradox in regard to the host range of infectivity of EBV and the presence of the virus in epithelial cells. The EBV is presently considered the best candidate for a human tumor virus. The association of EBV with both BL and NPC is supported by biochemical, immunological, seroepidemiological, and tumor induction studies performed in many laboratories since the original finding by Epstein and co-workers.

III. BIOLOGY OF THE EPSTEIN-BARR VIRUS

The lack of a fully permissive system made initial work with EBV difficult, a problem which continues to frustrate research even today. It was discovered, however, that some BL-derived cell lines spontaneously produce virus in a small (usually less than 10%) percentage of cells.[17] Sera from EBV antibody positive individuals have been used to elucidate the various antigens associated with the EBV replicative cycle.[17-19] A number of techniques were tried but by far the most useful assay employs fluorescein-conjugated antiserum in the direct, indirect, or anticomplementary immunofluorescence (IF) tests. When EBV infects B lymphocytes, the virus genome may become stably associated with the host cell either by integration into the host chromosome (integration in the classical sense has not been proven beyond doubt), by existing in the nucleus of the cell as a circular episomal element,[20,21] or in a condition where the bulk of EBV DNA is episomal with a small percentage actually integrated. The latter association seems to be the most plausible explanation of data published in the literature. It is of interest that studies performed using mouse fibroblast/Burkitt lymphoma hybrid cells indicate that the EBV genome, at least in this system, is not associated with any particular human chromosome.[22]

There are two distinct biological types of EBV. Virtually all isolates from producer cell lines or from patients shedding the virus are capable of transforming human and certain nonhuman primate B lymphocytes.[23-25] These viruses are not able to initiate lytic infections in superinfected EBV genome positive nonproducer cell lines, e.g., Raji. There is one ''strain'' of EBV which is derived from the HR-1 BL cell lines (HR-1 EBV) which is capable of inducing a lytic cycle in superinfected lymphoblastoid cells. It is of interest that the HR-1 EBV cannot transform lymphocytes.[25] After infection of B lymphocytes with transforming EBV in vitro, the cells are permanently ''immortalized'' into lymphoblastoid cell lines capable of indefinite growth.[23,24] Presumably, in vivo the EBV genome can become associated with the host B lymphocyte without causing ''immortalization'', thus establishing a ''latent'' infection, since infection with EBV can be lifelong without the manifestation of overt acute or malignant disease. In vitro, the virus can replicate in latently infected cells and subsequently transform other noninfected B lymphocytes in cell cultures.[23] The replication of EBV in vivo is thought to be restricted. The basis for the in vivo restriction is not precisely known, but is thought to involve elements of the host's immune response and possibly cellular mechanisms as well.[26-28] Evidence for this was obtained when a new cell surface antigen was detected in T-cell cytotoxicity assays.[29,30] B lymphocyte depleted peripheral blood lymphocytes and lymph node cells from IM patients exhibited specific in vitro cytotoxicity against a variety of EBV-infected cell lines, which did not always correlate with serologically detectable EBV membrane antigens.[27,30,31] This implies that the lymphocytes are recognizing a distinct surface antigen detectable only in the cytotoxicity assay. Hence the antigen has been tentatively designated as the lymphocyte detectable membrane antigen or LYDMA[30] and is presumably synthesized in EBV-infected cells at about the same time as the EBV nuclear antigen (EBNA).[7,32] T-cell reactivity to EBV-associated antigens has been demonstrated in lymphocytes isolated from NPC tumor biopsies and from draining lymph nodes, but was not found in peripheral blood lymphocytes from the same patients.[33,34] However, skin test reactivity to antigens associated with an NPC-derived cell line was shown to be increased in NPC patients as compared to non-NPC cancer controls.[35]

When EBV replicates, several virus-specific antigens are synthesized which can be detected by IF. These include the early antigen (EA)[17] which is compased of at least two components designated diffuse (D) and restricted (R) based on whether the antigen is found localized in the cytoplasm (R component) or found throughout the cell (D component) as well as the ability to retain IF reactivity after methanol fixation.[18] It is uncommon for healthy EBV seropositive individuals to have antibodies to EA, but patients with active EBV disease are usually positive. The virus capsid antigen (VCA) is generally found in cells synthesizing virus particles. It is a late virus protein and a structural component of the virus capsid.[36] The EBV membrane antigen (MA) is composed of at least two components, termed early (E-MA) and late (L-MA).[37] The E-MA is independent of virus DNA synthesis and can be found in some cells not producing virus. The L-MA appears only during the lytic cycle and after initiation of virus DNA synthesis.[37] Correlation of high anti-MA titers with the ability to neutralize EBV strongly suggests that MA is incorporated into the virus envelope,[38,39] and monoclonal antibody prepared against MA components has been shown to neutralize the virus.[40] The presence of the EBV genome in cells is always accompanied by the synthesis of EBNA, a nonhistone DNA-binding protein detected by the anticomplementary IF test, and is probably involved with regulation of the EBV genome and the transformed or latent state.[41-43]

Recognition of, and antibody titers against, these antigen types by patient sera can be characteristic for the type of EBV-related disease and can be of diagnostic and prognostic significance. Recent studies using the highly sensitive antibody-dependent cellular cytotoxicity assay (ADCC) against HR-1 EBV-infected Raji cells indicate that the antibodies to MA demonstrated by this technique may be of prognostic significance.[44] Using sera from African patients with NPC it was shown that patients surviving more than 2 years after diagnosis had significantly higher ADCC titers than those surviving less than 2 years.[44] In addition, there was an indication that high anti-VCA and the presence of anti-EA (IgA) antibody titers (elevated in advanced disease) were negatively correlated with ADCC titers.[44]

IV. THE ASSOCIATION OF EBV WITH EPITHELIAL CELLS

As previously discussed, the EBV has a very narrow host range in vitro. It is highly B-lymphcoyte tropic. However, we were able to show that certain NPC epithelial explant cultures were superinfectable with HR-1 EBV. However, not all specimens were superinfectable and this property seemed to correlate with the proportion of cells expressing EBNA.[45] We were also able to induce the virus to replicate in the tumor cells by exposing epithelial tumor cell explants to iododeoxyuridine (IUdR).[45] As mentioned above, NPC biopsy tissue is regularly positive for EBV DNA and *in situ* hybridization with cRNA has confirmed its presence in the malignant epithelial cells.[6]

In a later study it was shown that passage of NPC tumor(s) through athymic nude mice selected for the malignant epithelial cells with the apparent elimination of contaminating lymphoid cells (which are not neoplastic).[46] Tumor cells from the inoculated mice were found to be positive for EBNA, and could be induced with BUdR to produce virus.[46] The cells were confirmed as being predominantly human epithelial cells by chromosome analysis and electron microscopy.[46] In follow-up studies, some nude mouse-passaged NPC cells were found to spontaneously produce virus which was capable of transforming cord blood lymphocytes.[47]

Generally it has not been possible to find epithelial cells which are infectable with EBV. How EBV gets into the nasopharyngeal epithelial cells which become NPC tumors is yet unclear. The observation that infectious EBV is regularly found in oropharyngeal excretions of patients with IM, sometimes for prolonged periods after the onset of disease,[24] may be pertinent. Although the virus-producing cell type in the oropharynx has not been conclusively identified, it is conceivable that the epithelial cells are responsible for or contribute to the amount of excreted virus. There are data which support the concept that epithelial cells can be directly infected with EBV. One of these studies, already discussed, showed that NPC biopsy specimens could be infected with EBV.[45] In another study it was shown that normal nasopharyngeal epithelial cells derived from explant cell cultures from squirrel monkeys could also be infected, as demonstrated by electron microscopy (Figure 1) and by IF.[48] In addition, there is also a report of infection of normal nasopharyngeal tissue with EBV and the subsequent stimulation of epithelial cell growth, but this report has yet to be confirmed.[49] One of the problems in demonstrating the susceptibility of normal epithelial cells in vitro may be related to the fact that the cells are of necessity grown in vitro prior to infection, usually as an explant. It is known that primary epithelial cells taken from the nasopharynx differentiate very rapidly when grown in vitro. It is possible that the membrane changes taking place as a result of the process of differentiation may alter the expression of EBV receptors or eliminate them entirely. Thus, it is possible that manipulation of the cell culture

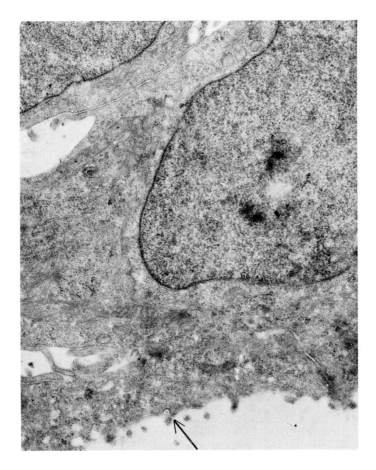

FIGURE 1. Electron photomicrograph of a squirrel monkey epithelial cell infected with EBV. The cells were exposed to virus at 4°C for 1 hr, then incubated at 37°C for 20 min. Note the penetration of an EBV particle (arrow) (magnification ×24,000). (From Glaser, R., Lang, C. M., Lee, K. J., Schuller, D. E., Jacobs, D., and McQuattie, C., *J. Natl. Cancer Inst.*, 64, 1085, 1980. With permission.)

medium — lowering calcium concentrations — might affect the modification of the membranes and the ability to show permissiveness for EBV infection. This, however, is speculation and remains to be shown.

Earlier data from Klein's laboratory[50] suggested that the EBV receptor was juxtaposed and possibly identical to the C3 receptor found on B lymphocytes; however, our laboratory and others have now shown that these two receptors are separate and distinct.[51-54] It is still conceivable that a nearby C3 receptor facilitates EBV adsorption and/or penetration and thus increases the apparent affinity of EBV for its true receptor. It is possible that epithelial cells may possess only the EBV receptor, or a partial receptor, and therefore are very difficult to infect. It is also possible that a population of epithelial cells in the nasopharynx possesses receptors for EBV, but quickly loses them in culture due to the in vitro growth conditions and their effects on cell differentiation, as already discussed. Still another possibility is that EBV positive B lymphocytes in the lymphoid-rich nasopharynx transfer the EBV genome to epithelial cells by cell fusion.[55] However, data supporting this kind of transfer are yet to be shown in vivo or in vitro.

V. AN IN VITRO MODEL FOR NPC

Thus far, it has not been possible to establish an EBV genome positive NPC tumor cell

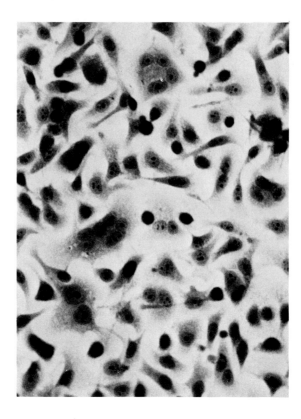

FIGURE 2.   Photomicrograph of H and E stained D98/HR-1 cells.
Note the epithelial morphology of the hybrid cells (magnification
× 527).

line, though many attempts have been made by workers in many laboratories. The reason
for this is not clear. An observation made in this laboratory is that perhaps terminal differentiation of the epithelial cells might take place, thereby rendering the cells unable to
propagate under the growth conditions used. One model system that has been used to study
the association and replication of EBV in epithelial cells has been the use of epithelial/
Burkett lymphoma somatic cell hybrids.[56,57] Work from our laboratory using such cells as
D98/HR-1 and D98/Raji, two epithelial hybrid cell lines (Figure 2), has yielded much
information regarding the replicative cycle of the virus.[58-61] Virus expression in such hybrid
cells is normally limited just to EBNA which is similar to nonproducer BL cells, e.g., Raji.
When the cells are exposed to IUdR, the virus is induced to replicate with the production
of EBV-specific EA, VCA, DNA, and virus particles (Figure 3).[56,57] Therefore, it has been
shown that once the EBV genome becomes associated with an epithelial-like cell, it can
replicate. This has now been confirmed by other techniques such as microinjection[62] and
by transfection with EBV DNA.[63,64] In addition, the D98/HR-1 hybrid cells presumably
have the receptor for EBV on the surface, since the cells are directly superinfectable with
HR-1 EBV.[51] In this particular case, the genetic information coding for the EBV receptor
is probably contributed by the BL parental cell line. Nevertheless, it clearly shows again
that if an epithelial-like cell has a proper receptor on the surface, it can be infected with
infectious EBV and the virus can replicate.

In another study it was shown that cells not normally possessing receptors for EBV can
express EBV antigens after artificial implantation of the receptor on the cell surface and
subsequent virus challenge.[65] Mouse lymphocytes implanted with EBV receptors and chal-

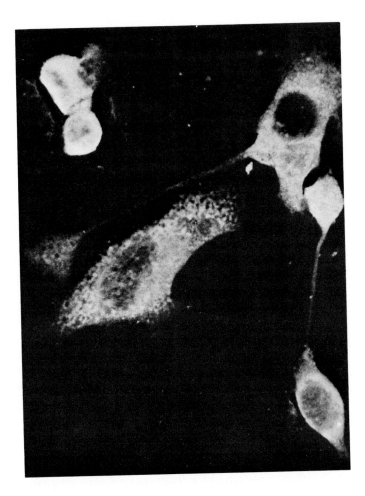

FIGURE 3. Photomicrograph of EA, VC IF positive D98/HR-1 cells after treatment with IUdR (magnification ×1000).

lenged with virus have been shown to undergo a complete viral replicative cycle.[66] Work in our laboratory and others continues to attempt the infection and transformation of epithelial cells with intact infectious EBV, whole EBV DNA, and cloned EBV DNA fragments in order to learn more about the replication of EBV, particularly in epithelial cells, and eventually to obtain a transformed epithelial cell line.

VI. HISTOLOGICAL CLASSIFICATION OF NASOPHARYNGEAL CARCINOMA

There has not been general agreement as to the classification of NPC into histological types.[67] However, the World Health Organization (WHO) has proposed that NPC be divided into three histological subtypes based on their predominant pattern using light microscopy. These are

1. Squamous cell carcinoma (keratinizing squamous cell carcinoma), WHO-1
2. Nonkeratinizing carcinoma, WHO-2
3. Undifferentiated carcinoma (undifferentiated carcinoma of the nasopharyngeal type, including lymphoepithelioma), WHO-3

Evidence to date suggests that Epstein-Barr-associated NPC is almost exclusively of type 3 and to a lesser extent, type 2. Occasionally we have found EBV DNA positive WHO-1 tumors, but the certainty of the histopathology could be questioned. Due to the lack of uniformity in typing these tumors, the significance of this finding is not clear, but it seems that the presence of EBV is most commonly limited to tumors of the poorly or undifferentiated type[68] (unpublished data from the authors' laboratory).

VII. THE USE OF ANTIBODY AND OTHER MARKERS TO DETECT NPC IN PATIENTS

Individuals with NPC of the appropriate histological type (EBV-related) exhibit increased serum levels of anti-EBV antibody, as compared to age-, sex,- and race-matched healthy controls and to other cancer groups. Since infection with EBV is so common, especially in areas of the world where NPC is prevalent, a high proportion of healthy individuals have detectable serum antibody to the virus;[69] therefore, the use of antibody levels as an indicator of disease, however useful, is still somewhat problematic. Nevertheless, the level of antibody is correlated in some cases with the development or stage of the disease and total tumor burden.[70,71] Thus, NPC patients with stage I disease may have almost normal levels of anti-EBV antibodies, but patients with advanced disease usually have greatly increased geometric mean titers (up to tenfold) against EBV VCA and the D component of EA.[70,71] The latter observation is of particular interest since normal seropositive individuals rarely exhibit this antibody to any great extent. Another unique feature of the antibody response in EBV-related NPC is the appearance of high levels of serum IgA directed against VCA and sometimes EA-D.[72] This also is rarely seen in normal individuals or control patients with other tumors. It is true that patients with other tumors of the head and neck and a variety of other diseases (both neoplastic and nonneoplastic) have increased anti-EBV antibody levels, occasionally including IgA antibody, but usually a higher percentage of NPC patients have the levels increased to such a striking and characteristic degree.

The presence of high levels of anti-EBV antibody is of some prognostic significance in that successfully treated patients show a gradual decline in antibody titers to normal levels,[70,73] and recurrence of disease often results in an increase in VCA and EA antibody titers which may precede the appearance of clinical symptoms, i.e., recurrence of the primary tumor or a metastatic tumor mass. An example of this antibody pattern is shown in Figure 4, which shows EBV antibody titers in a long-term study in a female NPC patient (NPC-3).[73] The tumor was classified as a lymphoepithelioma and was positive for EBV DNA (Figure 5).

In collaboration with Cheng,[61] the authors recently described an EBV-associated DNase enzyme. This enzyme can be detected in HR-1 EBV superinfected Raji cells and in IUdR-induced D98/HR-1 hybrid cells. With Cheng, they proceeded to assay for the presence of neutralizing antibody in serum from different kinds of patients against the EBV DNase as determined by the number of units of enzyme that could be neutralized in vitro.[74] The following sera and numbers were tested: 102 sera from normal young adults, of which 75 serum samples were EBV (VCA) positive, 58 IM sera, 119 NPC patients, which included patients from North America, China, and Taiwan, 62 Burkitt's lymphoma patients, 31 other lymphomas, and 103 other carcinomas. The results are shown in Table 1. Of the 102 normal sera examined, only 1 of them had high neutralizing activity; of 58 IM patients, only 4 (or 7%) were highly positive. Of 62 BL sera samples tested, only 15% of these were positive against the EBV DNase. The other groups assayed all had approximately the same amount of background neutralization as our controls, between 5 and 10% positive sera[74] (unpublished data). In studies presently underway with collaborative laboratories in the People's Republic of China, where NPC is very prevalent, the results continue to support the specificity of the antibody against DBV DNase with NPC. The reason for this specificity is not clear. It

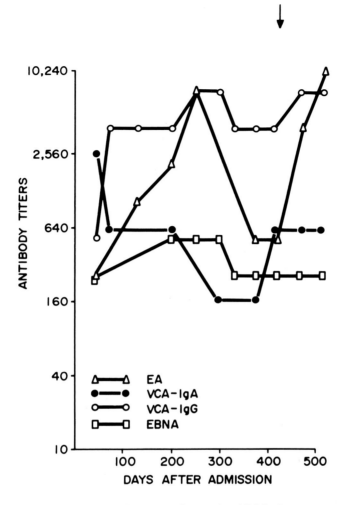

FIGURE 4. Serum antibody titers from patient NPC-3. Assays were performed on samples taken from the time of admission (surgery) to recurrence of tumor. (From Glaser, R., Nonoyama, M., Szymanowski, R. T., and Graham, W., *J. Natl. Cancer Inst.*, 64, 1317, 1980. With permission.)

remains to be seen, however, if the assay for this antibody may be useful for early diagnosis of the disease.

It has been shown by several workers that modified nucleosides and bases derived from the catabolism of transfer RNA can be detected in significant levels in the urine of cancer patients.[75,76] It has also been shown that the presence of these markers may be useful for prognostic and diagnostic purposes in patients with certain advanced cancers.[77,78] These kinds of studies have been extended to NPC study groups. In collaboration with Trewyn,[79] it has been found that elevated nucleosides can be detected in urine from at least North American NPC patients.[79] Preliminary data on urines from Chinese collaborating laboratories also support this finding. An example of the kind of data that has been obtained is shown in Figure 6, which shows the levels of nucleosides in the urine of the same patient that was discussed earlier (NPC-3). Clearly, several of the nucleosides were elevated and some continued to rise over the time period studied, until the patient died. It is not clear if the presumed alteration in metabolism of the NPC tumor cells is EBV related or solely a cellular function. The data obtained on a small number of NPC patients thus far indicate that it is

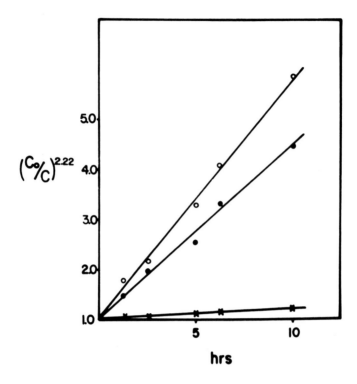

FIGURE 5.   DNA-DNA reassociation kinetics of NPC-3 tumor. ○ = NPC-3 tumor; ● = a mixture of EBV genome positive Raji cells + EBV genome negative BJA-B cells to make 10 genomes per cell; X = control BJA-B cells. (From Glaser, R., Nonoyama, M., Szymanowski, R. T., and Graham, W., *J. Natl. Cancer Inst.*, 64, 1317, 1980. With permission.)

Table 1
PRESENCE OF ANTIBODY TO EBV DNASE IN DIFFERENT PATIENT GROUPS

Patient group	Number tested	Percent positive
Normal	102	1
Infectious mononucleosis	58	7
NPC	119	94
BL	62	15
Other lymphomas	31	17
Leukemias	49	14
Other carcinomas	103	9

certainly worthwhile to examine this method further for potential usefulness for diagnosis of early-stage NPC and for monitoring progress of NPC patients while they are being treated. The difficulty in diagnosing early-stage NPC, which is very treatable with radiation therapy — e.g., along with the aggressive nature of the disease — underlines the importance of these and other types of studies to find markers which are useful for identifying early-stage NP patients.

VIII. SUMMARY

Epstein-Barr virus is a human herpes virus with proven oncogenic properties. It is well-

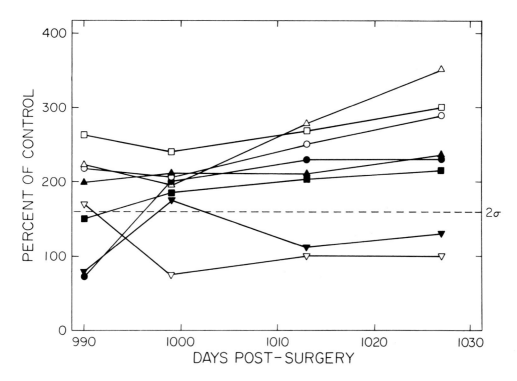

FIGURE 6. Excretion of nucleoside markers by patient NPC-3. The dashed line denotes the position of two standard deviations above normal for adenosine. Excretion levels above the dashed line are significant at the $p <$ 0.02 level. ● = pseudouridine; ▲ = 1, methyladenosine; ▼ = 5-methylcytidine; ■ = 2-pyridone-5-carboxamide-N′-ribofuranoside; ○ = 1-methylinosine, △ = 1-methylguanosine; ▽ = adenosine; □ = N^2,N^2-dimethyl-guanosine. (From Trewyn, R. W., Glaser, R., Kelly, D. R., Jackson, D. G., Graham, W. P., and Speicher, C. E., *Cancer*, 49, 2513, 1982. With permission.)

established as the cause of IM and an increasing amount of evidence indicates its close association with two human malignancies, African BL and NPC. In the laboratory, EBV is capable of transforming B lymphcoytes of humans and certain nonhuman primates into cell lines capable of indefinite growth. The EBV has been shown to be directly oncogenic when inoculated into cotton-top marmosets and to a lesser extent common marmosets and owl monkeys.[80,81] There is strong evidence for a very close association of EBV and NPC. The viral genome is regularly associated with NPC tumor cells and can be induced (in vitro) to undergo a full replicative cycle in these cells. The virus genome is capable of being expressed when introduced into epithelial and other cell types by a variety of means such as direct infection, cell fusion, transfection, and microinjection.

Patients with advanced NPC have greatly increased antibody titers to EBV antigens, of the IgG and IgA class, which is characteristic for the disease, and high levels of antibody detected by the DCC may indicate a favorable prognosis. T-cell reactivity to EBV-associated antigens has been demonstrated in patients with NPC but further work needs to be done. The reported transfer in vitro of reactivity to NPC tumor extracts using transfer factor (TF) from EBV seropositive donors is intriguing and should be pursued further, as possible adjunctive therapy with TF might be indicated in cases of NPC.[82] The presence of elevated serum levels of anti-EBV DNase antibody and abnormal nucleosides in the urine of NPC patients may prove useful in the early diagnosis of disease; however, additional research is needed in these areas.

The causal relationship of EBV to NPC is not yet totally clear, and there may be cofactors interacting at the virus/cell or host/virus infected cell level which ultimately determine the outcome of infection with EBV. For example, it may be that malaria in young African children plays a role in the induction of African BL by decreasing the effectiveness of the cellular immune response, thereby allowing the growth and establishment of EBV-transformed B lymphocytes and ultimately BL. At least two sets of cofactors are being considered in the case of NPC. One is the presence of carcinogens in the diet of certain high risk Chinese groups. The other is the possible influence of genetic factors, especially histocompatibility types.

It is hoped that continued research into the association of EBV and NPC will lead not only to a better understanding of the etiology and biology of NPC and other virus-associated tumors, but also to better and more useful diagnostic techniques which will result in greatly increased survival rates.

REFERENCES

1. **Nazerian, K.,** Marek's disease: a herpesvirus-induced malignant lymphoma of the chicken, in *Viral Oncology,* Klein, G., Ed., Raven Press, New York, 1980, 665.
2. **Mizell, M., Toplin, I., and Isaacs, J. J.,** Tumor induction in developing frog kidneys by a zonal centrifuge purified fraction of the frog herpes-type virus, *Science,* 165, 1134, 1969.
3. **Falk, L. A., Jr.,** Biology of *Herpesvirus saimiri* and *Herpesvirus ateles,* in *Viral Oncology,* Klein, G., Ed., Raven Press, New York, 1980, 813.
4. **Rapp, F. and Duff, R.,** Transformation of hamster embryo fibroblasts by herpes simplex virus types 1 and 2, *Cancer Res.,* 33, 1527, 1973.
5. **Aurelian, L., Schumann, B., Marcus, R. L., and Davis, H. J.,** Antibody to HSV-2 induced tumor specific antigens in serums from patients with cervical carcinoma, *Science,* 181, 161, 1973.
6. **Henle, G. and Henle, W.,** The virus as the etiologic agents of infectious mononucleosis, in *The Epstein-Barr Virus,* Epstein, M. A. and Achong, B. G., Ed., Springer-Verlag, New York, 1979, 297.
7. **Epstein, M. A. and Achong, B. G.,** Introduction: discovery and general biology of the virus, in *The Epstein-Barr Virus,* Epstein, M. A. and Achong, B. G., Eds., Springer-Verlag, New York, 1979, 1.
8. **Epstein, M. A. and Achong, B. G.,** The relationship of the virus to Burkitt's lymphoma, in *The Epstein-Barr Virus,* Epstein, M. A. and Achong, B. G., Eds., Springer-Verlag, New York, 1979, 321.
9. **Desgranges,, Wolf, H., de-Thé, G., Shanmugaratnam, K., Ellouz, R., Cammoun, N., Klein, G., and zur Hausen, H.,** Nasopharyngeal carcinoma. X. Presence of Epstein-Barr genomes in epithelial cells of tumours from high and medium risk areas, *Int. J. Cancer,* 16, 7, 1975.
10. **Nonoyama, M., Huang, H., Pagano, J. S., Klein, G., and Singh, S.,** DNA of Epstein-Barr virus detected in tissue of Burkitt's lymphoma and nasopharyngeal carcinoma, *Proc. Natl. Acad. Sci. U.S.A.,* 70, 3265, 1973.
11. **Glaser, R., Nonoyama, M., Szymanowski, R. T., and Graham, W.,** Epstein-Barr virus DNA positive North American nasopharyngeal carcinoma tumors, *J. Natl. Cancer Inst.,* 64, 1317, 1980.
12. **Lanier, P., Bender, T. R., Blot, W. J., Fraumeni, J. F., Jr., and Hurlburt, W. B.,** Cancer incidence in Alaska natives, *Int. J. Cancer,* 18, 409, 1976.
13. **Burkitt, D.,** A children's cancer dependent on climatic factors, *Nature (London),* 194, 232, 1962.
14. **Epstein, M. A., Achong, B. G., and Barr, Y. M.,** Virus particles in cultured lymphoblasts from Burkitt's lymphoma, *Lancet,* 1, 702, 1964.
15. **zur Hausen, H., Schulte-Holthausen, H., Klein, G., Henle, W., Henle, G., Clifford, P., and Santesson, L.,** EBV DNA in biopsies of Burkitt tumours and anaplastic carcinomas of the nasopharynx, *Nature (London),* 228, 1056, 1970.
16. **Wolf, H., zur Hausen, H., and Becker, V.,** EB virus genomes in epithelial nasopharyngeal carcinoma cells, *Nature (London), New Biol.,* 244, 245, 1973.
17. **Henle, W., Henle, G., Zajac, B. A., Pearson, G., Wajbke, R., and Scriba, M.,** Differential reactivity of human serums with early antigens induced by Epstein-Barr virus, *Science,* 169, 188, 1970.
18. **Henle, G., Henle, W., and Klein, G.,** Demonstration of two distinct components in the early antigen complex of Epstein-Barr virus-infected cells, *Int. J. Cancer,* 8, 272, 1971.
19. **Reedman, B. M. and Klein, G.,** Cellular localization of an Epstein-Barr virus (EBV)-associated complement-fixing antigen in producer and nonproducer lymphoblastoid cell lines, *Int. J. Cancer,* 11, 499, 1973.

20. **Nonoyama, M. and Pagano, J.,** Separation of Epstein-Barr virus DNA from large chromosomal DNA in nonvirus-producing cells, *Nature (London), New Biol.,* 238, 169, 1972.

21. **Lindahl, T., Adams, A., Bjursell, G., Bornkamm, W., Kaschka-Dierich, C., and John, U.,** Covalently closed circular duplex DNA of Epstein-Barr virus in a human lymphoid cell line, *J. Mol. Biol.,* 102, 511, 1976.

22. **Glaser, R., Nonoyama, M., Hampar, H., and Croce, C. M.,** Studies on the association of the Epstein-Barr virus genome and human chromosomes, *J. Cell. Physiol.,* 96, 319, 1978.

23. **Henle, W., Diehl, V., Kohn, G., zur Hausen, H., and Henle, G.,** Herpes-type virus and chromosome marker in normal leukocytes after growth with irradiated Burkitt cells, *Science,* 157, 1064, 1967.

24. **Miller, G., Niederman, J. C., and Andrews, L.,** Prolonged oropharyngeal excretion of Epstein-Barr virus after infectious mononucleosis, *N. Engl. J. Med.,* 288, 229, 1973.

25. **Miller, G., Robinson, J., Heston, L., and Lipman, M.,** Differences between laboratory strains of Epstein-Barr virus based on immortalization, abortive infection, and interference, *Proc. Natl. Acad. Sci. U.S.A.,* 71, 4006, 1974.

26. **Royston, I., Sullivan, J. L., Periman, P. O., and Perlin, E.,** Cell-mediated immunity to Epstein-Barr virus-transformed lymphoblastoid cells in acute infectious mononucleosis, *N. Engl. J. Med.,* 293, 1159, 1975.

27. **Rickinson, A. B., Crawford, D., and Epstein, M. A.,** Inhibition of the *in vitro* outgrowth of Epstein-Barr virus-transformed lymphocytes by thymus-dependent lymphocytes from infectious mononucleosis patients, *Clin. Exp. Immunol.,* 28, 72, 1977.

28. **Glaser, R., Farrugia, R., and Brown, N.,** Effect of the host cell on the maintenance and replication of Epstein-Barr virus, *Virology,* 69, 132, 1976.

29. **Svedmyr, E. and Jondal, M.,** Cytotoxic effector cells specific for B cell lines transformed by Epstein-Barr virus are present in patients with infectious mononucleosis, *Proc. Natl. Acad. Sci. U.S.A.,* 72, 1622, 1975.

30. **Jondal, M.,** Antibody-dependent cellular cytotoxicity (ADCC) against Epstein-Barr virus-determined membrane antigens. I. Reactivity in sera from normal persons and from patients with acute infectious mononucleosis, *Clin. Exp. Immunol.,* 25, 1, 1976.

31. **Britton, S., Andersson-Anvret, M., Gergely, P., Henle, W., Jondal, M., Klein, G., Sandstedt, B., and Svedmyr, E.,** Epstein-Barr virus immunity and tissue distribution in a fatal case of infectious mononucleosis, *N. Engl. J. Med.,* 298, 89, 1978.

32. **Pearson, G.,** Epstein-Barr virus: immunology, in *Viral Oncology,* Klein, G., Ed., Raven Press, New York, 1980, 739.

33. **Klein, E., Becker, S., Svedmyr, E., Jondal, M., and Vanky, F.,** Tumor infiltrating lymphocytes, *Ann. N.Y. Acad. Sci.,* 276, 207, 1976.

34. **Klein, E, Svedmyr, E., Jondal, M., and Vanky, F.,** Functional studies on tumor-infiltrating lymphocytes in man, *Isr. J. Med. Sci.,* 13, 747, 1977.

35. **Levine, P. H., de Thé, G., Brugere, J., Schwaab, G., Mourali, N., Herberman, R. B., Ambrosioni, J. C., and Reval, P.,** Immunities to antigens associated with a cell line derived from nasopharyngeal cancer (NPC) in non-Chinese NPC patients, *Int. J. Cancer,* 17, 155, 1976.

36. **Gergely, L., Klein, G., and Ernberg, I.,** Appearance of Epstein-Barr virus associated antigens in infected Raji cells, *Virology,* 45, 10, 1971.

37. **Ernberg, I., Klein, G., Kourilsky, F. M., and Silvestre, D.,** Differentiation between early and late membrane antigen on human lymphoblastoid cell lines infected with Epstein-Barr virus. I. Immunofluorescence, *J. Natl. Cancer Inst.,* 53, 61, 1974.

38. **Pearson, G. R., Dewey, F., Klein, G., Henle, G., and Henle, W.,** Relation between neutralization of Epstein-Barr virus and antibodies to cell membrane antigens induced by the virus, *J. Natl. Cancer Inst.,* 45, 989, 1970.

39. **Pearson, G. R., Henle, G., and Henle, W.,** Production of antigens associated with Epstein-Barr virus in experimentally infected lymphoblastoid cell lines, *J. Natl. Cancer Inst.,* 46, 1243, 1971.

40. **Thorley-Lawson, D. A. and Geilinger, K.,** Monoclonal antibodies against the major glycoprotein (gp350/220) of Epstein-Barr virus neutralize infectivity, *Proc. Natl. Acad. Sci. U.S.A.,* 77, 5307, 1980.

41. **Luka, J., Siegert, W., and Klein, G.,** Solubilization of the Epstein-Barr virus-determined nuclear antigen and its characterization as a DNA-binding protein, *J. Virol.,* 22, 1, 1977.

42. **Takada, K. and Osato, T.,** Analysis of the transformation of human lymphocytes by Epstein-Barr virus, *Intervirology,* 11, 30, 1979.

43. **Einhorn, L. and Ernberg, I.,** Induction of EBNA precedes the first cellular S-phase after EBV-infection of human lymphocytes, *Int. J. Cancer,* 21, 157, 1978.

44. **Pearson, G. R., Johansson, B., and Klein, G.,** Antibody-dependent cellular cytotoxicity against Epstein-Barr virus-associated antigens in African patients with nasopharyngeal carcinoma, *Int. J. Cancer,* 22, 120, 1978.

45. **Glaser, R., de-Thé, G., Lenoir, G., and Ho, J. H. C.,** Superinfection of epithelial nasopharyngeal carcinoma cells with Epstein-Barr virus, *Proc. Natl. Acad. Sci. U.S.A.*, 73, 960, 1976.
46. **Trumper, P. A., Epstein, M. A., Giovanella, B. C., and Finerty, S.,** Isolation of infectious EB virus from the epithelial tumour cells of nasopharyngeal carcinoma, *Int. J. Cancer*, 20, 655, 1977.
47. **Crawford, D. H., Epstein, M. A., Bornkamm, G. W., Achong, B. G., Finerty, S., and Thompson, J. L.,** Biological and biochemical observations on isolates of EB virus from the malignant epithelial cells of two nasopharyngeal carcinomas, *Int. J. Cancer*, 24, 294, 1979.
48. **Glaser, R., Lang, M., Lee, K. J., Schuller, D. E., Jacobs, D., and McQuattie, C.,** Attempt to infect normal nasopharyngeal epithelial cells with the Epstein-Barr virus, *J. Natl. Cancer Inst.*, 64, 1085, 1980.
49. **Huang, D. P., Ho, H. C., Ng, M. H., and Lui, M.,** Possible transformation of nasopharyngeal epithelial cells in culture with Epstein-Barr virus from B95-8 cells, *Br. J. Cancer*, 35, 630, 1977.
50. **Jondal, M., Klein, G., Oldstone, M. B. A., Bokish, V., and Yefenof, E.,** Surface markers on human B and T lymphocytes. VIII. Association between complement and Epstein-Barr virus receptors on human lymphoid cells, *Scand. J. Immunol.*, 5, 401, 1976.
51. **Glaser, R., Lenoir, G., Ferrone, S., Pellegrino, M. A., and de-Thé, G.,** Cell surface markers on epithelial-Burkitt hybrid cells superinfected with Epstein-Barr virus, *Cancer Res.*, 37, 2291, 1977.
52. **Hutt-Fletcher, L., Fowler, E., Simmons, J., Feighny, R., Lambris, J. D., and Ross, G. D.,** Characterization of Raji cell extract that binds the Epstein-Barr virus, *Int. Workshop on Herpesviruses*, Esculapio Publish. Co., Bologna, Italy, 1981, 270.
53. **Patel, P. and Menezes, J.,** Epstein-Barr virus (EBV)-lymphoid cell interactions. I. Quantification of EBV particles required for the membrane immunofluorescence assay and the comparative expression of EBV receptors on different human B, T and null cell lines, *J. Gen. Virol.*, 53, 1, 1981.
54. **Schwaber, J. F., Klein, G., Ernberg, I., Rosen, A., Lazarus, H., and Rosen, F. S.,** Deficiency of Epstein-Barr virus (EBV) receptors on B lymphocytes from certain patients with common varied agammaglobulinemia, *J. Immunol.*, 124, 2191, 1980.
55. **Bayliss, G. J. and Wolf, H.,** Epstein-Barr virus-induced cell fusion, *Nature (London)*, 287, 164, 1980.
56. **Glaser, R. and Rapp, F.,** Rescue of Epstein-Barr virus from somatic cell hybrids of Burkitt lymphoblastoid cells, *J. Virol.*, 10, 288, 1972.
57. **Glaser, R., Nonoyama, M., Decker, B., and Rapp, F.,** Synthesis of Epstein-Barr virus antigens and DNA in activated Burkitt somatic cell hybrids, *Virology*, 55, 62, 1973.
58. **Glaser, R., Ogino, T., Zimmerman, J., Jr., and Rapp, F.,** Thymidine kinase activity in Burkitt lymphoblastoid somatic cell hybrids after induction of the EB virus, *Proc. Soc. Exp. Biol. Med.*, 142, 1059, 1973.
59. **Mele, J., Glaser, R., Nonoyama, M., Zimmerman, J., and Rapp, F.,** Observations on the resistance of Epstein-Barr virus DNA synthesis to hydroxyurea, *Virology*, 62, 101, 1974.
60. **Miller, R., Glaser, R., and Rapp, F.,** Studies of an Epstein-Barr virus-induced DNA polymerase, *Virology*, 76, 494, 1977.
61. **Cheng, Y. C., Chen, J. Y., Hoffmann, P. J., and Glaser, R.,** Studies on the activity of DNase associated with the replication of the Epstein-Barr virus, *Virology*, 100, 334, 1980.
62. **Graessman, A., Wolf, H., and Bornkamm, G. W.,** Expression of Epstein-Barr virus genes in different cell types after microinjection of viral DNA, *Proc. Natl. Acad. Sci. U.S.A.*, 77, 433, 1980.
63. **Stoerker, J., Parris, D., Yajima, Y., and Glaser, R.,** Pleiotropic expression of Epstein-Barr virus DNA in human epithelial cells, *Proc. Natl. Acad. Sci. U.S.A.*, 78, 5882, 1981.
64. **Miller, G., Grogan, E., Heston, L., Robinson, J., and Smith, D.,** Epstein-Barr viral DNA: infectivity for human placental cell, *Science*, 212, 452, 1981.
65. **Volsky, D. J., Shapiro, I. M., and Klein, G.,** Transfer of Epstein-Barr virus receptors to receptor-negative cells permits virus penetration and antigen expression, *Proc. Natl. Acad. Sci. U.S.A.*, 77, 5453, 1980.
66. **Volsky, D. J., Klein, G., Volsky, B., and Shapiro, I. M.,** Production of infectious Epstein-Barr virus in mouse lymphocytes, *Nature (London)*, 293, 399, 1981.
67. **Shanmugaratnam, K.,** Histological typing of nasopharyngeal carcinoma, in *Nasopharyngeal Cancer: Etiology and Control*, de-Thé, G. and Ito, Y., Eds., WHO Publ. No. 20, International Agency for Research on Cancer, Lyon, 1978, 3.
68. **Andersson-Anvret, M., Klein, G., Forsby, N., and Henle, W.,** The association between undifferentiated nasopharyngeal carcinoma and Epstein-Barr virus shown by correlated nucleic acid hybridization and histopathological studies, in *Nasopharyngeal Cancer: Etiology and Control*, de-Thé, G. and Ito, Y., Eds., WHO, Publ. No. 20, International Agency for Research on Cancer, Lyon, 1978, 347.
69. **Levine, P. H., Wallen, W. C., Ablashi, D. V., Granlund, D. J., and Connelly, R.,** Comparative studies on immunity to EBV-associated antigens in NPC patients in North America, Tunisia, France and Hong Kong, *Int. J. Cancer*, 20, 332, 1977.
70. **Henle, W., Ho, H. C., Henle, G., and Kwan, H. C.,** Antibodies to Epstein-Barr virus related antigens in nasopharyngeal carcinoma. Comparison of active cases and long term survivors, *J. Natl. Cancer Inst.*, 51, 361, 1973.

71. **Henle, W., Ho, J. H. C., Henle, G., Chau, J. C. W., and Kwan, H. C.,** Nasopharyngeal carcinoma: significance of changes in Epstein-Barr virus related antibody patterns following therapy, *Int. J. Cancer,* 20, 663, 1977.

72. **Henle, G. and Henle, W.,** Epstein-Barr virus-specific IgA serum antibodies as an outstanding feature of nasopharyngeal carcinoma, *Int. J. Cancer,* 17, 1, 1976.

73. **de Schryver, A., Klein, G., Henle, W., and Henle, G.,** EB virus associated antibodies in Caucasian patients with carcinoma of the nasopharynx and in long term survivors after treatment, *Int. J. Cancer,* 13, 319, 1974.

74. **Cheng, Y. C., Chen, J. Y., Glaser, R., and Henle, W.,** Frequency and levels of antibodies to Epstein-Barr virus-specific DNase are elevated in patients with nasopharyngeal carcinoma, *Proc. Natl. Acad. Sci. U.S.A.,* 77, 6162, 1980.

75. **Borek, E. and Kerr, S. J.,** Atypical tRNAs in tumor tissue, *Adv. Cancer Res.,* 16, 163, 1972.

76. **Gehrke, C. W., Kuo, K. C., Davis, G. E., Suits, R. D., Waalkes, T. P., and Borek, E.,** Quantitative high performance liquid chromatography of nucleosides in biological materials, *J. Chromatogr.,* 150, 455, 1978.

77. **Waalkes, T. P. and Borek, E.,** The biochemical assessment of the malignant status in man: aspects related to tRNA modification, in *Biological Characterization of Human Tumors,* Vol. 3, Davis, W. and Maltoni, C., Eds., Excerpta Medica Int. Congr. Ser. No. 375, Elsevier, New York, 1975, 15.

78. **Waalkes, T. P., Gehrke, C. W., Zummalt, R. W., Chang, S. Y., Lakings, D. B., Tormex, D. C., Ahmann, D. L., and Moertel, C. G.,** The urinary excretion of nucleosides of tRNA by patients with advanced cancer, *Cancer,* 36, 390, 1975.

79. **Trewyn, R. W., Glaser, R., Kelly, D. R., Jackson, D. G., Graham, W. P., and Speicher, C. E.,** Elevated nucleoside excretion by patients with nasopharyngeal carcinoma: preliminary diagnostic/prognostic evaluations, *Cancer,* 49, 2513, 1982.

80. **Miller, G., Shope, T., Coope, D., Waters, L., Pagano, J., Bornkamm, G. W., and Henle, W.,** Lymphoma in cotton-top marmosets after inoculation with Epstein-Barr virus: tumor incidence, histologic spectrum, antibody responses, demonstration of virus DNA and characterization of viruses, *J. Exp. Med.,* 145, 948, 1977.

81. **Rabin, H., Wallen, W. , Neubauer, R. H., and Epstein, M. A.,** Comparisons of surface markers on herpesvirus-associated lymphoid cells of nonhuman primates and established human lymphoid cell lines, in *Comparative Leukemia Research 1973,* Ito, Y. and Dutcher, R. M., Eds., S. Karger, Basel, 1975, 367.

82. **Brandes, L. J. and Goldenberg, G.,** In vitro transfer of cellular immunity against nasopharyngeal carcinoma using transfer factor donors with Epstein-Barr virus antibody activity, *Cancer Res.,* 34, 3095, 1974.

Chapter 9

STUDIES ON THE RELATIONSHIP BETWEEN EPSTEIN-BARR VIRUS (EBV) AND NASOPHARYNGEAL CARCINOMA (NPC) IN CHINA

Y. Zeng

TABLE OF CONTENTS

I.   Introduction 188

II.   Epidemiology of NPC in China 188

III.   Detection of Antibody to EB Virus by the Microcomplement Fixation Test ... 191

IV.   Detection of Antibodies to EB Virus by the Immunofluorescence Test 191

V.   New Techniques for Detection of EBV Antibody, Antigen, and DNA 192
        A.   Immunoenzymatic Test 192
        B.   Immunoautoradiography 193
        C.   Anticomplement Immunoenzymatic (ACIE) Test 193
        D.   Blot Hybridization for the Detection of EBV DNA Repeats 193

VI.   Serological Mass Survey and Follow-Up Studies 194
        A.   Serological Mass Surveys in Zangwu County 194
        B.   Serological Mass Surveys in Wuzhow City 194
        C.   Relationship between EBV Antibody and Histological Changes of Naso-
            pharyngeal Mucosa 194

VII.   Establishment of Lymphoblastoid Cell Lines with Giant Group A Marker
        Chromosome 195

VIII. Establishment of an Epithelioid Cell Line from NPC Patients 195

IX.   Does EBV Play a Causative Role in the Development of NPC? 195

X.   Control and Prevention of NPC 196
        A.   Early Detection and Treatment of NPC 196
        B.   Interferon for Treatment and Prevention 196
        C.   Prevention with Retinoids 197
        D.   Conclusion 197

References 198

I. INTRODUCTION

Nasopharyngeal carcinoma (NPC) is extremely rare in Europe, North America, Oceania, and Latin America. The incidence rate is below 1 per 100,000 per annum. It is slightly higher in African countries such as Tunisia, Algeria, Morocco, Sudan, and Kenya; the exact incidence is not well-known, but may reach 2 to 7 per 100,000 of the general population a year.[3] NPC is very common in southern China and in southeast Asia. Since 1958, the epidemiology of NPC in China had been studied.[7] An investigation of causal factors of the tumor deaths during 1970 to 1972 was made in China, excluding Taiwan province.[1] From these surveys, a geographic distribution of NPC for the nation was delineated. Since Old et al.[19] first demonstrated the serological relationship between EBV and NPC by means of the immunodiffusion test, much data in the literature has indicated the close association of EBV and NPC. Studies on this problem were started in 1973 in China. We put our emphasis on the early detection of NPC by the combination of different viro-immunological tests with clinical, cytological, and histological examination. Early-stage NPC including carcinoma *in situ* could be detected. It is possible that NPC can be controlled through early detection and early treatment even when the exact etiological factors have not yet been elucidated.

II. EPIDEMIOLOGY OF NPC IN CHINA

According to the data provided by investigations on the cause of death for the whole country,[1] the distribution of NPC showed very significant geographical variations. The average death rate from NPC was 1.88 per 100,000: 2.49 for males and 1.27 for females, respectively. As shown in Figure 1, among the 29 provinces and cities surveyed, all except 6 (Guangdong, Guangsi, Fujian, Hunan, Jiangxi, and Zhejiang) were below the average. Among the 453 counties and cities of 5 southern provinces (Table 1), the area of the highest NPC death rate was Szehui of Guangdong province, being as high as 15.84. There were 23 counties and cities with NPC death rates above 9; 21 of these 23 counties belong to Guangdong province, most of which are located in Shaozhing, Fushan, and Guangzhou districts in the central part of Guangdong. Pinsiang and Zangwu were two other high risk counties of Guangxi province. There were 85 counties and cities with NPC death rates above 6. In addition to the 28 counties of the above-mentioned Shaozhing, Fushan, and Guangzhou districts, there were several contiguous counties such as Hui-Yang, Zhangiang, and Shaoguan districts of Guangdong; Wuzhow, Yuling, and Guilin of the eastern part of Guangxi as well as a portion of the counties belonging to the Zhenzhow district in the south of Hunan province. All these places formed a geographically unique high risk area including the central part of Guangdong and eastern part of Guangxi with incidence gradually sloping off eccentrically.

The proportion of NPC death to all tumor deaths as a whole in the 29 provinces and cities has been 3.11% for males and 2.34% for females, ranking seventh and ninth in prevalence for males and females, respectively (Figure 1). Nevertheless, in Guangdong and Guangxi the NPC death rate ranked third for males and fourth for females. In Guangdong, the ratio to all tumor deaths was 15.29% for males and 12.20% for females; for Guangxi the figures were 11.5 and 10.34%, respectively. Furthermore, the death rate for NPC in Szehui county was not only the highest among the whole country but has also ranked first among all tumor deaths both for males and females since 1970, being 31.03 and 21.12%, respectively. The mortality or incidence rate of NPC has been quite stable.

The sex ratio ($\delta:\female$) was 1.92:1, ranging from 1.09:1 to 2.51:1. No significant difference was found between the high and low risk areas.

The age-specific mortality curves for the whole country and for the highest risk county,

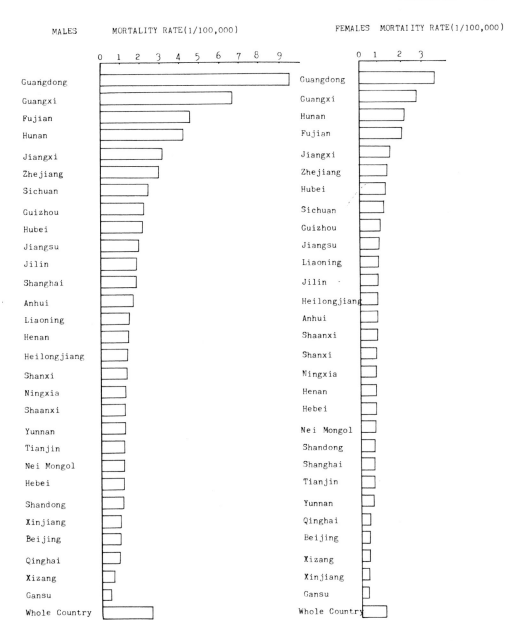

FIGURE 1. Age-adjusted mortality rates from nasopharynx cancer by province, municipality, and autonomous region.

Szehui, were similar (Figure 2). Both showed a fairly steep rise after 20 years of age and continue to rise steadily after 50 years of age. The death rates rose continuously up to the 80-year age group with no tendency to decline. But in some counties and cities such as Zangwu county and Wuzhou city, the mortality or incidence rate of NPC decreased in persons over 50 years of age.

Genetic factors may play a role in the development of NPC; epidemiological evidence has established definite racial risk centers for NPC in those areas where people mainly speak the Guanzhou dialect. Investigations of Guandonese immigrants within or out of the country revealed a similar pattern. Simons et al.[22] indicated that certain HL-A profiles were associated with increased risk for NPC. This needs to be further studied in China.

Table 1
NUMBER OF COUNTIES WITH MORTALITIES OF
NPC IN FOUR GRADIENTS

Province	Counties and cities investigated	Age/sex-adjusted mortality rate (per 100,000 population)			
		9	6—8	3—5	3
Kwangtung	107	21	29	52	5
Kwangsi	85	2	18	38	27
Hunan	103	0	12	54	37
Fukien	67	0	2	33	32
Kiangsi	91	0	1	23	67
Total	453	23	62	200	168

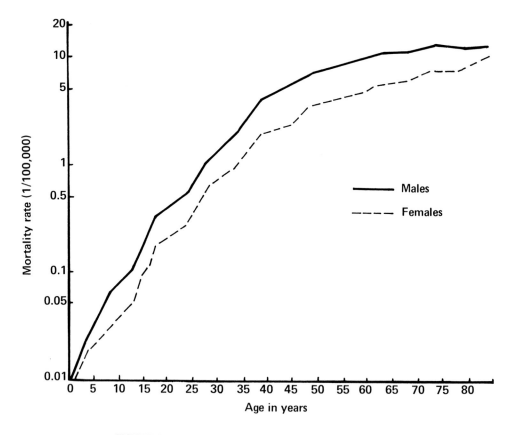

FIGURE 2.   Age-specific mortality curve of nasopharynx cancer.

Environmental carcinogens or promoters may also play a role in NPC development is suggested by the fact that the U.S.-born Chinese have a lower risk for the disease than those who immigrated from China.[9] Polycyclic aromatic hydrocarbon compounds and diethyl-nitrosamine have induced NPC in rats,[25] but no epidemiological evidence has yet been found in human beings. A number of case control studies failed to define any occupational or dietary factor which could be associated with NPC risk.

III. DETECTION OF ANTIBODY TO EB VIRUS BY THE MICROCOMPLEMENT FIXATION TEST

In early work,[2,27] complement fixing antibody to EB virus was determined in sera from NPC patients, patients with other tumors, and normal individuals. The rate of high antibody titer ($\geq 1:320$) and the geometric mean titer (GMT) of antibody in NPC patients were 61.8% and 1:331.4, respectively, both being higher than in the other two groups. After radiotherapy, complement fixing antibody remained at a rather high titer for a relatively long period of time. The antibody level in NPC patients remained about the same before and within 3 years after radiotherapy, but decreased slightly in NPC patients surviving 3 to 6 years after radiotherapy and markedly in NPC patients surviving 7 to 15 years. The difference in complement fixing titers in persons with nasopharyngeal hyperplastic lesions and normal individuals was also significant. This indicates that NPC is closely related to EBV infection.

Complement fixing antibody to EBV was also tested in high NPC risk areas (Zhungshan county and Guangzhow city of Guangdong) as well as low risk areas (Lufeng and Wuhua counties of Guangdong, and Beijing). Of a total of 2300 normal sera, 2080 were positive (titer $\geq 1:10$). The positive rate was 90.4% with a GMT of 1:52.8. The positive rate of antibody in the above various groups was relatively high, from 87 to 94%, showing no great difference. The positive rate reached 90 to 100% in the age group of 3 to 5 years. This indicates that the age of primary infection by EBV in different areas is similar. De-Thé et al.[3] reported that 97% of Ugandans and 20% of Singapore Chinese in the 2- to 3-years age group and about 60% of Singapore Chinese in the 3- to 5-years age group were EBV antibody positive. So Chinese in China have earlier EBV infection than Singapore Chinese, but later than Ugandans. As NPC occurs more frequently in persons above 20 years of age, it can be seen from Figure 3 that the antibody titers of a healthy population over 20 in the high risk areas were significantly higher than those in the low risk areas. This kind of variation may indicate that the EB virus is more active in people living in high NPC risk areas and this might be related to the occurrence of NPC.

IV. DETECTION OF ANTIBODIES TO EB VIRUS BY THE IMMUNOFLUORESCENCE TEST

Henle and Henle[5] reported that antibodies to EB virus in sera from NPC patients can be detected by immunofluorescence. The positive rate of EA/IgG, VCA/IgA, and EA/IgA antibody were 80, 93, and 73%, respectively. These antibodies were also detected in China;[10] 96% of NPC patients had EA/IgG antibody with a GMT of 1:22.7 and 81.0% had VCA/IgA antibody with a GMT of 1:13.6, whereas less than 6% of sera from patients with malignant tumor other than NPC and from normal subjects had these antibodies with a GMT of 1:1,25-1.46. Wu and Yao[32] reported that the positive rate of EA/IgG antibody ($\geq 1:10$) from NPC patients, with tumor other than NPC, patients with chronic inflammation of nasopharyngeal mucosa, and normal subjects were 79, 14.6, 4.9, and 0%, respectively. Similar results were obtained in Beijing and seven provinces and cities including high NPC risk provinces (Guangdong, Guangxi, Hunan, and Fujian). There was no marked difference in VCA/IgA antibody positive rates and GMT in different clinical stages, indicating the usefulness of this technique in the early detection of NPC.[36]

The level of IgA antibody to VCA declined gradually with increasing survival time of NPC patients after radiotherapy. Only 30% of NPC patients had this antibody at a very low titer (GMT, 1:2.8) 4 to 8 years after radiotherapy. When these patients suffered from recurrence or distant metastasis, this antibody increased again and reached its original level. On the other hand, 75.5% of NPC patients still had EA/IgG antibody with GMT of 1:4.5 4 to 18 years after radiotherapy. Therefore, serological follow-up of VCA/IgA antibody,

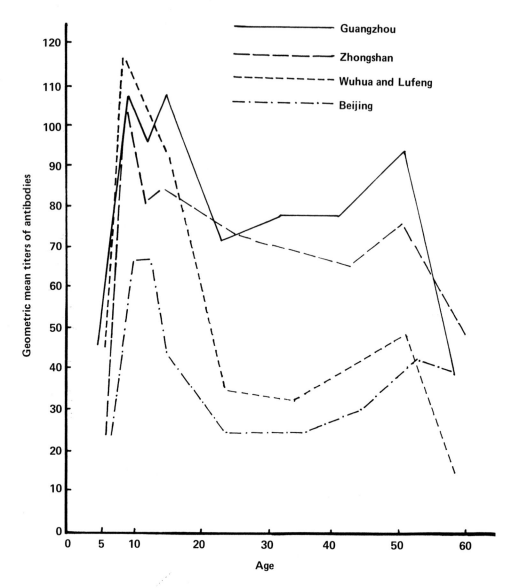

FIGURE 3.   Geometric mean titers of antibodies to EBV tested by complement fixation method in the population in high and low risk areas of NPC.

but not EA/IgG antibody, may provide prognostic information for NPC patients after radiotherapy.

V. NEW TECHNIQUES FOR DETECTION OF EBV ANTIBODY, ANTIGEN, AND DNA

The antibodies to EB virus were mainly detected by immunofluorescence tests in the literature. This technique requires fluorescence microscopes and is not convenient for NPC field study. Due to these problems we tried to establish a simpler and more sensitive test for NPC field work.

A. Immunoenzymatic Test[16]

An immunoenzymatic test was established by conjugating the antihuman IgA antibody with horseradish peroxidase instead of fluorescent dye. Sera from NPC patients, patients with other malignant tumors, and normal subjects were tested for VCA/IgA antibody to EB virus by this test. The positive rate of IgA antibody in NPC patients was 92 to 98%, but less than 6% in the other two groups. As compared to the indirect immunofluorescence test, the immunoenzymatic test is simpler and more sensitive, and can be more conveniently used in the NPC field work.

The positive rates of this antibody in saliva from NPC patients and from persons having VCA/IgA antibody in sera were 71.7 and 32%, respectively, by immunoenzymatic test. Therefore, saliva cannot be used for the diagnosis of NPC instead of serum, but positive VCA/IgA antibody in saliva is helpful for the diagnosis of NPC.[44]

B. Immunoautoradiography

The immunoautoradiograph was established in the laboratory by using ^{125}I-labeled anti-human IgA antibody for the detection of EBV VCA/IgA antibody in sera from NPC patients, patients with other malignant tumor, and normal subjects. The GMT of this antibody in these three groups were 1:3,259, 1:7.1, and 1:3.2, respectively. The highest level of antibody in normal individuals was 1:160. So a titer of 1:640 and higher was considered positive. The positive rates of the above three groups were 97.3, 1.7, and 0%.[14] Although it is rather complicated and too sensitive, 85.7% of NPC patients had this antibody ($\geq$1:2.5) in saliva detectable by this test.[15] Therefore, the immunoenzymatic test was widely used in routine tests for the serological diagnosis and screening of NPC.

C. Anticomplement Immunoenzymatic (ACIE) Test

An ACIE test was developed by conjugating the antihuman C3 antibody with horseradish peroxidase. EBNA (EB nuclear antigen) could be detected by this test in all cell lines related to EB virus, as well as in NPC cells, but not in cells from unrelated conditions. Antibody to EBNA could also be detected by this test. This test is sensitive and does not require a fluorescence microscope.[20]

Exfoliated cells collected by negative pressure suction from the nasopharynx of patients with poorly differentiated and undifferentiated carcinoma, and of suspected NPC patients, were examined for EBNA by means of the ACIE test.[38] Among the 79 NPC patients, all had EBNA-positive carcinoma cells, while the positive rates of cytological and histological examinations were only 87.3 and 91.1%, respectively. No EBNA was found in tumor cells from patients with malignant and benign tumors of head and neck other than NPC, nor was it found in nasopharyngeal epithelial cells of dead fetuses. These findings show that the ACIE test is specific and sensitive and can be used for the early detection of NPC, especially in combination with serological methods for the detection of antibodies to EB virus. Beside the finding of EBNA in NPC cells, EBNA can also be found in normal ciliated columnar epithelial cells and hyperplastic cells of the nasopharynx. This result seems to rule out the hypothesis that EB virus is a passenger virus only infecting malignant cells.

The ACIE test was further applied to detect NPC from VCA/IgA antibody positive individuals in the high risk area. Carcinoma cells with EBNA were found in 4 out of 64 antibody positive individuals; cytological and histological examination also showed poorly differentiated stage I carcinoma in these 4 cases. The interval between the first positive serology and diagnosis of NPC was 8 to 9 months. No further elevation of VCA/IgA antibody appeared during this period. These results further established the value of the ACIE test for the detection of early-stage NPC.[39]

D. Blot Hybridization for the Detection of EBV DNA Repeats

Blot hybridization was used for the detection of EBV DNA repeats in collaboration with de-Thé et al.[4] Among the 56 VCA/IgA antibody positive persons EBV DNA was detected in 3 out of 4 biopsies from NPC patients confirmed histologically and in 12 IgA antibody positive individuals with no evidence of NPC, but in none of the 7 biopsies from IgA negative individuals.[4] The presence of EBV markers in the nasopharyngeal mucosa as well as VCA/IgA antibody enables us to characterize precancerous conditions.

VI. SEROLOGICAL MASS SURVEY AND FOLLOW-UP STUDIES

A. Serological Mass Surveys in Zangwu County

From 1978 to 1980, 148,029 persons aged 30 and over were screened in Zangwu county of Guangxi Autonomous Region by the immunoenzymatic method; 3533 were found to have VCA/IgA antibody to EB virus. Among these, 55 cases were diagnosed histologically as NPC; 1 was carcinoma *in situ*, 12 were in stage I, 19 in stage II, 17 in stage III, and 6 in stage IV. After 1 to 3 years of follow-up study, 32 additional NPC cases were diagnosed: 10 in stage I, 9 in stage II, 11 in stage III, and 2 in stage IV. Altogether 87 NPC cases were detected from 3533 VCA/IgA antibody positive persons; the detection rate was 2462.5 per 100,000. This was 82 times higher than the incidence in the general population of the same age group.[34,35,37]

B. Serological Mass Surveys in Wuzhow City

In order to reduce the NPC mortality rate by early detection, a serological mass survey was carried out in Wuzhow city which is a NPC high risk area. Wuzhow city is located in the center of Zangwu county with a population of 170,000. The mean yearly incidence of NPC was 17/100,000 for 1975 to 1978. In the first stage study, sera were obtained from 12,932 persons of the 40- to 59-year age group; the positive rate of VCA/IgA antibody was 5.3%. Thirteen NPC patients were detected from 680 VCA/IgA antibody positive individuals by using the combination methods (immunoenzymatic test; anticomplement immunoenzymatic test; clinical, cytological, and histological examination). The detection rate of NPC from 12,932 persons examined was 100.5 per 100,000 and that from 680 VCA/IgA antibody positive individuals was 1900 per 100,000, which was twice and 38 times higher, respectively, than the incidence in the general population of the same age group for 1975 to 1978 in Wuzhow city. These results indicate that VCA/IgA antibody screening in combination with other tests and examination is valuable in the early detection of NPC, and that it might be possible to reduce the mortality rate of NPC by treating them in their early stage. These results also suggest that EB virus is closely associated with NPC.[40]

C. Relationship between EBV Antibody and Histological Changes of Nasopharyngeal Mucosa

VCA/IgA antibody positive persons were examined clinically. Biopsies were taken from those diagnosed clinically with NPC or suspected of having NPC, those having some lesions in the nasopharynx, and those without lesions in the nasopharynx but with a high antibody titer. The frequency of atypical hyperplasia and atypical metaplasia in the nasopharyngeal mucosa from NPC patients and from antibody positive normal individuals was higher than in antibody negative normal individuals. The GMT of VCA/IgA antibody in sera from the NPC group, atypical hyperplasia, and atypical metaplasia group were also higher than those in the simple hyperplasia and simple metaplasia group. After an 8- to 37-month follow-up study, the detection rates of NPC from the atypical hyperplasia and atypical metaplasia group, and from the simple hyperplasia, simple metaplasia, and normal mucosa group, were 27 and 2.6%, respectively. These results indicate that there is a close relationship between VCA/IgA antibody, atypical hyperplasia, atypical metaplasia, and NPC, and that EB virus might play an important role in the development of these histological and cancerous changes of nasopharyngeal mucosa.[13]

VII. ESTABLISHMENT OF LYMPHOBLASTOID CELL LINES WITH GIANT GROUP A MARKER CHROMOSOME

Lymphoblastoid cell lines were established from carcinoma tissue of NPC patients in Beijing, Shanghai, and Guangdong in 1973 to 1974.[11] Group A marker chromosome was detected only in lymphoblastoid cell lines from NPC patients. With the exception of one lymphoblastoid cell line derived from a normal donor, the group A marker chromosome could not be found in the cell lines from other sources, including P3HR-1, B95-8, Raji, and lymphoblastoid lines from tonsils and so on. The submetacentric group A chromosome was formed by translocation of the short arm of chromosome 3, breaking at the point near to, or even involving, its centromere, to the distal light band region of the long arm of chromosome 1. Group A marker chromosome was also found in biopsies from NPC and suspected NPC patients. These results suggest that the group A marker chromosome might be associated with NPC.[31]

Two strains of cytomegalovirus (CMV) were isolated from 16 NPC carcinoma tissues from which lymphoblastoid cell lines were also established. CMV can cause transformation of human cells, whether it plays any causative role together with EB virus in the development of NPC needs further study.[11]

VIII. ESTABLISHMENT OF AN EPITHELIOID CELL LINE FROM NPC PATIENTS

In order to further investigate the relationship between EBV and NPC, extensive attempts have been made to establish a permanent epithelial cell line from an NPC patient, but no successful results were reported prior to 1975. An epithelioid cell line (CNE-1) and a fusiform cell line (CNf-1) were established in 1975 from tumor biopsy material from a patient with NPC which was histologically diagnosed as a well-differentiated squamous cell carcinoma. Based on studies of the cell growth pattern, chromosome analysis, heterotransplantation, and electron microscopy, these two cell lines were considered to be squamous carcinoma cells, and the fusiform cells might have originated from the epithelioid cells. No EB virus particle, EBNA, or early antigen could be detected in these two cell lines.[12] De-Thé et al.[4] have recently reported that 3 out of 5 well-differentiated carcinoma showed EB virus DNA sequence by a very sensitive blot hybridization test. Thus the CNE-1 and CNf-1 cells lines should be further tested by this sensitive test.

Using the 3H-Tdr incorporation inhibition test, the cytotoxic effect of lymphocytes obtained from NPC patients and other malignancies, from patients with nonmalignant diseases, and from normal subjects was studied in vitro against NPC target cells (CNE-1 cell line). The cell line (Eca 109) derived from esophageal cancer was used as a control. The positive rates of cytotoxic effect of lymphocytes from different groups mentioned above were 82, 10, 18, and 6%, respectively. Only 4% of NPC patients had cytotoxic lymphocytes to Eca 109 cells. The incidence of cytotoxic effect of lymphocytes from NPC patients was found to be related to the radiotherapy and the clinical course. It decreased from 82 to 23% within 3 months after radiotherapy. It again increased to 70% when the patients had distant metastases or recurrent disease. These results suggest that some tumor-associated antigen might exist on the surface of NPC cells and that the cytotoxic effect of lymphocytes from NPC patients might be tumor-specific to a certain degree. This problem needs further study.[17]

IX. DOES EBV PLAY A CAUSATIVE ROLE IN THE DEVELOPMENT OF NPC?

The serological relationship between nasopharyngeal carcinoma and EB virus was first demonstrated by Old et al.[19] using immunodiffusion. It was shown subsequently by indirect immunofluorescence that NPC patients had various antibodies to EB virus and the antibody spectra and titers were clearly related to the total tumor mass.[5] Furthermore, EB virus DNA and EBNA have been regularly demonstrated in epithelial tumor cells of NPC,[18,30,45] and EB virus production has been demonstrated in the epithelial tumor cells passed in nude mice.[24]

In addition to the above data, our studies have presented evidence that EB virus is closely associated with NPC:

1. The positive rate of complement fixing antibody to EB virus in sera from the general population in NPC high and low risk areas showed no great difference. However, the GMT of antibody in healthy populations above 20 years old in high risk areas was significantly higher than that in low risk areas. These data indicate that EB virus is more active in the persons living in high NPC risk areas.
2. The positive rate of VCA/IgA antibody in sera from the general population increased with increasing age. This is probably due to some internal or external factors stimulating the activation of EB virus.
3. There is a close relationship between the presence of VCA/IgA antibody and the atypical hyperplasia, atypical metaplasia, and NPC. Thus EB virus might play an important role in the development of histological and cancerous changes of naso-pharyngeal mucosa.
4. EBNA was not only found in NPC carcinoma cells but also in normal epithelial cells from NPC patients or normal individuals. The hypothesis of EB virus as a passenger present only in NPC cells seems to be highly improbable.
5. EBV DNA internal repeats were detected in NPC carcinoma cells and nasopharyngeal mucosa from VCA/IgA antibody positive individuals without evidence of tumor.
6. The detection rate of NPC from VCA/IgA antibody positive individuals was 38 to 82 times higher than the incidence of NPC in the general population of the same age group, and VCA/IgA antibody could be detected 8 to 37 months before the diagnosis of NPC.

All of these data strongly suggest that EB virus plays a causative role in the development of NPC, but the EB virus is not the unique factor. It is necessary to study the role of environmental and genetic factors, and its relation to EBV in the development of NPC.

X. CONTROL AND PREVENTION OF NPC

A. Early Detection and Treatment of NPC

The treatment of NPC is mainly a matter of radiotherapy. It is very efficient, particularly for NPC in its early stages. In general the 5-year survival rate of NPC after radiotherapy is about 30 to 40%. Ho[6] reported that in stage I and stage II the survival rate was about 70%, and Shanghai Cancer Hospital reported a survival rate up to 92% for stage I patients.[21] As mentioned above, by combination of all the methods for the detection of NPC in their early stages, satisfactory results were obtained in Wuzhow city. All NPC patients were detected in stage I and stage II, and 70% were in stage I. Therefore, serological mass survey, periodical follow-up study, and education of the public on the early signs of the disease are very essential in high NPC risk populations, and if all patients are treated in their early stages, the mortality rate can certainly be reduced, even before the etiology of NPC has been clarified.

B. Interferon for Treatment and Prevention

Interferon has been shown to have antiviral and antitumor activities. Treaner et al.[23]

reported that a patient with advanced-stage NPC showed complete regression of tumor after treatment with fibroblast interferon, but no success was obtained for other NPC patients. Hence it would be logical to postulate that interferon would be more effective for the treatment of NPC patients in their early stages or for the prevention of NPC development in VCA/IgA antibody positive individuals. An early-stage NPC patient was treated with human leukocyte interferon by our research group and temporary regression of tumor occurred.[28]

More early-stage NPC patients are being treated with leukocyte interferon provided by Cantell. At the same time, attempts have been made to study the antiviral activity of interferon in vitro by using B95-8 cells and Raji cells carrying EBV genome. An unexpected result was obtained in that interferon showed enhancement of spontaneous VCA-EA induction in B95-8 cells and EA induction in Raji cells.[41] The enhancing activity of interferon could be partially inhibited by retinoids. We do not know whether the enhancing activity of interferon for EA and VCA induction is favorable or not for the treatment of NPC patients with interferon. In our experience, there was no change of EB virus-specific IgG and IgA antibody level in the sera of NPC patients before and after treatment with interferon for 10 weeks, and the tumor showed either temporary or progressive regression (unpublished data). Thus, the enhancing activity of interferon might not be harmful for the NPC patient treated with interferon. Alternatively the enhancing activity might cause the activation of EB virus in NPC carcinoma cells and lead to a lytic infection which might be favorable for the NPC patient. If interferon is effective for the treatment of early NPC, the next step is to try to apply interferon for the possible prevention of NPC in VCA/IgA antibody positive individuals.

C. Prevention with Retinoids

Yamamoto et al.[33] first reported that retinoic acid interferes with EB virus EA induction in Rajic cells treated with TPA. Ito et al.[8] also reported that increase in EBV EA and VCA in Raji and P3HR-1 cells treated with croton oil and *n*-butyrate was markedly inhibited by retinoic acid and retinoids. Although treatment of experimental animals with vitamin A and retinoids inhibits tumor, vitamin A is highly toxic after long-term administration and cannot be used clinically. However, synthesis of vitamin A derivatives with low toxicity has been accomplished. Such retinoids, made in China (7901) and by Hoffmann-La Roche, (Ro10-9359) were tested for inhibitory effect on EBV induction for possible use in the prevention of NPC.[42] The results further confirmed that EA induction by croton oil and *n*-butyrate could be inhibited markedly by both retinoids 7901 and Ro10-7359. Since retinoid 7901 has a lower toxicity than Ro10-9359, which has been used in clinical trials, it appears that 7901 could also be used clinically.

The field studies showed that NPC patients could be detected from the VCA/IgA antibody positive individuals, but there remains a large number of VCA/IgA antibody positive persons without evidence of tumor. Because vitamin A and its derivatives have shown effective inhibition of EBV induction and antitumor effect, administration of retinoids to VCA/IgA antibody positive individuals might prevent EBV activation and possibly NPC. Clinical trials are being carried out in the field.

D. Conclusion

Viroimmunological tests for the detection of EBV IgA antibody in the serum and EBV marker in the nasopharyngeal mucosa in combination with clinical, cytological, and histological examination are valuable for the early detection of NPC. Serology has become a routine test widely used for the detection of NPC in China. This should lead to the better control of NPC through early treatment. The present evidence suggests that EB virus plays an important role in the development of NPC. Successful intervention against the possible causal factors of this cancer may provide further evidence for their relationship. Studies on intervention against EB virus by retinoids and interferon are in progress.

REFERENCES

1. Coordination Group of Study on Nasopharyngeal Carcinoma in China, Preliminary study on epidemiology of nasopharyngeal carcinoma in southern 5 provinces of China, *J. Guangdong Cancer Control,* 22, 23, 1978.

2. Department of Microbiology and Cancer Hospital of Zhongshan Medical College, Department of Virology of Cancer Institute, Department of Tumor Viruses of Institute of Virology; and Cancer Institute of Zhongshan County, Investigation of Epstein-Barr Virus complement-fixing antibody levels in sera of patients with nasopharyngeal carcinoma and nasopharyngeal mucosal hyperplasia, *Chinese J. Ear, Nose, Throat,* 93, 359, 1980.

3. **De-Thé, G., Ho, C. H. C., Muir, C.,** Nasopharyngeal carcinoma, in *Viral Infections of Human,* Evans, A. S., Ed. Plenum Press, New York, 1976, 539.

4. **De-Thé, G., Desgranges, C., Zeng, Y., Wang, P. C., Bornkamm, G. W., Zhu, J. S., and Shang, M.,** Search for pre-cancerous lesions and EBV markers in the nasopharynx of IgA positive individuals, 11th Int. Symp. Nasopharyngeal Carcinoma, Düsseldorf, West Germany, October 1980.

5. **Henle, G. and Henle, W.,** Epstein-Barr Virus-specific IgA serum antibodies as an outstanding feature of nasopharyngeal carcinoma, *Int. J. Cancer,* 17, 1, 1976.

6. **Ho, J. H. C.,** The natural history and treatment of nasopharyngeal carcinoma (NPC), in *Oncology,* Vol, 4, Proc. 10th Int. Cancer Congr., Lee-Clarm, R., Cumeley, R. W., McCay, J. E., and Copeland, M., Eds., Year Book Medical, Chicago, 1970, 1.

7. **Hu, M. X.,** The epidemiological study on nasopharyngeal carcinoma in China, IUAC Training Course on Epidemiology of Cancer, Beijing, 1979.

8. **Ito, Y., Kishishita, M., Morigak, T., Yanase, S., and Hirayama, T.,** Induction and intervention of EB virus antigens in human lymphoblastoid cell lines: a simulation model for study of cause and prevention of nasopharyngeal carcinoma and Burkitt lymphoma, 11th Int. Symp. Nasopharyngeal Carcinoma, Düsseldorf, West Germany, October 1980.

9. **King, H. and Haenszel, K.,** Cancer mortality among foreign and native born Chinese in the United States, *J. Chron. Dis.,* 26, 623, 1972.

10. Laboratory of Tumor Viruses of Cancer Institute, Laboratory of Tumor Viruses of Institute of Epidemiology, Department of Radiotherapy of Cancer Institute, Department of Otolaryngology of Beijing Worker-Peasant-Soldier Hospital, Detection of EB virus-specific serum IgG and IgA antibodies from patients with nasopharyngeal carcinoma, *Acta Microbiol. Sin.,* 18, 253, 1978.

11. Laboratory of Tumor Viruses of Cancer Institute, Laboratory of Tumor Viruses of Institute of Epidemiology, and Department of Microbiology of Zhongshan Medical College, Establishment of lymphoblastoid cell lines and isolation of cytomegolovirus from nasopharyngeal carcinoma, *Chinese J. Ear, Nose, Throat,* 1, 14, 1978b.

12. Laboratory of Tumor Viruses of Cancer Institute, Laboratory of Tumor Viruses of Institute of Epidemiology, Department of Radiotherapy of Cancer Institute, and Laboratory of Cell Biology of Cancer Institute, Chinese Academy of Medical Sciences, Establishment of an epithelioid cell line and a feesiform cell line from a patient with nasopharyngeal carcinoma, *Sci. Sin.,* 21, 127, 1978.

13. **Li, E. J., Tan, B. F., Zeng, Y. I., Wang, P. Z., Zhong, J. M., D. H., Zhu, J. S., Liu, Y. X., Wei, J. N., and Pan, W. J.,** Some change observed on nasopharyngeal mucosa of persons showing EB IgA/VCA antibody positive, *J. Guangxi Med.,* in press.

14. **Liu, Z. R., Shan, M., Zeng, Y., Han, Z. S., Dai, H. J., Hu, Y. L., Cao, G. R., and Dong, W. P.,** Immunoradioautography and its application in the detection of anti-EBV IgA antibody in NPC patients, *Kexne Tongbao,* 24, 715, 1979a.

15. **Liu, Z. R., Shan, M., Zeng, Y., Dai, H. J., and Du, R. S.,** Application of immunoradioautograph for detection of IgA/VCA antibody in saliva from patients with NPC, *Chinese J. Med. Exam.,* 2, 197, 1979b.

16. **Liu, Y. X., Zeng, Y., Dong, W. P., and Gao, G. R.,** Detection of EB virus specific IgA antibody from patients with nasopharyngeal carcinoma by immunoenzymatic method, *Chinese J. Oncol.,* 1, 8, 1979.

17. **Liu, Y. Z., Zhao, W. P., Hu, R. L., and Zeng, Y.,** The cytotoxic effect of lymphocytes from patients with nasopharyngeal carcinoma (NPC) against a NPC epithelioid cell line, *Chinese J. Oncol.,* 3, 1, 1981.

18. **Nonoyama, M. and Pagano, J. S.,** Homology between EBV DNA and viral DNA from Burkitt's lymphoma and nasopharyngeal carcinoma determined by DNA-DNA reassociation, *Kinetics Nature (London),* 242, 44, 1973.

19. **Old, L. J., Boyes, E. A., Oettgen, H. F., De Harven, E., Geering, G., Williamson, B., and Clifford, P.,** Precipitating antibody in human serum to an antigen present in cultured Burkitt's lymphoma cells, *Proc. Natl. Acad. Sci. U.S.A.,* 56, 1699, 1966.

20. **Pi, G. H., Zeng, Y., Zhao, W. P., and Zhang, Q.,** Development of an anticomplement immunoenzyme test for detection of EB Virus nuclear antigen (EBNA) and antibody to EBNA, *J. Immunol. Methods,* 44, 73, 1981.

21. Shanghai Tumor Hospital, Treatment of NPC with Radiotherapy, 4th Natl. Conf. NPC, Changshai, 1979.

22. **Simons, M. J., Wee, G. B., Day, N. E., Chan, S. H., Shanmugaratnam, K., and De-Thé, G.,** Immunogenetic aspects of nasopharyngeal carcinoma. IV. Probable identification of an HL-A second antigen associated with a high risk for NPC, *Lancet,* 1, 142, 1975.

23. **Treaner, J., Niethammer, D., Dannecker, G., Hagmann, R., Neef, V., and Hofschneider, P. H.,** Successful treatment of nasopharyngeal carcinoma with interferon, *Lancet,* i, 817, 1980.

24. **Trumper, P. A., Epstein, M. A., and Finerty, S.,** Isolation of infectious EB virus from the epithelial tumor cells of nasopharyngeal carcinoma, *Int. J. Cancer,* 20, 655, 1972.

25. Tumor Laboratory of Hunan Medical College, Experimental study on nasopharyngeal carcinoma in rat induced by diethylnitrosamine, *Res. Data of Hunan Med. Coll.,* 1, 21, 1977.

26. Tumor Control Team of Zhongshan County, Department of Microbiology of Zhongshan Medical College, Department of Virology of Cancer Institute, Department of Tumor Viruses of Institute of Epidemiology, Chinese Academy of Medical Sciences, A study on the complement-fixing antibody to EB virus in groups of normal individuals in Guangdong Province and Beijing, *Chinese J. Ear, Nose, Throat,* 1, 23, 1975.

27. Tumor Control Team of Zhongshan County, Department of Microbiology of Zhongshan Medical College, Laboratory of Tumor Viruses of Cancer Institute and Institute of Epidemiology of Chinese Academy of Medical Sciences, A study on the complement fixing antibody to EB virus in groups of normal individuals in Guangdong province and Beijing, *Chinese J. Ear, Nose, Throat,* 1, 23, 1978.

28. **Wang, P. C., Deng, H., Wu, S. H., Wang, L. Z., Zeng Y., and Hu, Y. T.,** Preliminary treatment of nasopharyngeal carcinoma with human interferon, *Interferon Sci. Memoranda,* April 1981, A1071/2.

29. **Wei, J. N., Zhang, S., Tung, S. Z., and Huang, Z. L.,** Detection of EB virus IgA/VCA antibody in sera from patient with nasopharyngeal carcinoma, *Guangxi Yi Xue,* 6, 5, 1980.

30. **Wolf, H., Zur Hansen, H., and Becker, V.,** EB viral genomes in epithelial nasopharyngeal carcinoma cells, *Nature (London), New Biol.,* 244, 245, 1973.

31. **Wu, B., Wu, Y. G., Li, Y. W., Zeng, Y., Wu, M., Zhao, Z. H., and Gong, C. H.,** Study of giant group A marker chromosome in several Burkitt's lymphoma and lymphoblastoid cell lines with Epstein-Barr Virus from different origins, *Chinese Med. J.,* 93, 400, 1980.

32. **Wu, X. X. and Yao, Z. S.,** Clinical application of serology for diagnosis of nasopharyngeal carcinoma, *Shanghai Med.,* 3, 10, 1978.

33. **Yamamoto, N., Birter, K., and Zur Hansens, H.,** Retinoic acid inhibition of Epstein-Barr induction, *Nature (London),* 278, 553, 1979.

34. **Zeng, Y., Liu, Y. X., Liu, Z. Y., Zhen, S. W., Wei, J. N., Zhu, J. S., and Zai, H. J.,** Application of immunoenzymatic method and immunoautoradiographic method for the mass survey of nasopharyngeal carcinoma, *Chinese J. Oncol.,* 1, 2, 1979a.

35. **Zeng, Y., Liu, Y. X., Wei, J. N., Zhu, J. S., Cai, S. L., Wang, P. Z., Zhong, J. M., Li, R. C., Pan, W. J., Li, E. J., and Tan, B. F.,** Serological mass survey of nasopharyngeal carcinoma, *Acta Acad. Med. Sin.,* 1, 123, 1979b.

36. **Zeng, Y., Zhang, M., Liu, Z. R., Zheng, Y. H., Du, R. S., Li, X. H., Gan, B. W., Hu, M. G., Zhen, M., He, S. A., and Mu, G. P.,** Detection of IgA antibody to EB virus VCA from patients with nasopharyngeal carcinoma by immunofluorescence test, *Chinese J. Oncol.,* 1, 81, 1979c.

37. **Zeng, Y., Liu, Y. X., Liu, Z. R., Zhen, S. W., Wei, J. N., Zhu, J. S., and Zai, H. S.,** Application of an immunoenzymatic method and an immunoautoradiographic method for a mass survey of nasopharyngeal carcinoma, *Intervirology,* 13, 162, 1980a.

38. **Zeng, Y., Pi, G. H., Zhang, Q., Shen, S. J., Zhao, M. L., Ma, J. L., and Dong, H. J.,** Application of anticomplement immunoenzymatic method for the detection of EBNA in carcinoma cells and normal epithelial cells from nasopharynx, 11th Int. Symp. Nasopharyngeal Carcinoma, Düsseldorf, West Germany, October 1980.

39. **Zeng, Y., Zhen, S. J., Dan, H., Ma, T. L., Zhang, Q., Zhu, J. S., Zheng, T. R., and Tan, B. F.,** Detection of early stage NPC from IgA/VCA antibody positive individuals by anticomplement immunoenzymatic method, *Acta Acad. Med. Sin.,* 4, 254, 1982.

40. **Zeng, Y., Zhang, L. G., Li, H. Y., Jan, M. G., Zhang, Q., Wu, Y. C., Wang, Y. S., and Su, G. R.,** Serological mass survey for early detection of NPC in Wuzhow city, *Int. J. Cancer,* 29, 139, 1982.

41. **Zeng, Y., Zhong, J. M., De-Thé, G., Wu, S. H., Hou, Y. T., and Miao, X. O.,** Enhancement of spontaneous VCA-EA induction in B95-8 cells and EA induction in Raji cells treated with human lenhocyte interferon, *Intervirology,* 18, 33, 1982.

42. **Zeng, Y., Zhon, H. M., and Yu, S. P.,** Inhibitory effect of retinoids on Epstein-Barr virus induction in Raji cells, *Intervirology,* 16, 29, 1982.

43. Zhangjiang Medical College, Diagnosis of nasopharyngeal carcinoma by cytological examination of exfoliated cells taken by negative pressure suction, *Chinese Med. J.,* 1, 45, 1976.

44. **Zhong, J. M., Zeng, Y., Liu, Y. X., Wei, J. N., Pi, G. H., Zhu, J. S., Mao, Y. K., and Zhan, J. Y.,** Detection of EBV IgA/CA antibody to in saliva from patients with nasopharyngeal carcinoma and normal subjects, *J. Epidemiol.,* 1, 255, 1980.

45. **Zur Hansen, H., Zchulte Holthausen, H., Klein, G., Henle, W., Henle, G., Clifford, P., and Santessoni, L.,** EBV DNA in biopsies of Burkitt tumors and anaplastic carcinomas of the nasopharynx, *Nature (London),* 228, 1056, 1970.

Chapter 10

NASAL CAVITY CARCINOGENS: POSSIBLE ROUTES OF METABOLIC ACTIVATION

Stephen S. Hecht, Andre Castonguay, and Dietrich Hoffmann

TABLE OF CONTENTS

I.   Introduction 202

II.   *N*-Nitrosodiethylamine 202

III.   *N*-Nitrosodiethanolamine 203

IV.   *N*-Nitrosomorpholine 204

V.   *N*-Nitrosopyrrolidine 205

VI.   *N'*-Nitrosonornicotine and 4-(Methylnitrosamino)-*1*-(3-Pyridyl)-*1*-Butanone: To-
        bacco-Specific Nitrosamines 207

VII.   *p*-Cresidine (2-Methoxy-5-Methylbenzenamine)................................209

VIII.   Phenacetin 210

IX.   Dioxane 211

X.   Hexamethylphosphoramide...212

XI.   Thio-TEPA...214

XII.   1,2-Dibromoethane...215

XIII.   Dimethylcarbamoyl Chloride..215

XIV.   Bis(Chloromethyl)Ether 217

XV.   Vinyl Chloride 217

XVI.   Epichlorohydrin 218

XVII.   Formaldehyde 219

XVIII. Nickel and Nickel Compounds 220

XIX.   Isopropyl Oils..220

XX.   3,4,5-Trimethoxycinnamaldehyde 221

Acknowledgments 223

References 223

I. INTRODUCTION

A variety of chemicals induce nasal cavity cancer in experimental animals. Many of these compounds also give tumors in other organs, depending on the species and route of administration. In almost every case, studies on the metabolic conversion of these compounds to reactive intermediates that can covalently bind to cellular macromolecules (metabolic activation) have been carried out in tissues other than the nasal cavity. Thus, the mechanisms of metabolic activation of nasal cavity carcinogens are really not known. In this chapter, some of the major metabolic pathways that could possibly be involved in carcinogenesis by a representative group of nasal cavity carcinogens will be outlined. This includes various nitrosamines, industrial solvents, alkylating agents, haloalkanes and haloalkenes, and miscellaneous substances such as *p*-cresidine, phenacetin, nickel, formaldehyde, and isopropyl oils. These compounds were chosen because of their structural diversity and, in many cases, their environmental importance.

II. *N*-NITROSODIETHYLAMINE

N-Nitrosodiethylamine is commonly detected in air, water, various foods, and tobacco smoke.[1] It is a potent carcinogen which has induced tumors in at least 18 different species.[2] Its principal target organ in mice and rats is generally the liver, but nasal cavity tumors have been observed in certain cases.[3-5] However, in Syrian Golden hamsters it predominantly induces tumors of the nasal cavity, larynx, and trachea.[6,7] In one study, a total dose of only 6 mg (60 μmol) induced respiratory tract tumors in 29 of 35 Syrian Golden hamsters.[7] A high incidence of respiratory tract tumors was also induced by as little as 15 μg *N*-nitrosodiethylamine administered as a single injection to newborn hamsters.[8] Of the nitrosamines considered in this chapter, *N*-nitrosodiethylamine is the most carcinogenic to the hamster nasal cavity.[6] *N*-Nitrosomorpholine, *N*-nitrosopyrrolidine, and 4-(methylnitrosamino)-*1*-(3-pyridyl)-*1*-butanone are less carcinogenic than *N*-nitrosodiethylamine but more active than *N'*-nitrosonornicotine.[9-12] The least active among these compounds is *N*-nitrosodiethanolamine. We estimate that *N*-nitrosodiethylamine is about 200 times as potent as *N*-nitrosodiethanolamine to the Syrian Golden hamster nasal cavity.[13]

The metabolism of *N*-nitrosodiethylamine is typical of the structurally simple dialkylnitrosamines. An important process is α-hydroxylation to yield the unstable α-hydroxy *N*-nitrosomine (1) which decomposes to acetaldehyde (2) and ethyldiazonium hydroxide (3) as shown in Figure 1. The former has been identified as a microsomal metabolite of *N*-nitrosodiethylamine in liver.[14-16] The latter is unstable and reacts with H_2O and other cellular nucleophiles including DNA bases. The major product of *N*-nitrosodiethylamine metabolism in vivo is CO_2; 3 hr after treatment with 0.4 to 5.0 mg/kg of the nitrosamine, 40 to 60% is exhaled as CO_2.[17,18] β-Hydroxylation of *N*-nitrosodiethylamine has not been reported.

The major DNA adduct formed as a consequence of metabolism of *N*-nitrosodiethylamine is 7-ethylguanine. However, a more important event in carcinogenesis may be formation of O^6-ethylguanine. Studies on the related carcinogens *N*-ethyl-*N*-nitrosourea and *N*-nitrosodimethylamine indicate that the O^6-alkylguanines persist in target tissues and, because of their miscoding properties, may be critical adducts.[19] The removal of O^6-ethylguanine from

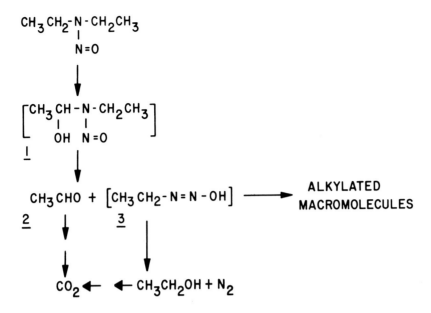

FIGURE 1.   Metabolic α-hydroxylation of *N*-nitrosodiethylamine.

DNA is an enzymatic process which takes place very rapidly in rat liver after low doses of *N*-nitrosodiethylamine.[18] O^2-Ethyl- and O^4-ethylthymidine are also formed in rat liver following administration of *N*-nitrosodiethylamine, and it has been suggested that these minor adducts may be important in carcinogenesis.[20]

Very little data are available concerning the metabolism and DNA binding of *N*-nitrosodiethylamine in the nasal cavity. However, it has been shown that nasal cavity tissue of C57Bl mice was more efficient than any other tissue examined in converting *N*-nitrosodiethylamine to CO_2.[21] This is apparently the only report to date of nitrosamine metabolism by isolated nasal cavity tissue. Radioactivity was also incorporated into the acid-insoluble material of the nasal cavity tissue in this in vitro study. It is difficult to assess the importance of this observation in carcinogenesis by *N*-nitrosodiethylamine since the nasal cavity is not a target tissue in C57Bl mice.[22] The distribution of the enzyme systems which remove O^6-ethylguanine, and possibly other lesions, from DNA in the nasal cavity and other tissues is likely to play an important role in carcinogenesis by *N*-nitrosodiethylamine as well as other nitrosamines.

III. *N*-NITROSODIETHANOLAMINE

N-Nitrosodiethanolamine has been detected in a variety of products including industrial cutting fluids, cosmetics, pesticides, tobacco, and tobacco smoke.[23-27] The major target organ of *N*-nitrosodiethanolamine in the rat is the liver although nasal cavity tumors are also observed.[28-30] However, in the Syrian Golden hamster *N*-nitrosodiethanolamine induces nasal cavity and tracheal tumors, as is characteristic of a number of nitrosamines.[31] These tumors are induced by *N*-nitrosodiethanolamine regardless of whether the route of administration is subcutaneous injection, oral swabbing, or skin painting.[13] This organ specificity is typical of nitrosamines and suggests that particular characteristics of the hamster trachea and nasal cavity mucosa, such as the ability to efficiently metabolize nitrosamines, may be involved in carcinogenesis at these sites. The lowest total dose of *N*-nitrosodiethanolamine to induce nasal cavity tumors in hamsters was 6.7 mmol.[13] It is therefore a considerably weaker carcinogen for the nasal cavity than any of the other nitrosamines considered in this chapter.

In the rat, *N*-nitrosodiethanolamine is excreted largely unchanged (70 to 79%) in the urine.[32] This is in contrast to the structurally related compounds *N*-nitrosodiethylamine and *N*-nitrosomorpholine which are both extensively metabolized and are also much more potent carcinogens. In fact, *N*-nitrosodiethanolamine is a major urinary metabolite of *N*-nitrosomorpholine, as described below. There have been no reports of identified metabolites of *N*-nitrosodiethanolamine. By analogy to other nitrosamines, it might be expected that *N*-nitrosodiethanolamine would undergo α-hydroxylation to give 2-hydroxyethyl adducts of DNA bases.

However, this has not been demonstrated. It has been suggested that sulfate esters of β-hydroxynitrosamines such as *N*-nitrosodiethanolamine could undergo solvolysis to give electrophilic oxadiazolium ions.[33] Further studies on the mechanism of action of *N*-nitrosodiethanolamine are clearly necessary.

IV. *N*-NITROSOMORPHOLINE

N-Nitrosomorpholine has been detected as a contaminant in crankcase emissions from diesel engines, in rubber manufacturing factories, and in chewing tobacco.[34-36] It is readily formed by nitrosation of morpholine, in vitro and in vivo.[37-39] Like *N*-nitrosopyrrolidine, the principal target organs of *N*-nitrosomorpholine are the liver in the rat and the nasal cavity mucosa and trachea in the Syrian Golden hamster. Nasal cavity tumors have also been observed in BD rats after i.v. injection of *N*-nitrosomorpholine.[9,28,37] However, *N*-nitrosomorpholine is apparently a more powerful nasal cavity carcinogen in the hamster than is *N*-nitrosopyrrolidine.[9,10]

Metabolic studies on *N*-nitrosomorpholine have been performed in the rat,[40-44] and are summarized in Figure 2. As in the case of *N*-nitrosopyrrolidine, a major pathway is α-hydroxylation leading to (2-hydroxyethoxy)acetaldehyde (7) in vitro and to (2-hydroxyethoxy)acetic acid (10) as a major urinary metabolite. These products are formed by reaction of H$_2$O with the electrophilic diazohydroxide (4). β-Hydroxylation of *N*-nitrosomorpholine occurs to a greater extent than of *N*-nitrosopyrrolidine (see Section V), possibly because of the oxygen in the ring system. The major urinary product of β-hydroxylation is *N*-nitroso-2-hydroxyethylglycine (9). Another major urinary metabolite of *N*-nitrosomorpholine is *N*-nitrosodiethanolamine (3). The latter is not converted to a significant extent to (9).

The role of α-hydroxylation as the activation step in rat liver carcinogenesis by *N*-nitrosomorpholine is supported by comparative carcinogenicity and metabolism studies of *N*-nitrosomorpholine and 3,3,5,5-tetradeutero-*N*-nitrosomorpholine in which the α-hydrogens are substituted by deuteriums. The latter was shown to be significantly less carcinogenic to the rat liver than was *N*-nitrosomorpholine.[45] The extent of formation of (2-hydroxyethoxy)-acetic acid by α-hydroxylation was approximately one fifth as great in the metabolism of 3,3,5,5-tetradeutero-*N*-nitrosomorpholine as in the metabolism of *N*-nitrosomorpholine. In contrast, the extents of formation of *N*-nitroso-(2-hydroxyethyl)glycine from β-hydroxylation and of *N*-nitrosodiethanolamine were the same in the metabolism of both the deuterated and undeuterated nitrosamines.[44] These results strongly indicate that α-hydroxylation is the major activation pathway of *N*-nitrosomorpholine in the rat.

Unfortunately, no analogous data are available with respect to the Syrian Golden hamster nasal cavity. If similar mechanisms operate, one might expect a reduction in tumor yield in the nasal cavity of hamsters treated with 3,3,5,5-tetradeutero-*N*-nitrosomorpholine. As in the case of *N*-nitrosopyrrolidine, one can speculate that an ultimate carcinogen of *N*-nitrosomorpholine such as (4) might be formed by metabolism of the nitrosamine in the nasal cavity mucosa. It is unlikely that reactive species such as (1) or (4) could be transported to the nasal cavity as such. However, one cannot exclude the possibility that these intermediates could be formed in the liver, conjugated, transported to other tissues, and deconjugated.

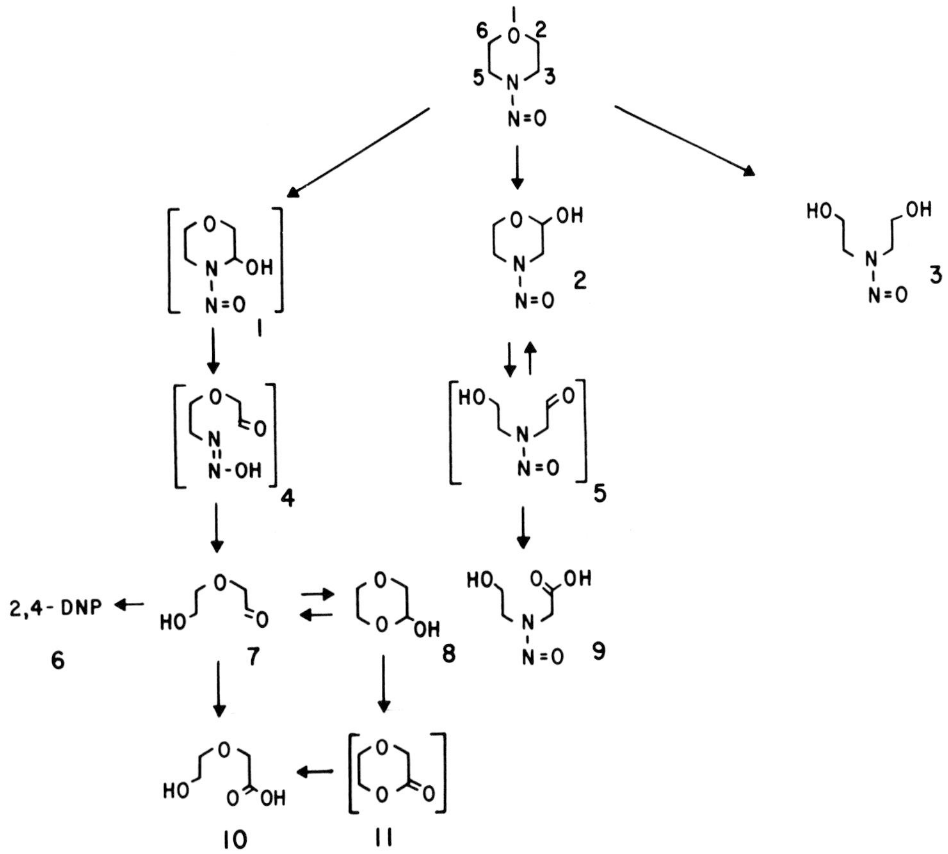

FIGURE 2.   Metabolism of *N*-nitrosomorpholine in the Fischer 344 rat.

There is presently no available evidence on this question. As in the case of other nitrosamines, differing rates of DNA repair of specific adducts in target and nontarget tissues may also be involved in nasal cavity carcinogenesis by *N*-nitrosomorpholine.

V. *N*-NITROSOPYRROLIDINE

N-Nitrosopyrrolidine is a frequent contaminant in cooked bacon and other processed meats and is found in main- and sidestream tobacco smoke.[46-48] It induces primarily liver tumors in rats, in contrast to the structurally related compound, *N'*-nitrosonornicotine, which gives mainly tumors of the esophagus and nasal cavity.[28,49,50] However, in the Syrian Golden hamster its target organs are the trachea and nasal cavity.[10]

The metabolism of *N*-nitrosopyrrolidine has been investigated in vitro and in vivo, mainly in the rat.[51-53] Known metabolic transformations are summarized in Figure 3. The major pathway appears to be α-hydroxylation leading to the unstable α-hydroxy-*N*-nitrosopyrrolidine (1). This compound undergoes ring opening to the electrophilic diazohydroxide (4), a potential ultimate carcinogen of *N*-nitrosopyrrolidine. Compound (4) is trapped by H_2O to give the major microsomal metabolite of *N*-nitrosopyrrolidine, 4-hydroxybutyraldehyde (6) which exists primarily as 2-hydroxytetrahydrofuran (7). These metabolites are further oxidized in vivo to give 4-hydroxybutyrate (9) and butyrolactone (10) as urinary metabolites. Oxidation of (9) leads to CO_2, the major metabolite of *N*-nitrosopyrrolidine in the rat. Other metabolites of *N*-nitrosopyrrolidine in the rat include 3-hydroxy-*N*-nitrosopyrrolidine (2) and 2-pyrrolidinone (3).

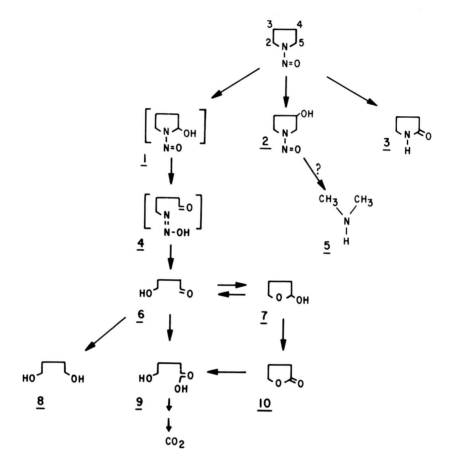

FIGURE 3.   Metabolism of *N* -nitrosopyrrolidine in the rat.

The role of diazohydroxide (4) as a possible ultimate carcinogen of *N*-nitrosopyrrolidine is suggested by the observation that synthetic precursors to this electrophile are mutagenic toward *Salmonella typhimurium* without enzymatic activation.[54-56] In addition, liver preparations from rats or hamsters pretreated with compounds which induce α-hydroxylation of *N*-nitrosopyrrolidine are generally more effective than control preparations in converting it to a mutagen.[57,58] Rates of metabolic α-hydroxylation of *N*-nitrosopyrrolidine are higher in tracheal rings isolated from chronic ethanol-consuming hamsters than from control hamsters. This observation also supports the role of α-hydroxylation as an activation mechanism of *N*-nitrosopyrrolidine in the hamster trachea since its carcinogenicity in this organ is increased in the ethanol-consuming hamster.[10,59] It is not known whether similar changes occur in the Syrian Golden hamster nasal cavity which also has increased sensitivity to *N*-nitrosopyrrolidine in the ethanol-consuming hamster.[10]

Further studies on *N*-nitrosopyrrolidine metabolism in the hamster nasal cavity are clearly needed in order to determine the basis for its organospecificity. Based on results in other tissues and with other nitrosamines, it is likely that *N*-nitrosopyrrolidine is metabolized in the hamster nasal cavity and is converted to DNA damaging intermediates such as (4) (Figure 3). Particular DNA adducts may be resistant to repair mechanisms in the nasal cavity tissues. It will be difficult to establish this until the structures of the DNA adducts have been elucidated.

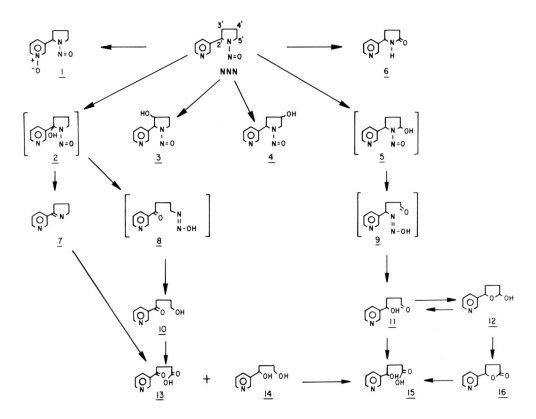

FIGURE 4.   Metabolism of *N*'-nitrosonornicotine in the Fischer 344 rat.

VI. *N*'-NITROSONORNICOTINE AND 4-(METHYLNITROSAMINO)-*1*-(3-PYRIDYL)-*1*-BUTANONE: TOBACCO-SPECIFIC NITROSAMINES

N'-Nitrosonornicotine (NNN) (see Figure 4) and 4-(methylnitrosamino)-*1*-(3-pyridyl)-*1*-butanone (NNK (1), Figure 5) are tobacco-specific nitrosamines which were detected in μg amounts in chewing tobacco and in main- and sidestream smoke of cigarettes and cigars.[60-62] Of all the known *N*-nitrosamines found in the respiratory environment, tobacco-specific nitrosamines are the most prevalent.

The hepatocyte primary culture/DNA repair test revealed that both nitrosamines damaged DNA.[63] In mice, NNN and NNK induced lung adenomas and carcinomas,[64,65] NNK being 30 times more potent than NNN.[66] After administration of NNN in drinking water, rats developed esophageal papillomas and carcinomas, and nasal cavity carcinomas.[49,67] When administered subcutaneously, NNN and NNK induced papillomas and neuroblastomas of the nasal cavity. The NNK-treated rats also developed tumors of the liver and lung.[50] These results suggested that NNN can be activated by esophageal tissues and acted locally. NNN and NNK administered subcutaneously, intraperitoneally, or by cheek pouch swabbing induced nasal cavity carcinomas in Syrian Golden hamsters.[10-12,68] Lungs and trachea are also target organs of NNK.[11] The histogenesis of NNN- and NNK-induced tumors has been discussed in detail in Chapter 4.

The metabolism of NNN and NNK by mice, rats, and hamsters was investigated in order to propose mechanisms for their activation and deactivation. Urinary metabolites were isolated and identified by liquid and gas chromatography, mass spectrometry, and comparison with synthetic reference compounds.[11,69-73] The major urinary metabolites excreted by NNN-treated Fischer 344 rats were 4-hydroxy-4-(3-pyridyl)butyric acid (15, Figure 4) *N*'-nitro-

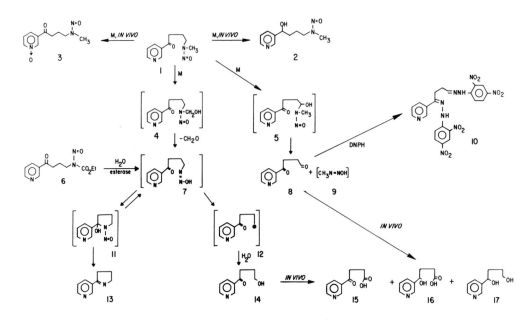

FIGURE 5.   Metabolism of 4-(methylnitrosamino)-*1*-(3-pyridyl)-*1*-butanone in the Fischer 344 rat.

sonornicotine *N*-oxide (1), and 4-oxo-4-(3-pyridyl)butyric acid (13). The metabolites nor-cotinine (6), 5-(3-pyridyl)tetrahydrofuran-2-one (16), myosmine (7), 3′-hydroxy-*N*′-nitrosonornicotine (3), and 4′-hydroxy-*N*′-nitrosonornicotine (4) were present in small amounts (0.1 to 5%). The compounds 4-hydroxy-*1*-(3-pyridyl)-*1*-butanone (10) and 2-hydroxy-5-(3-pyridyl)tetrahydrofuran (12) were not detected in urine but were formed in vitro by incubating NNN with rat liver microsomes. The microsomal metabolism of NNN and other nitrosamines in various tissues is most likely mediated by multiple forms of cytochrome P-450.[74] Various nitrosamines including NNN bind to cytochrome P-450 and change its spectral absorption.[57,75,76] Metyrapone, an inhibitor of cytochrome P-450 oxidation, reduces the metabolism of *N*-nitrosodibutylamine to CO_2 in the nasal mucosa.[77]

The formation of the metabolites (13) and (15) (Figure 4) can be explained by α-carbon hydroxylation of NNN. The initially formed 2′-hydroxyNNN (2) and 5′-hydroxyNNN (3) would decompose to oxodiazohydroxides (8) and (9) which could lose nitrogen and hydroxide ion to give the corresponding oxocarbonium ions. Whether the ultimate carcinogens of NNN are the oxodiazohydroxides (8) and (9), or the corresponding diazonium or carbonium ions has still to be determined. These reactive species react with water to give the intermediates (10) and (12), but they can also alkylate nucleic acids. Specific alkylated deoxyribonucleo-sides could induce miscoding during DNA replication leading to tumor formation. Human liver microsomes metabolized NNN to (10) and (12) in vitro indicating that human liver enzymes can activate NNN to potential ultimate carcinogens.[78]

In order to confirm the 2′- and 5′-hydroxylation of NNN as activating processes, the reactive intermediate (8) was generated by hydrolysis of 4-(*N*-carbethoxy-*N*-nitrosamino)-*1*-(3-pyridyl)-*1*-butanone (6), Figure 5) or 2′-acetoxyNNN. After treatment with hog liver esterase, (6) reacted with water to give the keto alcohol (10) (Figure 4) or (14) (Figure 5)[56] or with ^{14}C-labeled guanosine to give a 7-alkylguanosine.[79] Keto alcohol (10) and myosmine (7) were also produced via the oxodiazohydroxide (8) by hydrolysis of 2′-acetoxyNNN. The oxodiazohydroxide (9) was formed as an intermediate by hydrolysis of another model com-pound: 5′-acetoxyNNN. This reaction catalyzed by hog liver esterase gave 2-hydroxy-5-(3-pyridyl)-tetrahydrofuran (12) as its main product.[56] The mutagenicity of the nitrosourethane (6) (Figure 5), 2′-acetoxyNNN, and 5′-acetoxyNNN observed in the *S. typhimurium* (TA 100) assay is consistent with the hypothesis that NNN is activated by α-carbon hydroxylation.[69]

Identification of the urinary metabolites of Fischer 344 rats treated with NNK showed that this tobacco-specific *N*-nitrosamine was metabolized by α-carbon hydroxylation (Figure 5). The three intermediates myosmine (13), 4-hydroxy-*1*-(3-pyridyl)-*1*-butanone (14), and 4-oxo-4-(3-pyridyl)butanal (8) were observed in vitro and were not detected in urine extracts.[71] Further oxidation and/or reduction of (8) and (14) in vivo resulted in the formation of the urinary metabolites diol (17), keto acid (15), and hydroxy acid (16).

Methyl hydroxylation of NNK leads to the diazohydroxide (7) which is also formed by 2′-hydroxylation of NNN. α-Methylene hydroxylation of NNK gives the methyldiazohydroxide (9), a reactive intermediate in the metabolic activation of *N*-nitrosodimethylamine. In that respect, it is interesting to note that both NNN and NNK induce nasal cavity tumors in rats while both NNK and *N*-nitrosodimethylamine induce liver tumors.[50,80]

Oxidation of NNK to the rapidly excreted NNK-*N*-oxide (3) is an effective metabolic deactivation process. Injection of this *N*-oxide in A/J mice induced ten times less lung adenomas per animal than NNK and four times less adenomas than ethyl carbamate.[66] The *N*-oxide (3) accounts for 3% of the dose administered by gavage to Fischer 344 rats.[71]

Reduction of the NNK carbonyl which gives the hydroxy nitrosamine (2) is a major metabolic process in vivo (Fischer 344 rats)[71] as well as in experimental animal and human tissues cultured in vitro.[66,79] This reduction seems to be in dynamic equilibrium with the oxidation of the hydroxyl group of (2). In cultured human tissues this equilibrium favors the formation of (2).

Autoradiographic studies[81-82a] have shown that [2′-¹⁴C]NNN or its metabolites accumulated in tracheobronchial and nasal mucosa, liver, submaxillary salivary glands, and esophagus of mouse and rat. Radioactivity in the nasal, tracheobronchial, and esophageal mucosa was tissue bound. This accumulation can be attributed to the high rate of metabolism of the nasal cavity mucosa. In Syrian Golden hamsters treated with [2′-¹⁴C]NNN or [1-¹⁴C]NNK, high levels of tissue-bound radioactivity were detected in liver, lungs, kidneys, and adrenal glands.[11] Binding of radiolabeled NNN to melanin-rich tissues such as eye and hair of C57BL mice and Syrian Golden hamsters has also been observed by whole body autoradiography. Slow release of the nitrosamines from the melanin followed by metabolic activation in target tissues could result in long-term exposure to the ultimate carcinogen. Metabolism and DNA alkylation studies with cultured nasal mucosa of the ethmoturbinates could assess the ability of this tissue to activate tobacco-specific nitrosamines to their reactive species. Modes of DNA alkylation by the ultimate carcinogens and persistence of various alkylated nucleotides should be investigated.

VII. *p*-CRESIDINE (2-METHOXY-5-METHYLBENZENAMINE)

p-Cresidine is used as an intermediate in the manufacturing of dyes and pigments. Its estimated use in the U.S. from 1971 to 1976 was about 590,000 lb annually. *p*-Cresidine given at the 5000- or 10,000-ppm levels in their diets induced tumors of the nasal cavity, urinary bladder, and liver in Fischer-344 rats.[83,84] Tumors of the bladder and liver, but not of the nasal cavity, were also observed in B6C3F1 mice treated with *p*-cresidine.[83]

Several aromatic amines with methyl or methoxy groups ortho to the amine functionality are more carcinogenic than the corresponding unsubstituted compounds or than those with meta and para substitutents. For example, *o*-toluidine is more carcinogenic than aniline, and *o*-anisidine is a fairly potent bladder carcinogen in rats.[85,86] In contrast, *p*-anisidine and *p*-toluidine are only weakly carcinogenic or inactive.[85,87] Since *p*-cresidine has a methoxy group ortho to the amino group, its mechanism of activation may in some way be similar to those of *o*-toluidine and *o*-anisidine. However, no metabolic studies have been reported on *p*-cresidine.

Many aromatic amines are activated by formation of hydroxamic acid esters or hydroxylamines which dissociate to electrophilic nitrenium ions that react with DNA.[88,89] It is likely that the metabolic activation of *p*-cresidine involves *N*-oxidation. In the metabolism of *o*-toluidine, *N*-oxidation is a relatively minor pathway, but the resulting metabolites are mutagenic toward *S. typhimurium*.[90,91] The major metabolites of *o*-toluidine in vivo in the rat result from oxidation of the para position and conjugation. This is probably a detoxification process. Oxidation at the para position of *p*-cresidine might be inhibited by the neighboring methyl group. This could result in a relatively greater proportion of *N*-oxidation. The activity in the nasal cavity mucosa for conjugation of metabolites of aromatic amines could be a major factor in their carcinogenicity, but no relevant studies have been performed.

VIII. PHENACETIN

Phenacetin (1), (Figure 6), is widely used as an analgesic and antipyretic agent and is frequently combined with aspirin and caffeine. It is produced in many countries including West Germany, France, Japan, and the U.S., and has been incriminated as a possible carcinogen in the renal pelvis of man.[91a]

When activated by hamster liver S-9, (1) has been reported to be mutagenic in the *S. typhimurium* (TA 100) assay.[92,93] Phenacetin induced chromosome aberrations in Chinese hamster fibroblasts and sister-chromatid exchanges in Sprague-Dawley rats.[94,95]

Carcinogenicity studies of phenacetin have raised considerable controversy. Fischer 344 rats and B6C3F1 mice fed with high doses of aspirin, phenacetin, and caffeine showed no evidence of neoplasia.[96] Long-term carcinogenicity studies of phenacetin in Sprague-Dawley rats,[97] Berlin-Druckrey rats,[98] C57BL/6 mice,[99] and dogs[93,96,97-100] were also negative. Nevertheless, Isaka et al.[101] observed adenomas and carcinomas of the nasal cavity and carcinomas of the urinary passages in Sprague-Dawley rats fed with phenacetin for 18 mon. Johansson and Angervall[102] have reported urothelial hyperplasia of the renal pelvis in female Sprague-Dawley rats fed with phenacetin for 28 months. Considering the long debate over the validity of the last two studies,[99,103,104] confirmation of the carcinogenicity of phenacetin in Sprague-Dawley rats is highly desirable.

Oxidative deethylation by cytochrome P-450 is the main metabolic pathway of phenacetin in rats, rabbits, guinea-pigs, and ferrets. The resulting *N*-acetyl-*p*-aminophenol (acetaminophen) (3) or its conjugates (*O*-sulfate or *O*-glucuronide) are excreted in the urine.[105,106] Deethylation by hamster liver microsomes shows a deuterium isotope effect for the α-methylene position of the ethoxy group ($K_h/K_d = 1.86$).[107] Various enzyme inducers such as 3-methylcholanthrene and benzo [a] pyrene as well as dried Brussels sprouts increase the *O*-dealkylation of phenacetin.[108-112] In humans, the ratio of the plasma concentration of total acetaminophen (3) to phenacetin (1) is increased by cigarette smoking or by a diet containing charcoal-broiled beef.[110,113]

N-Hydroxylation of acetaminophen by a cytochrome P-450 isolated from hamster liver microsomes would yield the unstable intermediate (9) which spontaneously dehydrates to the *N*-acetylquinone imine (13), a known arylating agent.[114-116]

Hinson et al.[117,118] proposed that phenacetin was activated directly to an arylating metabolite by formation of phenacetin-3,4-epoxide (2). This epoxide could tautomerize to the hemiacetal of quinone imine (7), which upon hydrolysis could give *N*-acetylquinone imine (13). Alternatively, deethylation of the epoxide (7) would form acetaminophen-3,4-epoxide (8) which would rearrange to (13).

Phenacetin undergoes *N*-deacylation to a greater extent in rat (21% of the dose) and ferret (13%) than in guinea pig (7%) and rabbit (4%).[119] The resulting *p*-phenetidine (4) could readily oxidize hemoglobin and be responsible for the occurrence of methaemoglobinaemia after administration of phenacetin to the rat. Further hydroxylation of (4) in the rat gave 2-hydroxy-*p*-phenetidine (5).[105]

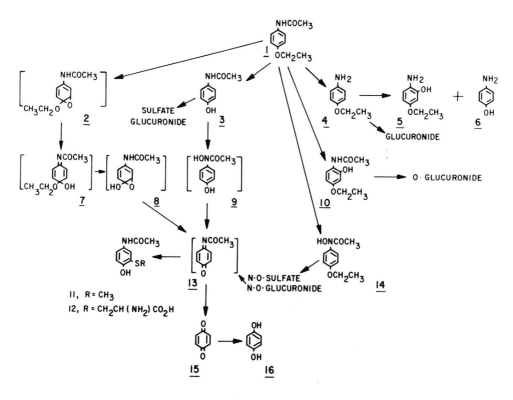

FIGURE 6. Some aspects of the metabolism of phenacetin.

N-Hydroxylation has been proposed as the initial activation step of phenacetin to a carcinogen and nephrotoxic agent.[120-122] This reaction is catalyzed by hamster liver microsomes.[114] The stable metabolite *N*-hydroxy phenacetin (14) is mutagenic after rat or hamster liver S-9 activation and induces hepatomas in the rat.[124-126] It is transformed to the unstable conjugates, phenacetin *N,O*-sulfate, and phenacetin *N,O*-glucuronide which subsequently decompose to *N*-acetylbenzoquinone imine (13).[116,127] This reactive intermediate can covalently bind to glutathione or bovine serum albumin.[128] Hydrolysis of (13) to *p*-benzoquinone (15) followed by reduction would yield hydroquinone (16), the minor urinary metabolite of phenacetin which is nephrotoxic in rats.[120-123] Like *N*-hydroxy-2-acetylaminofluorene, *N*-hydroxyphenacetin can be activated by rabbit liver acyltransferase or by sulfate conjugation resulting in binding to transfer RNA.[129]

IX. DIOXANE

Dioxane, a widely employed solvent, is a weak nasal cavity carcinogen in the rat. Dioxane administered in the drinking water (0.75 to 1.0%) induced nasal cavity tumors in 6 of 120 rats given total doses of between 104 to 256 g.[130] In a dose-response study, only the 1% level was effective; administration of 0.1 or 0.01% dioxane in drinking water did not lead to treatment-related tumors.[131] In a National Cancer Institute bioassay, dioxane was administered in concentrations of either 1.0 or 0.5% (V/V) in the drinking water to groups of Osborne-Mendel rats and B6C3F1 mice. It was carcinogenic at both doses in both sexes of rats, inducing squamous cell carcinomas of the nasal turbinates. Dioxane also causes hepatocellular tumors in rats and mice.[131,131a,133] Exposure of rats to dioxane by inhalation failed to induce tumors.[132]

The metabolism of dioxane has been studied in the rat in vivo (see Figure 7). The major

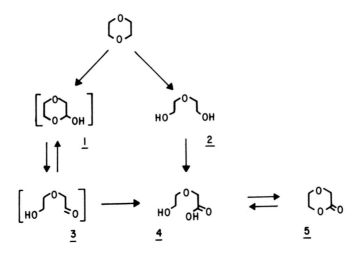

FIGURE 7.   Metabolism of dioxane in the rat.

urinary metabolite has been identified as either (2-hydroxyethoxy)acetic acid (4) or the corresponding cyclic lactone, dioxan-2-one (5) depending on the method of isolation.[134,135] This metabolite may have been formed by initial α-hydroxylation of dioxane to give the lactol (1) which could be oxidized either directly or via its acyclic tautomer (3) to (4) or (5). Attempts to isolate (1) or (3) as a metabolite of dioxane have not been described. Alternatively, dioxane may undergo ring cleavage to diethylene glycol (2) which is then oxidized to (4) or (5). While (2) has not been detected as a urinary metabolite of dioxane, it is rapidly converted metabolically to (4) or (5).[134]

It has been suggested that the weak carcinogenicity of dioxane may be due in part to the metabolite dioxan-2-one (5). Preliminary studies indicated that (5) is more toxic than dioxane but its carcinogenicity has not been reported.[136] The only other potential metabolite having electrophilic character is the hydroxyaldehyde (3), but this would exist predominantly as the lactol (1). Of course unidentified metabolites such as peroxy derivatives could also be involved in dioxane carcinogenesis, but no evidence has been obtained to support this suggestion.[136]

It is interesting that the metabolites of dioxane are the same ones that are formed in the α-hydroxylation of the potent carcinogen N-nitrosomorpholine (see Figure 2). However, in the case of N-nitrosomorpholine, (2-hydroxyethoxy)acetaldehyde is generated by reaction of a highly electrophilic diazohydroxide with H_2O. No corresponding electrophile is formed from dioxane even though the end products of metabolism are similar. The greater carcinogenicity of N-nitrosomorpholine than of dioxane is undoubtedly due to the metabolic formation of a potent electrophile, such as diazohydroxide (4) (Figure 2).

X. HEXAMETHYLPHOSPHORAMIDE

Hexamethylphosphoramide (HMPA) is widely used as a solvent in the polymer industry and in organic reactions in research laboratories.[136] It is also an effective chemosterilant for the control of insects.[138-140] It is produced in Japan, Western Europe, and the U.S.[141]

HMPA induces mutagenic effects in *Drosophila melanogaster* but not in the *S. typhimurium* mutation assay.[142] In the cell transformation assay, Ashby et al.[143] observed a positive response with HMPA, but a negative response with the phenyl analogue of HMPA. These authors concluded that the methyl groups of HMPA are activated and react with genetic material. HMPA also inhibits spermatogenesis in rats and rabbits.[144]

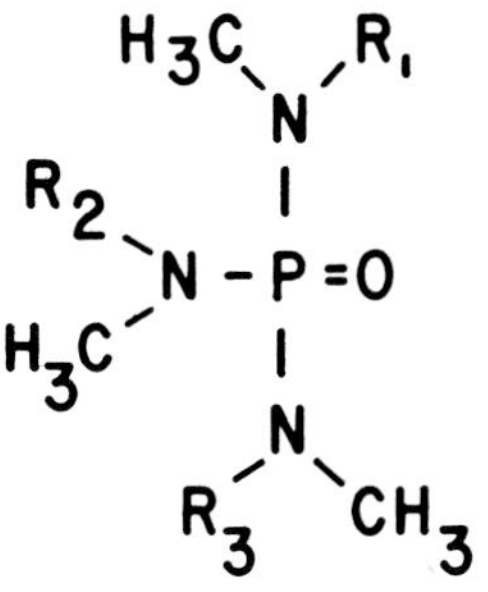

$$H_3C \diagdown_{N} \diagup R_1$$

(chemical structure of hexamethylphosphoramide core with substituents R_1, R_2, R_3, $N-P=O$, and CH_3 groups)

$\underline{1}$ $R_1 = R_2 = R_3 = CH_3$, HMPA

$\underline{2}$ $R_1 = H$, $R_2 = R_3 = CH_3$, PMPA

$\underline{3}$ $R_1 = R_2 = H$, $R_3 = CH_3$

$\underline{4}$ $R_1 = R_2 = R_3 = H$

FIGURE 8. Some metabolites of hexamethylphosphoramide.

The long-term inhalation toxicity and carcinogenicity of HMPA were evaluated in Charles River strain CD rats. The animals were exposed to 0, 50, 400, and 4000 ppb of HMPA, 6 hr/day, 5 days/week. After 8 months of treatment, rats of the highest exposure groups had developed squamous cell carcinomas originating from the epithelial lining of the nasal turbinate bones and penetrating into the brain. The incidence of those tumors was dose related and no tumors were observed in the 50-ppb dose group.[145] Male Sherman rats fed with diets containing HMPA developed reticulum cell sarcoma or lymphosarcoma of the lung.[145] Oral administration of HMPA to rats also induced severe bronchiectasis and bronchopneumonia.[147]

HMPA undergoes a sequence of demethylations in vivo to N,N',N''-trimethylphosphoramide (4), (Figure 8). Rats and mice injected intraperitoneally with ^{32}P-labeled HMPA excreted 87% of the radioactive dose in the urine within 13 hr.[148] Two urinary metabolites, pentamethylphosphoramide (PMPA) (2) and tetramethylphosphoramide (3), were isolated by extraction and thin-layer chromatography. The major metabolite PMPA is considerably less toxic than HMPA and is degraded to tetramethylphosphoramide (3) and trimethylphosphoramide (4).[148] HMPA is detected unchanged in cow milk following oral administration.[149]

Formation of ^{14}C-labeled formaldehyde during incubation of ^{14}C-HMPA with rat liver slices suggests that HMPA is metabolized by a sequence of oxidative dealkylations.[148] Unlike the related compound triethylenephosphoramide (TEPA), HMPA is not degraded to inorganic phosphate by the mouse.[144,148]

The fact that nasal cavity tumors are induced by inhalation but not by oral administration indicates that HMPA can be activated by the nasal mucosa to an ultimate carcinogen. Jones and Bertram[148] suggested that methyl oxidation would convert HMPA to an active hydroxymethyl intermediate having a carbinolamine function. Oxidation of HMPA by the nasal cavity mucosa could generate formaldehyde which is a nasal cavity carcinogen in rats (see Section XVII).

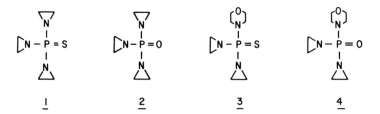

FIGURE 9.   Structures of Thio-TEPA (1), TEPA (2), OPSPA (3), and MEPA (4).

XI. THIO-TEPA

Thio-TEPA (1), (Figure 9) is a phosphine sulfide derivative which was commonly used in the U.S. as an antineoplastic agent in the 1950s and 1960s.[150] Although thio-TEPA is an effective insect chemosterilant, it has not been marketed as such.[151]

Thio-TEPA induces lung tumors in A/He mice but is 20 times less active than uracil mustard.[152] The carcinogenicity of thio-TEPA was also demonstrated by intraperitoneal injection to Sprague-Dawley rats and B6C3F1 mice. Rats developed neuroepitheliomas and nasal carcinomas and squamous cell carcinomas of the skin or ear canal. Adenocarcinomas of the uterus occurred in mice.[148] Thio-TEPA is also carcinogenic in BR46 rats.[154]

The occurrence of acute leukemia among patients with ovary, breast, or lung cancer who were treated with thio-TEPA has suggested that there is an increased risk of acute leukemia associated with long-term (13 to 60 months) treatment.[155-157]

After i.v. or oral administration of thio-TEPA to dogs, the sulfur of thio-TEPA is rapidly (less than 60 min) exchanged for oxygen to give TEPA (2). Less than 0.4% of the administered dose of thio-TEPA is recovered in the 24-hr urine and only 8 to 15% is recovered as TEPA. Treatment of the dogs with β-diethylaminoethyl diphenylpropyl acetate (SKF-525A) prior to administration of thio-TEPA delays the conversion of thio-TEPA to TEPA and is accompanied by increased toxicity. While thio-TEPA, which is lipid soluble, is degraded by most tissue homogenates, the water soluble TEPA is relatively unaffected.[158] Rats metabolize extensively and rapidly ^{32}P-labeled thio-TEPA to TEPA, 70% of the radioactive dose being excreted in the 18-hr urine.[159] When thio-TEPA labeled with ^{14}C was administered, 94 to 98% of the dose was recovered in the 24-hr urine, less than 2% in the feces and less than 3% as CO_2 in the expired air.[160]

The mouse has the unique ability to rapidly and effectively degrade ^{32}P thio-TEPA to inorganic phosphate which is excreted in the urine (90% of the radioactive dose). Radiochromatography of the plasma indicated that the first metabolic step was formation of TEPA.[159] A few percent of the dose administered was recovered in the urine as an organic phosphorus compound which upon hydrolysis yielded inorganic phosphate.[161]

Data on the absorption and plasma levels of ^{14}C-thio-TEPA administered orally to cancer patients are erratic. This is probably due to the instability of the drug in weak acid solution and to the difference in the gastric acidity among patients.[158,162] The total radioactivity excreted in the urine ranged between 24 and 84% of the administered dose, and TEPA was detected only in trace amounts (0.3%).[162] Bateman et al.[163] demonstrated that the blood radioactivity was associated with the protein fraction and observed considerable localization of radioactivity in the adrenals following intravenous injection of ^{14}C-thio-TEPA.

OPSPA (3) which is an analogue of thio-TEPA is metabolized to MEPA (4), morpholine, and inorganic phosphate after administration of ^{32}P or ^{14}C-labeled OPSPA to rats or humans.[164] These results suggest that one metabolic pathway of thio-TEPA could be the cleavage of the nitrogen phosphorous bond with formation of the intermediate, aziridine.

The study of Benckhuijen[165] on the stability of thio-TEPA in acid medium has suggested intramolecular alkylation of the sulfur following protonation of the aziridine ring. It is possible that a similar process could occur in vivo after oral administration.

XII. 1,2-DIBROMOETHANE

1,2-Dibromoethane is employed as a soil fumigant and as a lead scavenger in gasoline. It appears to act as a carcinogen mainly at the site of application. Thus, it has been shown to induce squamous cell carcinomas of the stomach in rats and mice when administered by intragastric intubation.[166,167] It causes skin tumors in mice when applied repeatedly to mouse skin,[168] and induces nasal cavity tumors in rats and mice when administered by inhalation.[169] In subchronic inhalation assays with 1,2-dibromoethane, rats and mice developed squamous cell metaplasia, hyperplasia, and cytomegaly of the respiratory nasal turbinates.[170]

The metabolism of 1,2-dibromoethane has been studied in vivo and in vitro in the rat. Some aspects of this work are outlined in Figure 10. Conjugation with glutathione is an important metabolic pathway leading initially to (2), followed by hydrolysis to S-(2-hydroxyethyl)glutathione (5). Traces of S,S'-ethylene bisglutathione (3) are also formed. S-(2-hydroxyethyl)cysteine (6) and the mercapturic acid (7), as well as the corresponding S-oxides, have been identified as urinary metabolites of 1,2-dibromoethane in the rat. Carbon dioxide is also produced from 1,2-dibromoethane, apparently by way of (6) and its S-oxide. These reactions are most likely detoxification pathways for 1,2-dibromoethane.[171-173]

In microsomal systems, bromoacetaldehyde (4) has been identified as a metabolite of 1,2-dibromoethane.[174] The formation of this metabolite in vivo or its involvement in the eventual excretion of (7) have not been established. Bromoacetaldehyde may result from direct hydroxylation of 1,2-dibromoethane to give the unstable bromohydrin (1) or it may be formed by oxidation of 2-bromoethanol. However, the latter has not been observed as a metabolite of 1,2-dibromoethane. Another possible route to bromoacetaldehyde is dehydrohalogenation to vinyl bromide, oxidation to its epoxide, and rearrangement.[175] Regardless of its mode of formation, bromoacetaldehyde would appear to be important in the macromolecular binding of 1,2-dibromoethane, which has been demonstrated in vivo and in vitro.[175-177]

The in vitro binding of 1,2-dibromoethane to protein and to salmon sperm DNA requires microsomal oxidation.[174,175] However, bromoacetaldehyde reacts with DNA and protein in the absence of an activating system. Its rates of reaction with these macromolecules exceed those of 2-bromoethanol.[177] Haloacetaldehydes form bridged derivatives with nucleic acid bases, e.g., $1,N^2$-ethenoguanosine, $1,N^6$-ethenoadenosine, and $3,N^4$-ethenocytidine.[178,179] Such adducts (see Figure 14) could be involved in carcinogenesis by 1,2-dibromoethane. The observation that 1,2-dibromoethane affects primarily the tissue to which it is applied suggests that the relevant activation processes take place in that tissue. Thus, it appears likely that oxidation of 1,2-dibromoethane to bromoacetaldehyde and macromolecular binding can occur in the nasal cavity after exposure by inhalation. However, these processes have not yet been demonstrated.

XIII. DIMETHYLCARBAMOYL CHLORIDE

Dimethylcarbamoyl chloride (DMCC, (1), Figure 11) is a highly reactive derivative of carbamic acid. It is used as a chemical intermediate in the production of the drugs pyrodistigmine bromide, neostigmine bromide, and neostigmine methosulfate, and in the preparation of carbamate pesticides in West Germany, U.K., and U.S.[180] The ethyl analogue of DMCC, diethylcarbamoyl chloride (DECC) (2), is extensively used in the production of the antifilarial drug, diethyl carbamazine citrate.[181] In microbial and bacterial mutagenicity assays, both DMCC and DECC are positive without enzymatic activation, DECC being somewhat weaker than DMCC.[182,183]

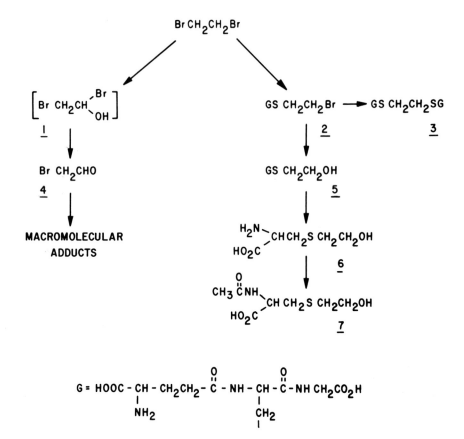

FIGURE 10.   Some aspects of the metabolism of 1,2-dibromoethane.

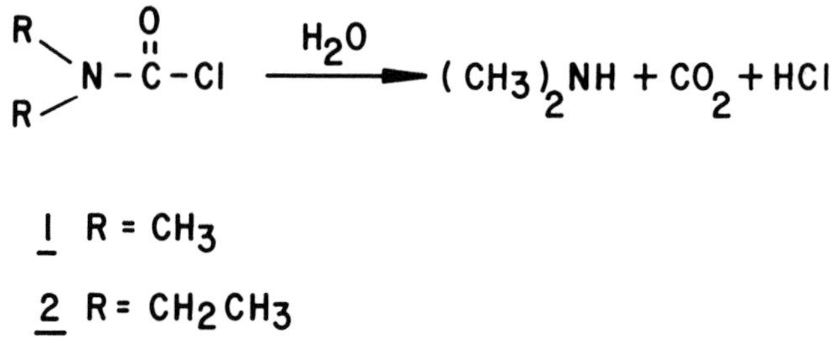

$$ \underset{R}{\overset{R}{\diagdown}} N - \overset{\overset{O}{\parallel}}{C} - Cl \quad \xrightarrow{\ H_2O\ } \quad (CH_3)_2NH + CO_2 + HCl $$

1 R = CH$_3$

2 R = CH$_2$CH$_3$

FIGURE 11.   Hydrolysis of dimethylcarbamoyl chloride (1) and diethylcarbamoyl chloride (2).

DMCC is considered as one of the most potent direct-acting acylating carcinogens, its carcinogenic activity on mouse skin being greater than that of bis-chloromethylether or β-propiolactone. Skin painting of ICR/Ha Swiss mice with DMCC caused a high incidence of skin papillomas and carcinomas. A few lung papillomas were also observed.[184] After subcutaneous injection of DMCC, a high incidence of local sarcomas was reported.[184]

An inhalation carcinogenicity study was undertaken with rats and male Syrian Golden hamsters. The animals were exposed to 1 ppm of DMCC, 6 hr/day, 5 days/week for life. After 625 days, 75% of the hamsters had developed squamous cell carcinomas of the nasal cavity. Rats showed increased sensitivity to DMCC due to irritation and died earlier than hamsters.[185]

$$CI-CH_2-O-CH_2-CI \qquad CI-CH_2-O-CH_3$$

$$\underline{1} \qquad\qquad\qquad \underline{2}$$

FIGURE 12.   Structures of bis(chloromethyl)ether (1) and chloromethyl methyl ether (2).

DMCC is rapidly hydrolyzed in water to form dimethylamine, hydrochloric acid, and carbon dioxide, its half-life being 6 min. Bis-(chloromethyl)ether and epichlorohydrin are also direct-acting carcinogens with half-lives of 0.5 and 1000 min in hydrolysis. Inhalation studies in Sprague-Dawley rats suggest a positive relationship between rates of hydrolysis and carcinogenic potency in the respiratory tract.[186] Both DMCC and DECC react with DNA in vitro to give the corresponding O^6-dialkylcarbamoylde-oxyguanosine and 2-amino-N^6-dialkyldeoxyadenosine. These adducts could be involved in carcinogenesis by DMCC and DECC.[187]

XIV. BIS(CHLOROMETHYL)ETHER

The high risk of laboratory workers exposed to bis(chloromethyl)ether (BCME, (1), Figure 12) for lung cancer, and predominately for oat-celled carcinomas, has been documented.[188,189] Workers handling chloromethyl methyl ether (2), which contains 1 to 8% of BCME, also have an increased risk for lung cancer.[190,191] In a long-term inhalation experiment with 0.1 ppm BCME, nasal cavity tumors were induced in 26 of 200 Sprague-Dawley rats.[192] Inhalation of low doses of BCME (1 ppm) led to an increased incidence of lung adenomas in mice.[193] BCME is highly genotoxic as a tumor initiator as well as a complete carcinogen on mouse skin.[194-196] In model studies, it has been shown that traces of hydrochloric acid and formaldehyde in air can lead to BCME formation in an equilibrium.[197]

BCME is known to be an in vitro alkylating agent of exceptional reactivity.[189,197] In water it hydrolyzes to formaldehyde and hydrochloric acid. Either BCME or its hydrolysis product, formaldehyde, could react with DNA. Model studies on the reaction of calf thymus DNA with ^{14}C-BCME and with ^{14}C-formaldehyde have shown that DNA alkylation with BCME is quite different from that obtained with formaldehyde. BCME is bound to DNA to a greater extent than is formaldehyde.[198] At present, however, we are lacking details as to the site of the binding of BCME to DNA and to other cellular macromolecules.

XV. VINYL CHLORIDE

Vinyl chloride is a major industrial chemical. It is estimated that in the U.S. alone about 4 million tons are produced annually.[199] Vinyl chloride is primarily used for the synthesis of homo- and copolymer resins. Workers exposed to the monomer have an increased risk for cancer of the liver, brain, lung, and hemolymphopoietic system. Similar carcinogenic effects were reported in mice, rats, and hamsters.[200]

In an inhalation study, 62 male and 62 female rats were exposed to an atmosphere containing 5000 ppm of vinyl chloride. After 4, 13, 26, and 52 weeks, 10 rats of each sex were killed and thoroughly examined. Of the rats examined after 52 weeks of inhalation, 5 females and 2 males had carcinoma of the olfactory epithelium.[244]

Vinyl chloride (1), (Figure 13), is metabolized by microsomal mixed-function oxidases to chloroethylene oxide (2) which rearranges to chloroacetaldehyde (3). The latter can be oxidized to chloroacetic acid (4). Chloroethylene oxide, chloroacetaldehyde, and chloroacetic acid react directly with glutathione or enzymatically via glutathione S-transferase to form

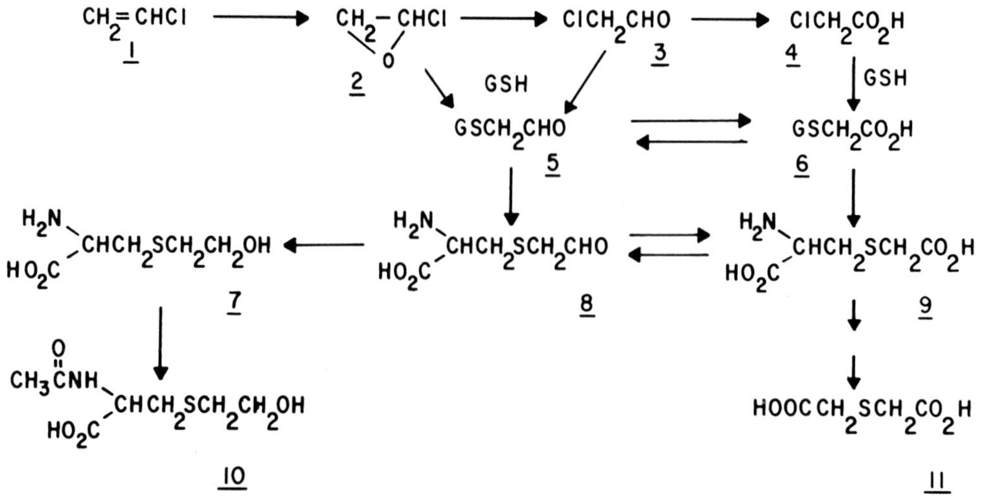

FIGURE 13.   Metabolism of vinyl chloride (1). GSH = glutathione.

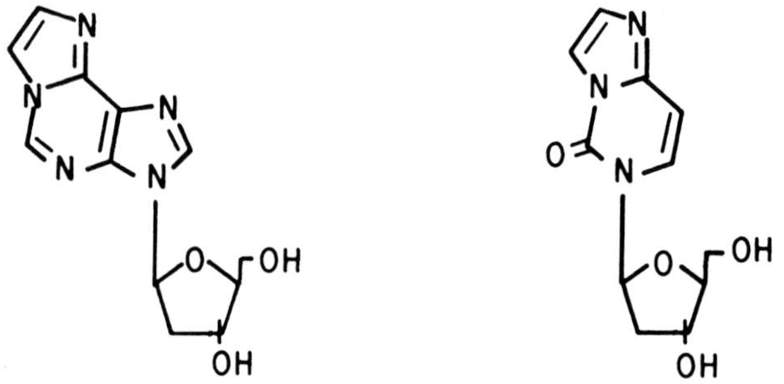

FIGURE 14.   Structures of 1,N ⁶-ethenoadenosine (1) and 3,N ⁴-ethenocytidine (2).

S-formylmethyl glutathione (5) or *S*-carboxymethylglutathione (6), respectively. Urinary excretion products include *N*-acetyl-*S*-(2-hydroxyethyl)cysteine (10), *S*-(carboxyme-thyl)cysteine (9), and thiodiglycolic acid (11).[200-203]

Both in vitro and in vivo experiments have shown that the metabolically activated form(s) of vinyl chloride react(s) with nucleic acid bases.[203-205] After enzymatic hydrolysis of the modified DNA or RNA, 9-(β-D-2'-deoxyribofuranosyl)imidazo[2,1-i]purine (1,*N*⁶-ethen-oadenosine; (1), Figure 14) and 1-(β-D-2'-deoxyribofuranosyl)imidazo[1,2-c]-pyrimid-2(1H)-one (3,*N*⁴-ethenocytidine; (2)) were isolated. The imidazole ring in these nucleoside analogs shields two normal hydrogen bonding positions and is expected to interfere with the normal Watson Crick base pairing. It has been hypothesized that these adducts of chloroethylene oxide and/or chloroacetaldehyde with the DNA bases may represent promutagenic le-sions.[196,206] The same adducts may be involved in carcinogenesis by 1,2-dibromoethane (see Section XII).

XVI. EPICHLOROHYDRIN

Epichlorohydrin is a volatile liquid which is primarily used for production of synthetic glycerol and for epoxy resins. As a carcinogen it appears to act mainly at the site of application. In Swiss mice receiving 2 mg epichlorohydrin as a tumor initiator on skin and 2.5 μg tetradecanoyl phorbol acetate (TPA) thrice weekly as tumor promoter, 9 out of 30 animals developed papilloma of the skin during the 385-day experiment. In the control group treated only with TPA, 3 out of 30 mice developed skin papilloma.[207] Upon weekly subcutaneous application of 1 mg of epichlorohydrin for up to 83 weeks, 6 out of 50 mice developed local sarcoma compared to only 1 sarcoma-bearing animal in a group of 50 mice receiving the solvent tricaprylin alone.[207]

The carcinogenicity of the direct-acting alkylating agent epichlorohydrin in inhalation experiments was demonstrated in a short-term exposure of noninbred Sprague-Dawley rats to 100 ppm and lifetime exposure of the rats to 30 ppm of the agent.[243] Thirty exposures to 100 ppm epichlorohydrin resulted in malignant squamous cell carcinomas of the nasal cavity in 15 out of 140 rats and respiratory tract papillomas in 3 rats. At 30 ppm, lifetime exposure of 100 rats yielded 1 malignant squamous carcinoma of the nasal cavity and 1 nasal papilloma. Lifetime exposure to 10 ppm epichlorohydrin produced no nasal or respiratory tract tumors, thus strengthening the dose-rate effect observed for the higher concentrations. Single 6-hr exposure of the Sprague-Dawley rats to epichlorohydrin established the median lethal concentration as 360 ppm.

Men at two plants who were exposed to epichlorohydrin had increased occurrence of deaths due to respiratory cancer (8 observed, 4.7 expected) and leukemia (2 observed, 0.4 expected). This excessive cancer incidence, however, was not statistically significant.[208]

Epichlorohydrin reacts with nucleophiles, such as alcohols and amines, primarily at the more reactive epoxide site, although reactions involving the chlorine are also known to occur. In vitro assays have demonstrated that epichlorohydrin is an alkylating agent.[209] At this time data on the in vivo alkylation by epichlorohydrin are not available. However, it is possible that it reacts with DNA to give cyclic nucleoside adducts.

XVII. FORMALDEHYDE

People may be exposed to formaldehyde in industry and in laboratories. Formaldehyde is also present in automotive exhaust and other combustion products, urban air, and tobacco smoke, as well as in indoor environments polluted with tobacco smoke or with vapors from urea-formaldehyde foams.[210,211] Exposure to trace amounts of formaldehyde may lead to irritation of the eye, the skin, and the respiratory tract, or cause headaches.

Epidemiological studies have so far not correlated exposure to formaldehyde and cancer in man.[212] In mice and Syrian Golden hamsters, formaldehyde induces hyperplasia and squamous cell metaplasia in the bronchial epithelium.[213,214] Swenberg et al.[215] exposed 120 male and 120 female rats each to 0, 2, 6, and 15 ppm formaldehyde vapors for 6 hr/day, 5 days/week. In an interim report after 18 months of exposure the authors reported carcinoma of the nasal cavity in the rats exposed to 15 ppm formaldehyde. At that time, 44 of the 240 rats had died and an additional 40 were sacrificed. Of these 84 rats, 36 had developed squamous cell carcinoma in the nasal turbinals. According to a second interim report, after 24 months exposure of the rats to formaldehyde a total of 93 animals in the 15-ppm group had developed squamous cell carcinoma of the nasal turbinals and 2 rats had respiratory carcinoma. In the 6-ppm group 2 out of 240 rats had developed carcinoma of the nasal turbinals and 2 out of 240 B6C3F1 mice exposed for up to 24 months to 15 ppm formaldehyde had developed carcinoma of the nasal turbinals.[216] The above-cited formaldehyde inhalation study has been criticized because viral infection of the salivary glands was found at the 12th month in all groups of rats. Although one cannot discount the contribution of the viral infection to the development of the nasal carcinoma in the rats, formaldehyde must be held strongly suspect as the major causative agent for the development of these carcinomas.[217]

The major route of biotransformation of formaldehyde is its oxidation to formic acid followed by further oxidation to carbon dioxide and water.[218] Application of radiolabeled formaldehyde to rats by the oral or intraperitoneal route resulted in 40 and 82%, respectively, of the label being exhaled as carbon dioxide. The remaining label was found in urine as methionine, serine, and as an adduct from cysteine and formaldehyde.[219,220] Investigations of formaldehyde distribution by whole body autoradiography are discussed by Brittebo and Tjälve in Chapter 11.

Formaldehyde reacts with DNA to yield adducts which are thought to involve the formation of labile methylol products. The latter can be easily removed or react further to form stable methylene bridges involving either amino groups of proteins or DNA.[221] Chemical structures of the DNA adducts are not known.

XVIII. NICKEL AND NICKEL COMPOUNDS

Nickel is most likely an essential trace element for the nutrition of man and animals.[222] It is commonly detected in food (≤ 7.6 ppm), drinking water (≤ 75 μg/1), and urban air (≤ 0.2 μg/m^3).[222,223] However, epidemiological studies have also demonstrated a high risk of cancer of the nasal cavity and lung for workers in nickel refineries (see Chapter 2, Volume II). Nickel has also been incriminated as one factor contributing to the increased risk of cancer of the lung in cigarette smokers. Since nickel is found not only in the particulate phase but also in the gaseous phase of cigarette smoke, it is presumably partially present as nickel carbonyl. In whole tobacco smoke, nickel concentrations reach up to 3 μg per cigarette.[224] Cigarette smoking has been discussed also as a cofactor for the increased lung cancer risk of nickel workers but not for cancer of the nasal cavity.[225]

Long-term inhalation exposure of rats to nickel carbonyl (Ni[CO]$_4$) has led to a few pulmonary malignancies.[222,226] Nickel subsulfide (Ni$_3$S$_2$) is the most potent metal carcinogen tested in laboratory animals. Upon inhalation of an aerosol of Ni$_2$S$_3$ for 78 weeks, 14 out of 570 rats developed malignant neoplasms of the lung.[227] Intramuscular injection of nickel subsulfide or nickel oxide induced rhabdomyosarcoma and fibrosarcoma in a high percentage of rats and mice.[222,223] A dose response relationship for local tumor induction after intramuscular injection of nickel subsulfide has been demonstrated in rats.[223] A number of other nickel compounds including nickel powder, carbonate, and hydroxide have also induced tumors in rats, mice, and hamsters.[222,223] Long-term inhalation experiments with nickel powder led to epidermoid lung lesions in 15 out of 50 rats and in some rats to inflammatory changes and mucosal ulcers in the paranasal sinuses.[228]

Under various conditions, Ni(II) can activate or inhibit numerous enzymatic reactions including the induction of benzo(a)pyrene hydroxylase activity in lung and liver of rats.[229] In order to elucidate the mechanisms of nickel carcinogenesis a number of in vivo and in vitro studies have been initiated.[230] Nickel(II) induces mispairing of bases in polynucleotide strands and decreases the fidelity of DNA replication by AMV-DNA polymerase. The inhibition of the DNA polymerase by carcinogenic nickel compounds has been demonstrated in rat embryo cells exposed to Ni$_2$S$_3$, whereas Ni(CO)$_4$ has been shown to inhibit RNA polymerase activity in rat hepatocytes.[231,232] These and other experimental data suggest that nickel carcinogenesis may be mediated by effects of Ni(II) on DNA and RNA synthesis with inhibition of DNA polymerase and RNA polymerase activities and with diminution of fidelity of DNA replication.

XIX. ISOPROPYL OILS

Workers in isopropyl alcohol manufacturing plants using the strong-acid process have an elevated risk of cancer of the paranasal sinuses and possibly of the larynx (see Chapter 5,

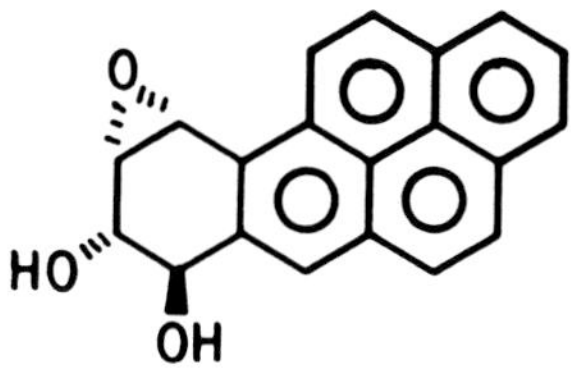

FIGURE 15. Structures of major ultimate carcinogens of benzo(a)pyrene (1) and 5-methylchrysene (2) and the major benzo(a)pyrene DNA adduct (3).

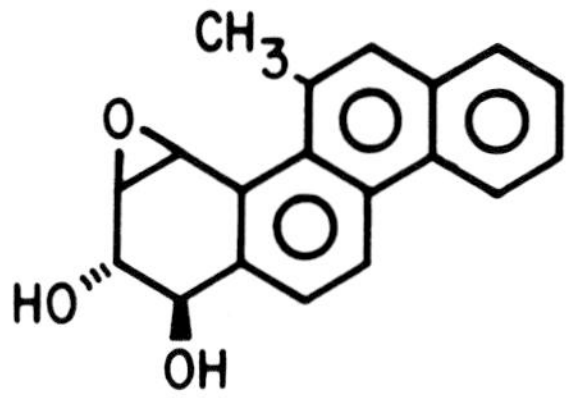

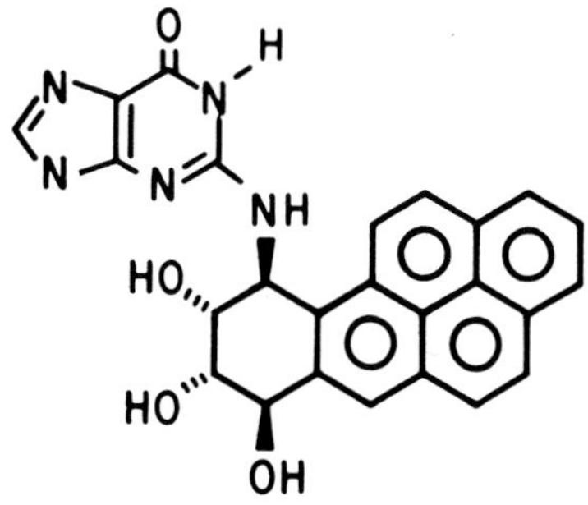

Volume I). The strong-acid process forms isopropyl oils as byproducts. These are considered to be the carcinogenic factors generated during the technical synthesis.[233] This concept is supported by the observation that the reaction products deriving from the strong-acid process, but not those from the weak-acid process, induce skin tumors in mice.[234] In two strains of mice a single application of 25 μℓ of isopropyl oils from the strong-acid process induced an increased incidence of lung adenomas.[234] Exposure of mice to an aerosol mist of isopropyl oils led to a small but statistically significant increase in lung tumors.[235]

In addition to tri- and tetrameric polypropylene, isopropyl oils from the strong-acid process contain alcohols, volatile aliphatic and aromatic hydrocarbons, and polynuclear aromatic hydrocarbons (PAH).[235] The nasal passage systems of experimental animals may be resistant to the carcinogenic action of certain PAH.[236] Nevertheless, a brief summary of the metabolic activation of genotoxic PAH is indicated, since most tissues are able to metabolize PAH and certain members of this class may be carcinogenic in the nasal cavity. A number of carcinogenic PAH are metabolically activated to dihydrodihydroxyepoxides in the angular ring of the bay region of the PAH.[237] This ultimate carcinogenic form is exemplified for benzo(a)pyrene (BaP) by 7,8-dihydroxy-9,10-epoxy-7,8,9,10-tetrahydroBaP (1), (Figure 15). In the case of methylated PAH a "bay-region" methyl group and a free peri-position, both adjacent to an unsubstituted angular ring, favor the metabolic activation through dihydro-dihydroxyepoxides. As an example, the ultimate carcinogenic form of 5-methylchrysene is shown in (2) of Figure 15.[238]

The dihydrodihydroxyepoxides may react with cellular macromolecules including DNA. The major BaP-DNA adduct in mouse skin is a reaction product of a single enantiomer of 7α,8β-dihydroxy-9β,10β-epoxy-7,8,9,10-tetrahydroBaP with the C-2 amino of guanosine[239] (3), (Figure 15).

XX. 3,4,5-TRIMETHOXYCINNAMALDEHYDE

Workers exposed to wood dust, especially those in the furniture industry, face an increased

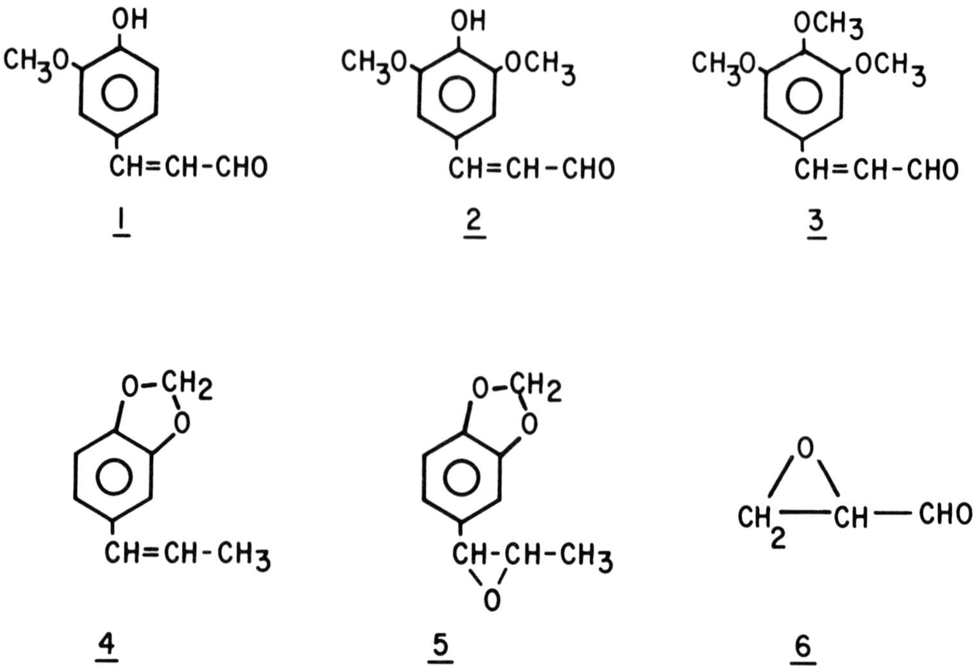

FIGURE 16.   Compounds related to 3,4,5-trimethoxycinnamaldehyde (3): coniferaldehyde (1), sinapaldehyde (2), isosafrole (4), epoxyisosafrole (5), and glycidal (6).

risk for cancer of the nasal cavity (see Chapter 5, Volume I). However, at present we do not know the nature of the tumorigenic agent(s) in wood dust. Schoental and Gibbard[240] hypothesized that methoxylation of certain lignin compounds with an α,β-unsaturated aldehyde group such as coniferyl aldehyde (1), (Figure 16) and sinapaldehyde (2) may lead to tumorigenic agents. Therefore, the authors synthesized 3,4,5-trimethoxycinnamaldehyde (3) as a representative compound and injected it into six male rats at a dose of 250 mg/kg. Of the four rats surviving 17 months after treatment, two developed carcinoma of the nasal cavity. Although this finding needs to be confirmed, it remains an important observation.

Since 3,4,5-trimethoxycinnamaldehyde has an α,β-unsaturated aldehyde group in m- and p-position to phenolic ether groups, its metabolism may be similar to that of the weak carcinogen isosafrole (4) which can be epoxidized to (5).[241] The structurally related epoxide of acrolein, glycidal (6), is a known animal carcinogen.[242] However, metabolism studies on 3,4,5-trimethoxycinnamaldehyde have not been reported. Further studies on the identification of the tumorgenic agent in wood dust are indicated.

Note Added in Proof

Two important recent studies[245,246] have demonstrated that the microsomal fractions of the nasal epithelium of the rat and the dog contain relatively high levels of cytochrome P-450 dependent monooxygenases. Levels of nasal epithelium cytochrome P-450 in the rat were higher on a per gram basis than in lung, but lower than in liver. The p-nitroanisole O-demethylase activity of rat nasal epithelial microsomes was greater than that observed in microsomes from liver or lung, but the aniline hydroxylase activity was intermediate between the liver and lung activities. The nasal epithelial P-450 systems of both rat and dog were able to metabolize hexamethylphosphoramide to formaldehyde. Cytochrome P-450 dependent monooxygenases are known to be involved in the metabolic activation of most of the nasal cavity carcinogens discussed in this review. Thus, the presence of this enzyme system in the nasal epithelium indicates that many of the metabolic pathways illustrated in this chapter may also occur in the target tissue. Recently, this has been demonstrated for NNN and NNK.[247] An organ culture system for the short term maintenance of the rat nasal septum was developed. Using this system, it was demonstrated that both NNN and NNK were extensively metabolized by α-hydroxylation which is believed to be the mechanism of metabolic activation of these nasal carcinogens. In agreement with the studies described above, the metabolism of NNN and NNK was inhibited by addition to the cultures of metyrapone, a known inhibitor of cytochrome P-450 activity.

ACKNOWLEDGMENTS

This publication is dedicated to the founder of the American Health Foundation, Dr. Ernst L. Wynder, on the occasion of the tenth anniversary of the Naylor Dana Institute for Disease Prevention.

The authors thank Mrs. Connie Hickey, Mrs. Lorraine Landy, and Mrs. Bertha Stadler for their expert help in preparing this manuscript. Our studies on nitrosamine metabolism were supported by NCI Grants CA-21393 and CA-23901.

REFERENCES

1. International Agency for Research on Cancer, *IARC Monographs on the Evaluation of the Carcinogenic Risk of Chemicals to Humans: Some N-Nitroso Compounds*, Vol. 17, IARC, Lyon, 1978, 83.
2. **Schmähl, D. and Habs, M.**, Carcinogenicity of *N*-nitroso compounds. Species and route differences in regard to organotropism, *Oncology*, 37, 237, 1980.
3. **Hoffmann, F. and Graffi, A.**, Nasenhöhlentumoren bei Mäusen nach percutaner Diäthylnitrosaminapplikation, *Arch. Geschwulstforsch.*, 23, 274, 1964.
4. **Hoffmann, F. and Graffi, A.**, Carcinome der Nasenhöhle bei Mäusen nach Tropfung der Rückenhaut mit Diäthylnitrosamin, *Acta Biol. Med. Ger.*, 12, 623, 1964.
5. **Thomas, C.**, Zur Morphologie der Nasenhöhlentumoren bei der Ratte, *Z. Krebsforsch.*, 67, 1, 1965.
6. **Herrold, K. M. and Dunham, L. J.**, Induction of tumors in the Syrian hamster with diethylnitrosamine (*N*-nitrosodiethylamine), *Cancer Res.*, 23, 773, 1963.
7. **Montesano, R. and Saffiotti, U.**, Carcinogenic response of the respiratory tract of Syrian Golden hamsters to different doses of diethylnitrosamine, *Cancer Res.*, 28, 2197, 1968.
8. **Montesano, R. and Saffiotti, U.**, Carcinogenic response of the hamster respiratory tract to single subcutaneous administrations of diethylnitrosamine at birth, *J. Natl. Cancer Inst.*, 44, 413, 1970.
9. **Haas, A., Mohr, U., and Krüger, F. W.**, Comparative studies with different doses of *N*-nitrosomorpholine, *N*-nitrosopiperidine, *N*-nitrosomethylurea, and dimethylnitrosamine in Syrian Golden hamsters, *J. Natl. Cancer Inst.*, 51, 1295, 1973.
10. **McCoy, G. D., Hecht, S. S., Katayama, S., and Wynder, E. L.**, Differential effect of chronic ethanol consumption on the carcinogenicity of *N*-nitrosopyrrolidine and *N'*-nitrosonornicotine in male Syrian Golden hamsters, *Cancer Res.*, 41, 2849, 1981.
11. **Hoffmann, D., Castonguay, A., Rivenson, A., and Hecht, S. S.**, Comparative carcinogenicity and metabolism of 4-(methylnitrosamino)-*1*-(3-pyridyl)-*1*-butanone and *N'*-nitrosonornicotine in Syrian Golden hamsters, *Cancer Res.*, 41, 2386, 1981.
12. **Hilfrich, J., Hecht, S. S., and Hoffmann, D.**, A study of tobacco carcinogenesis. XV. Effects of *N'*-nitrosonornicotine and *N'*-nitrosoanabasine in Syrian Golden hamsters, *Cancer Lett.*, 2, 169, 1977.
13. **Hoffmann, D., Brunnemann, K. D., Rivenson, A., and Hecht, S. S.**, N-Nitrosodiethanolamine: analysis, formation in tobacco products and carcinogenicity in Syrian Golden hamsters, Bartsch, H., O'Neill, I. K., Castegnaro, M., and Okada, M., Eds., IARC Scientific Publ. No. 41, International Agency for Research on Cancer, Lyon, 1982, 299.
14. **Mizrahi, I. J. and Emmelot, P.**, The effect of cysteine on the metabolic changes produced by two carcinogenic *N*-nitrosodialkylamines in rat liver, *Cancer Res.*, 22, 339, 1962.

15. **Arcos, J. C., Bryant, G. M., Pastor, K. M., and Argus, M. F.,** Structural limits of specificity of methylcholanthrene-repressible nitrosamine N-dealkylases. Inhibition by analog substrates, *Z. Krebsforsch.,* 86, 171, 1976.

16. **Chan, I. Y., Dagani, D., and Archer, M. C.,** Kinetic studies on the hepatic microsomal metabolism of dimethylnitrosamine, diethylnitrosamine, and methylethylnitrosamine in the rat, *J. Natl. Cancer Inst.,* 61, 517, 1978.

17. **Heath, D. F.,** The decomposition and toxicity of dialkylnitrosamines in rats, *Biochem. J.,* 85, 72, 1962.

18. **Pegg, A. E. and Balog, B.,** Formation and subsequent excision of O^6-ethylguanine from DNA of rat liver following administration of diethylnitrosamine, *Cancer Res.,* 39, 5003, 1979.

19. **Pegg, A. E.,** Formation and metabolism of alkylated nucleosides: possible role in carcinogenesis by nitroso compounds and alkylating agents, *Adv. Cancer Res.,* 25, 195, 1977.

20. **Scherer, E., Timmer, A., and Emmelot, P.,** Formation by diethylnitrosamine and persistence of O^4-ethyl-thymidine in rat liver DNA *in vitro, Cancer Lett.,* 10, 1, 1980.

21. **Brittebo, E. B., Löfberg, B., and Tjälve, H.,** Sites of metabolism of N-nitrosodiethylamine in mice, *Chem. Biol. Interact.,* 34, 209, 1981.

22. **Diwan, B. A. and Meier, H.,** Carcinogenic effects of a single dose of diethylnitrosamine in three unrelated strains of mice: genetic dependence of the induced tumor types and incidence, *Cancer Lett.,* 1, 249, 1976.

23. **Zingmark, P. A. and Rappe, C.,** On the formation of N-nitrosodiethanolamine in a grinding fluid concentrate after storage, *Ambio,* 6, 237, 1977.

24. **Fan, T. Y., Goff, U., Song, L., Fine, D. H., Arsenault, G. P., and Biemann, K.,** N-Nitrosodiethanolamine in cosmetics, lotions, and shampoos, *Food Cosmet. Toxicol.,* 15, 423, 1977.

25. **Zweig, G., Selim, S., Hummel, R., Mittelman, A., Wright, D. P., Jr., Law, C., Jr., and Regelman, E.,** Analytical survey of N-nitroso contaminants in pesticide products, in *N-Nitroso Compounds: Analysis, Formation and Occurrence,* Walker, E. A., Griciute, L., Castegnaro, M., and Börzsonyi, M., Eds., IARC Scientific Publ. No. 31, International Agency for Research on Cancer, Lyon, 1980, 555.

26. **Schmeltz, I., Abidi, S., and Hoffmann, D.,** Tumorigenic agents in unburned processed tobacco: N-nitrosodiethanolamine and 1,1-dimethylhydrazine, *Cancer Lett.,* 2, 125, 1977.

27. **Brunnemann, K. D. and Hoffmann, D.,** Assessment of the carcinogenic N-nitrosodiethanolamine in tobacco products and tobacco smoke, *Carcinogenesis,* 2, 1123, 1981.

28. **Druckrey, H., Preussmann, R., Ivankovic, S., and Schmähl, D.,** Organotrope carcinogene Wirkungen bei 65 verschiedenen N-Nitroso Verbindungen an BD-Ratten, *Z. Krebsforsch.,* 69, 103, 1967.

29. **Preussmann, R., Habs, M., Schmähl, D., and Eisenbrand, G.,** Dose-response study on the carcinogenicity of N-nitrosodiethanolamine in male Sprague-Dawley rats, Bartsch, H., O'Neill, I. K., Castegnaro, M., and Okada, M., Eds., IARC Scientific Publ. No. 41, International Agency for Research on Cancer, Lyon, 1982, 591.

30. **Lijinsky, W., Reuber, M. D., and Manning, W. B.,** Potent carcinogenicity of nitrosodiethanolamine in rats, *Nature (London,)* 288, 589, 1980.

31. **Hilfrich, J., Schmeltz, I., and Hoffmann, D.,** Effects of N-nitrosodiethanolamine and 1,1-diethanolhydrazine in Syrian Golden hamsters, *Cancer Lett.,* 4, 55, 1977.

32. **Preussmann, R., Würtele, G., Eisenbrand, G., and Spiegelhalder, B.,** Urinary excretion of N-nitrosodiethanolamine administered orally to rats, *Cancer Lett.,* 4, 207, 1978.

33. **Michejda, C. J., Kroeger-Koepke, M. B., Koepke, S. R., and Sieh, D. H.,** Activation of nitrosamines to biological alkylating agents, in *N-Nitroso Compounds,* American Chemical Society Symp. Ser. 174, Scanlan, R. A. and Tannenbaum, S. R., Eds., American Chemical Society, Washington, D.C., 1981, chap. 1.

34. **Fajen, J. M., Carson, G. A., Rounbehler, D. P., Fan, T. Y., Vita, R., Goff, U. E., Wolf, M. H., Edwards, G. S., Fine, D. H., Reinhold, V., and Biemann, K.,** N-Nitrosamines in the rubber and tire industry, *Science,* 205, 1262, 1979.

35. **Goff, E. U., Coombs, J. R., Fine, D. H., and Baines, T. M.,** Determination of N-nitrosamines from diesel engine crankcase emissions, *Anal. Chem.,* 52, 1833, 1980.

36. **Brunnemann, K. D., Scott, J. C., and Hoffmann, D.,** N-Nitrosomorpholine and other volatile N-nitrosamines in snuff tobacco, *Carcinogenesis,* 3, 693, 1982.

37. International Agency for Research on Cancer, *IARC Monographs on the Evaluation of the Carcinogenic Risk of Chemicals to Humans: Some N-Nitroso Compounds,* Vol. 17, IARC, Lyon, 1978, 263.

38. **Mirvish, S. S.,** Formation of N-nitroso compounds: chemistry, kinetics, and *in vivo* occurrence, *Toxicol. Appl. Pharmacol.,* 31, 325, 1975.

39. **Sander, J. and Bürkle, G.,** Induktion maligner Tumoren bei Ratten durch gleichzeitige Verfütterung von Nitrit und sekundären Aminen, *Z. Krebsforsch.,* 73, 54, 1969.

40. **Stewart, B. W., Swann, P. F., Holsman, J. W., and Magee, P. N.,** Cellular injury and carcinogenesis. Evidence for alkylation of rat liver nucleic acids *in vivo* by N-nitrosomorpholine, *Z. Krebsforsch.,* 82, 1, 1974.

41. **Manson, D., Cox, P. J., and Jarman, M.,** Metabolism of *N*-nitrosomorpholine by the rat *in vivo* and by rat liver microsomes and its oxidation by the Fenton system, *Chem. Biol. Interactions*, 20, 341, 1978.

42. **Appel, K. E., Schrenk, D., Schwarz, M., Mahr, B., and Kunz, W.,** Denitrosation of *N*-nitrosomorpholine by liver microsomes; possible role of cytochrome P-450, *Cancer Lett.*, 9, 13, 1980.

43. **Süss, R.,** Zur Wirkungsweise der Nitrosamine, *Z. Naturforsch.*, 20b, 714, 1965.

44. **Hecht, S. S. and Young, R.,** Metabolic α-hydroxylation of *N*-nitrosomorpholine and 3,3,5,5-tetradeutero-*N*-nitrosomorpholine in the F-344 rat, *Cancer Res.*, 41, 5039, 1981.

45. **Lijinsky, W., Taylor, H. W., and Keefer, L. K.,** Reduction of rat liver carcinogenicity of 4-nitrosomorpholine by α-deuterium substitution, *J. Natl. Cancer Inst.*, 57, 1311, 1976.

46. **Fazio, T., Havery, D. C., and Howard, J. W.,** Determination of volatile *N*-nitrosamines in foodstuffs. I. A new cleanup technique for confirmation by GLC-MS. II. A continued survey of foods and beverages, IARC Scientific Publ. No. 31, Walker, E. A., Griciute, L., Castegnaro, M., and Børzsonyi, M., Eds., International Agency for Research on Cancer, Lyon, 1980, 419.

47. **Spiegelhalder, B., Eisenbrand, G., and Preussmann, R.,** Further studies on the occurrence of volatile and non-volatile nitrosamines in foods, IARC Scientific Publ. No. 31, Walker, E. A., Griciute, L., Castegnaro, M., and Børzsonyi, M., Eds., International Agency for Research on Cancer, Lyon, 1980, 457.

48. **Brunnemann, K. D., Yu, L., and Hoffmann, D.,** Assessment of carcinogenic volatile *N*-nitrosamines in tobacco and in mainstream and sidestream smoke from cigarettes, *Cancer Res.*, 37, 3218, 1977.

49. **Hoffmann, D., Raineri, R., Hecht, S. S., Maronpot, R., and Wynder, E. L.,** A study of tobacco carcinogenesis. XIV. Effects of *N'*-nitrosonornicotine and *N'*-nitrosoanabasine in rats, *J. Natl. Cancer Inst.*, 55, 977, 1975.

50. **Hecht, S. S., Chen, C. B., Ohmori, T., and Hoffmann, D.,** Comparative carcinogenicity in F-344 rats of the tobacco-specific nitrosamines, *N'*-nitrosonornicotine and 4-(*N*-methyl-*N*-nitrosamino)-*1*-(3-pyridyl)-*1*-butanone, *Cancer Res.*, 40, 298, 1980.

51. **Hecht, S. S., Chen, C. B., and Hoffmann, D.,** Evidence for metabolic α-hydroxylation of *N*-nitrosopyrrolidine, *Cancer Res.*, 38, 215, 1978.

52. **Hecker, L. I., Farrelly, J. G., Smith, J. H., Saavedra, J. E., and Lyon, P. E.,** Metabolism of the liver carcinogen *N*-nitrosopyrrolidine by rat liver microsomes, *Cancer Res.*, 39, 2679, 1979.

53. **Cottrell, R. C., Walters, D. G., Young, P. J., Phillips, J. C., Lake, B. G., and Gangolli, S. D.,** Studies of the urinary metabolites of *N*-nitrosopyrrolidine in the rat, *Toxicol. Appl. Pharmacol.*, 54, 368, 1980.

54. **Baldwin, J. E., Branz, S. E., Gomez, R. F., Kraft, P., Sinskey, A. J., and Tannenbaum, S. R.,** Chemical activation of nitrosamines into mutagenic agents, *Tetrahedron Lett.*, 333, 1976.

55. **Hecht, S. S., Chen, C. B., McCoy, G. D., and Hoffmann, D.,** Tobacco specific *N*-nitrosamines: occurrence, carcinogenicity, and metabolism, in *N-Nitrosamines*, American Chemical Society Symp. Ser. 101, Anselme, J. P., Ed., American Chemical Society, Washington, D. C., 1979, chap. 8.

56. **Hecht, S. S. and Chen, C. B.,** Hydrolysis of model compounds for α-hydroxylation of the carcinogens *N*-nitrosopyrrolidine and *N'*-nitrosonornicotine, *J. Org. Chem.*, 44, 1563, 1979.

57. **McCoy, G. D., Chen, C. B., Hecht, S. S., and McCoy, E. C.,** Enhanced metabolism and mutagenesis of nitrosopyrrolidine in liver fractions isolated from chronic ethanol-consuming hamsters, *Cancer Res.*, 39, 793, 1979.

58. **McCoy, G. D., Hecht, S. S., and McCoy, E. C.,** Comparison of microsomal inducer pretreatment on the *in vivo* α-hydroxylation and mutagenicity of *N*-nitrosopyrrolidine in rat and hamster liver, *Environ. Mutagen.*, 4, 221, 1982.

59. **McCoy, G. D., Katayama, S., Young, R., Wyatt, M., and Hecht, S. S.,** Influence of chronic ethanol consumption on the metabolism and carcinogenicity of tobacco related nitrosamines, Bartsch, H., O'Neill, I. K., Castegnaro, M., and Okada, M., Eds., IARC Scientific Publ. No. 41, International Agency for Research on Cancer, Lyon, 1982, 635.

60. **Hoffmann, D. and Adams, J. D.,** A study of tobacco carcinogenesis. XXIII. Carcinogenic tobacco specific *N*-nitrosamines in snuff and in the saliva of snuff dippers, *Cancer Res.*, 41, 4305, 1981.

61. **Hoffmann, D., Adams, J. D., Brunnemann, K. D., and Hecht, S. S.,** Assessment of tobacco-specific *N*-nitrosamines in tobacco products, *Cancer Res.*, 39, 2505, 1979.

62. **Hoffmann, D., Adams, J. D., Brunnemann, K. D., and Hecht, S. S.,** Formation, occurrence and carcinogenicity of *N*-nitrosamines in tobacco products, in *N-Nitroso Compounds*, American Chemical Society Symp. Ser. 174, Scanlan, R. A. and Tannenbaum, S. R., Eds., American Chemical Society, Washington, D.C., 1981, chap. 18.

63. **Williams, G. M. and Laspia, M. F.,** The detection of various nitrosamines in the hepatocyte primary culture/DNA repair test, *Cancer Lett.*, 6, 199, 1979.

64. **Boyland, E., Roe, F. J. C., and Gorrod, J. W.,** Induction of pulmonary tumours in mice by nitrosonornicotine, a possible constituent of tobacco smoke, *Nature (London)*, 202, 1126, 1964.

65. **Hecht, S. S., Chen, C. B., Hirota, N., Ornaf, R. M., Tso, T. C., and Hoffmann, D.,** Tobacco-specific nitrosamines: formation from nicotine *in vitro* and during tobacco curing and carcinogenicity in strain A mice, *J. Natl. Cancer Inst.,* 60, 819, 1978.

66. **Castonguay, A., Lin, D., Stoner, G. D., Radok, P., Furuya, K., Hecht, S. S., Schut, H. A. J., and Klaunig, J. E.,** Comparative carcinogenicity in A/J mice and metabolism by cultured mouse peripheral lung of *N'*-nitrosonornicotine, 4-(methylnitrosamino)-*1*-(3-pyridyl)-*1*-butanone and their analogues, *Cancer Res.,* in press.

67. **Singer, G. M. and Taylor, H. W.,** Carcinogenicity of *N '*-nitrosonornicotine in Sprague-Dawley rats, *J. Natl. Cancer Inst.,* 57, 1275, 1976.

68. **Hecht, S. S., Rivenson, A., and Hoffmann, D.,** unpublished data, 1981.

69. **Chen, C. B., Hecht, S. S., and Hoffmann, D.,** Metabolic α-hydroxylation of the tobacco-specific carcinogen, *N '*-nitrosonornicotine, *Cancer Res.,* 38, 3639, 1978.

70. **Chen, C. B., Fung, P. T., and Hecht, S. S.,** Assay for microsomal α-hydroxylation of *N '*-nitrosonornicotine and determination of the deuterium isotope effect for α-hydroxylation, *Cancer Res.,* 39, 5057, 1979.

71. **Hecht, S. S., Young, R., and Chen, C. B.,** Metabolism in the F-344 rat of 4-(*N*-methyl-*N*-nitrosamino)-*1*-(3-pyridyl)-*1*-butanone, a tobacco-specific carcinogen, *Cancer Res.,* 40, 4144, 1980.

72. **Hecht, S. S., Chen, C. B., and Hoffmann, D.,** Metabolic β-hydroxylation and *N*-oxidation of *N '*-nitrosonornicotine, *J. Med. Chem.,* 23, 1175, 1980.

73. **Hecht, S. S., Lin, D., and Chen, C. B.,** Comprehensive analysis of urinary metabolites of *N '*-nitrosonornicotine, *Carcinogenesis,* 2, 833, 1981.

74. **Lotlikar, P. D., Baldy, W. J., Jr., and Dwyer, E. N.,** Dimethylnitrosamine demethylation by reconstituted liver microsomal cytochrome P-450 enzyme system, *Biochem. J.,* 152, 705, 1975.

75. **Diaz Gomez, M. I. and Castro, J. A.,** Spectral changes resulting from the interaction of some *N*-alkyl nitrosamines and rat liver microsomes, *Experientia,* 33, 643, 1977.

76. **Appel, K. E., Ruf, H. H., Mahr, B., Schwarz, M., Rickart, R., and Kunz, W.,** Binding of nitrosamines to cytochrome P-450 of liver microsomes, *Chem. Biol. Interact.,* 28, 17, 1979.

77. **Brittebo, E. and Tjälve, H.,** Tissue-specificity of *N*-nitrosodibutylamine metabolism in Sprague-Dawley rats, *Chem. Biol. Interact.,* 38, 231, 1982.

78. **Hecht, S. S., Chen, C. B., McCoy, G. D., and Hoffmann, D.,** α-Hydroxylation of *N*-nitrosopyrrolidine and *N '*-nitrosonornicotine by human liver microsomes, *Cancer Lett.,* 8, 35, 1979.

79. **Castonguay, A.,** unpublished results.

80. **Magee, P. N. and Barnes, J. M.,** The production of malignant primary hepatic tumours in the rat by feeding dimethylnitrosamine, *Br. J. Cancer,* 10, 114, 1956.

81. **Waddell, W. J. and Marlowe, C.,** Localization of [^{14}C] -nitrosonornicotine in tissues of the mouse, *Cancer Res.,* 40, 3518, 1980.

82. **Brittebo, E. and Tjälve, H.,** Autoradiographic observations on the distribution and metabolism of *N'*-^{14}C-nitrosonornicotine in mice, *J. Cancer Res. Clin. Oncol.,* 98, 233, 1980.

82a. **Brittebo, E. and Tjälve, H.,** Formation of tissue-bound *N '*-nitrosonornicotine metabolites by the target tissues of Sprague-Dawley and Fischer rats, *Carcinogenesis,* 2, 959, 1981.

83. National Cancer Institute, Bioassay of *p*-cresidine for possible carcinogenicity, NCI Carcinogenesis Tech. Rep. Ser. No. 142, CAS No. 120-71-8, 1978.

84. **Reznik, G., Reznik-Schüller, H. M., Hayden, D. W., Russfield, A., and Krishna Murthy, A. S.,** Morphology of nasal cavity neoplasms in F-344 rats after chronic feeding of *p*-cresidine, an intermediate of dyes and pigments, submitted.

85. **Weisburger, E. K., Russfield, A. B., Homburger, F., Weisburger, J. H., Boger, E., van Dongen, C. G., and Chu, K. C.,** Testing of twenty-one environmental aromatic amines or derivatives for long-term toxicity or carcinogenicity, *J. Environ. Pathol. Toxicol.,* 2, 325, 1978.

86. National Cancer Institute, Bioassay of *o*-anisidine hydrochloride for possible carcinogenicity, NCI Tech. Rep. Ser. No. 89, CAS No. 134-29-0, DHEW Pub. No. (NIH) 78-1339, 1978.

87. National Cancer Institute, Bioassay of *p*-anisidine hydrocloride for possible carcinogenicity, NCI Tech. Rep. Ser. No. 116, CAS No. 20265-97-8, DHEW Publ. No. (NIH) 78-1371, 1978.

88. **Clayson, D. B. and Garner, R. C.,** Carcinogenic aromatic amines and related compounds, in *Chemical Carcinogens,* American Chemical Society Monograph 173, Searle, C. E., Ed., American Chemical Society, Washington, D.C., 1976, chap. 8.

89. **Miller, E. C. and Miller, J. A.,** The metabolism of chemical carcinogens to reactive electrophiles and their possible mechanism of action in carcinogenesis, in *Chemical Carcinogens,* American Chemical Society Monograph 173, Searle, C. E., Ed., American Chemical Society, Washington, D. C., 1976, chap. 16.

90. **Son, O. S., Everett, D. W., and Fiala, E. S.,** Metabolism of *o* -[methyl-^{14}C] toluidine in the F-344 rat, *Xenobiotica,* 10, 457, 1980.

91. **Hecht, S. S., El-Bayoumy, K., Tulley, L., and LaVoie, E.,** Structure-mutagenicity relationships of *N* -oxidized derivatives of aniline, *o*-toluidine, 2'-methyl-4-aminobiphenyl, and 3,2'-dimethyl-4-aminobiphenyl, *J. Med. Chem.*, 22, 981, 1979.

91a. International Agency for Research on Cancer, *IARC Monographs on the Evaluation of the Carcinogenic Risk of Chemicals to Humans: Some Pharmaceutical Drugs,* Vol. 24, IARC, Lyon, 1981, 135.

92. **Weinstein, D., Katz, M., and Kazmer, S.,** Use of a rat/hamster S-9 mixture in the Ames mutagenicity assay, *Environ. Mutagen,* 3, 1, 1981.

93. **Nagao, M., Sugimura, T., and Matsushima, T.,** Environmental mutagens and carcinogens, *Ann. Rev. Genet.*, 12, 117, 1978.

94. **Ishidate, M., Jr. and Odashima, S.,** Chromosome tests with 134 compounds on Chinese hamster cells *in vitro* — a screening for chemical carcinogens, *Mutat. Res.*, 48, 337, 1977.

95. **Granberg-Öhman, I., Johansson, S., and Hjerpe, A.,** Sister-chromatid exchanges and chromosomal aberrations in rats treated with phenacetin, phenazone and caffeine, *Mutat. Res.*, 79, 13, 1980.

96. National Cancer Institute, Bioassay of a mixture of aspirin, phenacetin and caffeine for possible carcinogenicity, NCI Carcinogenesis Tech. Rep. Ser. No. 67, Department of Health, Education and Welfare, Washington, D.C., 1978.

97. **Woodard, G., Post, K. F., Cockrell, K. O., and Cronin, M. T.,** Phenacetin — long-term studies in rats and dogs, *Toxicol. Appl. Pharmacol.*, 7, 503, 1965.

98. **Schmähl, D. and Reiter, A.,** Fehlen einer cancerogenen Wirkung beim Phenacetin, *Arzneim. Forsch.*, 4, 404, 1954.

99. **Macklin, A. W., Welch, R. M., and Cuatrecasas, P.,** Drug safety: phenacetin, *Science*, 205, 144, 1979.

100. **Studer, A. and Schärer, K.,** Langfristige Phenacetinbelastung am Hund mit Berücksichtigung der Leber- und Nierenpigmentierung, *Schweiz. Med. Wochenschr.*, 95, 933, 1965.

101. **Isaka, H., Yoshii, H., Otsuji, A., Koike, M., Nagai, Y., Koura, M., Sugiyasu, K., and Kanabayashi, T.,** Tumors of Sprague-Dawley rats induced by long-term feeding of phenacetin, *Gann,* 70, 29, 1979.

102. **Johansson, S. and Angervall, L.,** Urothelial changes of the renal papillae in Sprague-Dawley rats induced by long-term feeding of phenacetin, *Acta Pathol. Microbiol. Scand. Sect. A,* 84, 375, 1976.

103. **Vaught, J. B. and King, C. M.,** Phenacetin studies, *Science,* 206, 637, 1979.

104. **Macklin, A. W. and Welch, R. M.,** Phenacetin safety, *Science,* 207, 129, 1980.

105. **Dubach, U. C. and Raaflaub, J.,** Neue Aspekte zur Frage der Nephrotoxizität von Phenacetin, *Experientia,* 25, 956, 1969.

106. **Brodie, B. B. and Axelrod, J.,** The fate of acetophenetidin (phenacetin) in man and methods for the estimation of acetophenetidin and its metabolites in biological material, *J. Pharmacol. Exp. Ther.*, 97, 58, 1949.

107. **Nelson, S. D., Garland, W. A., Mitchell, J. R., Vaishnow, Y., Statham, C. N., and Buckpitt, A. R.,** Deuterium isotope effects on the metabolism and toxicity of phenacetin in hamsters, *Drug Metab. Dispos.*, 6, 363, 1978.

108. **Poppers, P. J., Levin, W., and Conney, A. H.,** Effect of 3-methylcholanthrene treatment on phenacetin *O* -dealkylation in several inbred mouse strains, *Drug Metab. Dispos.*, 3, 502, 1975.

109. **Conney, A. H., Sansur, M., Soroko, F., Koster, R., and Burns, J. J.,** Enzyme induction and inhibition in studies on the pharmacological actions of acetophenetidin, *J. Pharmacol. Exp. Ther.*, 151, 133, 1966.

110. **Pantuck, E. J., Hsiao, K-C., Maggio, A., Nakamura, K., Kuntzman, R., and Conney, A. H.,** Effect of cigarette smoking on phenacetin metabolism, *Clin. Pharmacol. Ther.*, 15, 9, 1974.

111. **Welch, R. M., Hughes, C. R., and Deangelis, R. L.,** Effect of 3-methylcholanthrene pretreatment on the bioavailability of phenacetin in the rat, *Drug Metab. Dispos.*, 4, 402, 1976.

112. **Pantuck, E. J., Hsiao, K-C., Loub, W. D., Wattenberg, L. W., Kuntzman, R., and Conney, A. H.,** Stimulatory effect of vegetables on intestinal drug metabolism in the rat, *J. Pharmacol. Exp. Ther.*, 198, 278, 1976.

113. **Pantuck, E. J., Hsiao, K-C., Conney, A. H., and Garland, W. A.,** Effect of charcoal-broiled beef on phenacetin metabolism in man, *Science,* 194, 1055, 1976.

114. **Hinson, J. A. and Mitchell, J. R.,** *N*-Hydroxylation of phenacetin by hamster liver microsomes, *Drug Metab. Dispos.*, 4, 430, 1976.

115. **Mitchell, J. R., Potter, W. Z., Hinson, J. A., Snodgrass, W. R., Timbrell, J. A., and Gillette, J. R.,** in *Handbook of Experimental Pharmacology,* Eichler, O., Farah, A., Herken, H., and Welch, A., Eds., Springer-Verlag, Berlin, 1975, 383.

116. **Calder, I. C., Creek, M. J., and Williams, P. J.,** *N*-Hydroxyphenacetin as a precursor of 3-substituted 4-hydroxyacetanilide metabolites of phenacetin, *Chem. Biol. Interact.*, 8, 87, 1974.

117. **Hinson, J. A., Nelson, S. D., and Mitchell, J. R.,** Studies on the microsomal formation of arylating metabolites of acetaminophen and phenacetin, *Mol. Pharmacol.*, 13, 625, 1977.

118. **Nelson, S. D., Vaishow, Y., Mitchell, J. R., Gillette, J. R., and Hinson, J. A.,** The use of ^{2}H and ^{18}O to examine arylating and alkylating pathways of phenacetin metabolism, *Proc. 3rd Int. Symp. Stable Isotopes,* Klein, E. and Klein, P. D., Eds., Academic Press, New York, 1979, 385.

119. **Smith, R. L. and Timbrell, J. A.,** Factors affecting the metabolism of phenacetin. I. Influence of dose, chronic dosage, route of administration and species on the metabolism of [1-^{14}C-acetyl]phenacetin, *Xenobiotica,* 4, 489, 1974.

120. **Nery, R.,** Some new aspects of the metabolism of phenacetin in the rat, *Biochem. J.,* 122, 317, 1971.

121. **Nery, R.,** The possible role of *N*-hydroxylation in the biological effects of phenacetin, *Xenobiotica,* 1, 339, 1971.

122. **Hinson, J. A., Andrews, L. S., and Gillette, J. R.,** Kinetic evidence for multiple chemically reactive intermediates in the breakdown of phenacetin *N-O* -glucuronide, *Pharmacology,* 19, 237, 1979.

123. **Calder, I. C., Creek, M. J., Williams, P. J., Funder, C. C., Green, C. R., Ham, K. N., and Tange, J. D.,** *N*-Hydroxylation of *p*-acetophenetidine as a factor in nephrotoxicity, *J. Med. Chem.,* 16, 499, 1973.

124. **Shudo, K., Ohta, T., Orihara, Y., Okamoto, T., Nagao, M., Takahashi, Y., and Sugimura, T.,** Mutagenicities of phenacetin and its metabolites, *Mutat. Res.,* 58, 367, 1978.

125. **Sawamura, M., Matsushima, T., and Sugimura, T.,** The utility of hamster S9-mix, mutagenicity of phenacetin and its analogs, Proc. Jpn. Cancer Assoc., 37th Annu. Meet., August 1978, 43.

126. **Calder, I. C., Goss, D. E., Williams, P. J., Funder, C. C., Green, C. R., Ham, K. N., and Tange, J. D.,** Neoplasia in the rat induced by *N*-hydroxyphenacetin metabolite of phenacetin, *Pathology,* 8, 1, 1976.

127. **Mulder, G. J., Hinson, J. A., and Gillette, J. R.,** Generation of reactive metabolites of *N*-hydroxyphenacetin by glucuronidation and sulfation, *Biochem. Pharmacol.,* 26, 189, 1977.

128. **Mulder, G. J., Hinson, J. A., and Gillette, J. R.,** Conversion of the *N-O*-glucuronide and *N-O*-sulfate conjugates of *N*-hydroxyphenacetin to reactive intermediates, *Biochem. Pharmacol.,* 27, 1641, 1978.

129. **Vaught, J. B., McGarvey, P. B., Lee, M.-S., Garner, C. D., Wang, C. Y., Linsmaier-Bedrar, E. M., and King, C. M.,** Activation of *N*-hydroxyphenacetin to mutagenic and nucleic acid-binding metabolites by acyltransfer, deacylation and sulfate conjugation, *Cancer Res.,* 41, 3424, 1981.

130. **Hoch-Ligeti, C., Argus, M. F., and Arcos, J. C.,** Induction of carcinomas in the nasal cavity of rats by dioxane, *Br. J. Cancer,* 24, 164, 1970.

131. **Kociba, R. J., McCollister, S. B., Park, C., Torkelson, T. R., and Gehring, P. J.,** 1,4-Dioxane. I. Results of a 2-year ingestion study in rats, *Toxicol. Appl. Pharmacol.,* 30, 275, 1974.

131a. National Cancer Institute, Bioassay of 1,4-dioxane for possible carcinogenicity, NCI Carcinogenesis Tech. Rep. Ser. No. 80, DHEW Publ. No. (NIH) 78-1330, Washington, D.C., 1978.

132. **Torkelson, T. R., Leong, B. K. J., Kociba, R. J., Richter, W. A., and Gehring, P. J.,** 1,4-Dioxane. II. Results of a 2-year inhalation study in rats, *Toxicol. Appl. Pharmacol.,* 30, 287, 1974.

133. **Argus, M. F., Arcos, J. C., and Hoch-Ligeti, C.,** Studies on the carcinogenic activity of protein-denaturing agents: hepatocarcinogenicity of dioxane, *J. Natl. Cancer Inst.,* 35, 949, 1965.

134. **Woo, Y.-T., Arcos, J. C., Argus, M. F., Griffin, G. W., and Nishiyama, K.,** Structural identification of *p*-dioxan-2-one as the major urinary metabolite of *p*-dioxane, *Naunyn-Schmiedeberg's Arch. Pharmacol.,* 299, 283, 1977.

135. **Braun, W. H. and Young, D. J.,** Identification of β-hydroxyethoxyacetic acid as the major urinary metabolite of 1,4-dioxane in the rat, *Toxicol. Appl. Pharmacol.,* 39, 33, 1977.

136. **Woo, Y.-T., Argus, M. F., and Arcos, J. C.,** Metabolism *in vivo* of dioxane: effect of inducers and inhibitors of hepatic mixed-function oxidases, *Biochem. Pharmacol.,* 25, 1539, 1977.

137. National Institute for Occupational Safety and Health, Background Information on Hexamethyl Phosphoric Triamide, U.S. Department of Health, Education and Welfare, Rockville, Md., 1975.

138. **Chang, S. C., Terry, P. H., and Borkovec, A. B.,** Insect chemosterilants with low toxicity for mammals, *Science,* 144, 57, 1964.

139. **Borkovec, A. B.,** in *Insect Chemosterilants,* Wiley-Interscience, New York, 1966.

140. **Terry, P. H. and Borkovec, A. B.,** Phosphoramides and thiophosporamides as insect chemosterilants, U.S. Patent 3,205,130, 1965.

141. International Agency for Research on Cancer, *IARC Monographs on the Evaluation of the Carcinogenic Risk of Chemicals to Man,* Vol. 15, IARC, Lyon, 1977, 211.

142. **Bemes, V. and Sram, R. J.,** Mutagenic activity of some pesticides in *Drosophila melanogaster, Ind. Med. Surg.,* 38, 442, 1969.

143. **Ashby, J., Styles, J. A., and Anderson, D.,** Selection of an in vitro carcinogenicity test for derivatives of the carcinogen hexamethylphosphoramide, *Br. J. Cancer,* 36, 564, 1977.

144. **Jackson, H. and Craig, A. W.,** Antifertility action and metabolism of hexamethylphosphoramide, *Nature (London),* 212, 86, 1966.

145. **Zapp, J. A., Jr.,** HMPA: a possible carcinogen, *Science,* 190, 422, 1975.

146. **Kimbrough, R. D. and Gaines, T. B.,** The chronic toxicity of hexamethylphosphoramide in rats, *Bull. Environ. Contam. Toxicol.,* 10, 225, 1973.

147. **Kimbrough, R. D. and Sedlak, V. A.,** Lung morphology in rats treated with hexamethylphosphoramide, *Toxicol. Appl. Pharmacol.,* 12, 60, 1968.

148. **Jones, A. R. and Bertram, J. S.,** The metabolism of hexamethylphosphoramide and hexamethylthio-phosphoramide, *Experientia,* 24, 326, 1968.

149. **Godfrain, J.-C., Rico, A. G., Lorgue, G., Burgat, V., Sy, M., Maillet, M., Megemont, C., Felix, C., Borrel, A., and Dumas, G.,** Contribution a l'etude, a l'aide de phosphore radioactif, du metabolisme de l'hexametapol ^{32}P (H.M.P.T.) chez les ovins et les bovins, *Rev. Med. Vet.,* 122, 371, 1971.

150. **Endicott, K. M.,** Current chemotherapy for cancer, *Modern Med.,* 260, 1957.

151. **Smith, C. N., Labrecque, G. C., and Borkovec, A. B.,** Insect chemosterilants, in *Annual Review of Entomology,* Vol. 9, Smith, R. F. and Mittler, T. E., Eds., Annual Reviews, Palo Alto, Calif., 1964, 269.

152. **Stoner, G. D., Shimkin, M. B., Kniazeff, A. J., Weisburger, J. H., Weisburger, E. K., and Gori, G. B.,** Tests for carcinogenicity of food additives and chemotherapeutic agents by the pulmonary tumor response in strain A mice, *Cancer Res.,* 33, 3069, 1973.

153. National Cancer Institute, Bioassay of thiotepa for possible carcinogenicity, NCI Tech. Rep. Ser. No. 58, DHEW Publ. No. (NIH) 78-1308, U.S. Government Printing Office, Washington, D.C., 1978.

154. **Schmähl, D. and Osswald, H.,** Experimentelle Untersuchungen über carcinogene Wirkungen von Krebs-Chemotherapeutica and Immunosuppressiva, *Arzneimittel-Forsch.,* 20, 1461, 1970.

155. **Greenspan, E. M. and Tung, B. G.,** Acute myeloblastic leukaemia after cure of ovarian cancer, *JAMA,* 230, 418, 1974.

156. **Allan, W. S. A.,** Acute myeloid leukaemia after treatment with cytostatic agents, *Lancet,* 2, 775, 1970.

157. **Perlman, M. and Walker, R.,** Acute leukaemia following cytotoxic chemotherapy, *JAMA,* 224, 250, 1973.

158. **Mellett, L. B. and Woods, L. A.,** The comparative physiological disposition of thio-TEPA and TEPA in the dog, *Cancer Res.,* 20, 524, 1960.

159. **Craig, A. W., Fox, B. W., and Jackson, H.,** Metabolic studies of ^{32}P-labelled triethylenethiophosphor-amide, *Biochem. Pharmacol.,* 3, 42, 1959.

160. **Boone, I. V., Rogers, B. S., and Williams, D. L.,** Toxicity, metabolism and tissue distribution of carbon-14 labeled *N,N',N''*-triethylenethiophosphoramide (thio-TEPA) in rats, *Toxicol. Appl. Pharmacol.,* 4, 344, 1962.

161. **Nadkarni, M. V., Goldenthal, E. I., and Smith, P. K.,** The distribution of radioactivity following administration of triethylene phosphoramide-^{32}P in tumor-bearing and control mice, *Cancer Res.,* 17, 97, 1957.

162. **Mellett, L. B., Hodzson, P. E., and Woods, L. A.,** Absorption and fate of ^{14}C-labelled *N,N',N''*-triethylenethiophosphoramide (thio-TEPA) in humans and dogs, *J. Lab. Clin. Med.,* 60, 818, 1962.

163. **Bateman, J. C., Carlton, H. N., Calvert, R. C., and Lindenblad, G. E.,** Investigation of distribution and excretion of ^{14}C-tagged triethylenethiophosphoramide following infection by various routes, *Int. J. Appl. Radiat.,* 7, 287, 1960.

164. **Maller, R. K. and Heidelberger, C.,** Studies on OPSPA. IV. Metabolism of OPSPA in the rat and human, *Cancer Res.,* 17, 296, 1957.

165. **Benckhuijen, C.,** Acid-catalysed conversion of triethyleneimine thiophosphoramide (thio-TEPA) to an SH compound, *Biochem. Pharmacol.,* 17, 55, 1968.

166. **Olson, W. A., Habermann, R. J., Weisburger, E. K., Ward, J. M., and Weisburger, J. H.,** Induction of stomach cancer in rats and mice by halogenated aliphatic fumigants, *J. Natl. Cancer Inst.,* 51, 1993, 1973.

167. **Weisburger, E. K.,** Carcinogenicity studies on halogenated hydrocarbons, *Environ. Health Perspect.,* 21, 7, 1977.

168. **Van Duuren, B. L., Goldschmidt, B. M., Loewengart, G., Smith, A. C., Melchionne, S., Seidman, I., and Roth, D.,** Carcinogenicity of halogenated olefinic and aliphatic hydrocarbons in mice, *J. Natl. Cancer Inst.,* 63, 1433, 1979.

169. National Cancer Institute, Inhalation bioassay of 1,2-dibromoethane for possible carcinogenicity, NCI Tech. Rep. No. 206, U.S. Department of Health and Human Services, Public Health Service, National Institutes of Health, Bethesda, Md., 1980.

170. **Reznik, G., Stinson, S. F., and Ward, J. M.,** Respiratory pathology in rats and mice after inhalation of 1,2-dibromo-3-chloropropane or 1,2-dibromoethane for 13 weeks, *Arch. Toxicol.,* 46, 233, 1980.

171. **Nachtomi, E., Alumot, E., and Bondi, A.,** The metabolism of ethylene dibromide in the rat: identification of detoxification products in urine, *Isr. J. Chem.,* 4, 239, 1966.

172. **Nachtomi, E.,** The metabolism of ethylene dibromide in the rat. The enzymatic reaction with glutathione in vitro and in vivo, *Biochem. Pharmacol.,* 19, 2853, 1970.

173. **Jones, A. R. and Edwards, K.,** The comparative metabolism of ethylene dimethanesulphonate and ethy-lenedibromide, *Experientia,* 24, 1100, 1968.

174. **Hill, D. L., Shih, T.-W., Johnston, T. P., and Struck, R. F.,** Macromolecular binding and metabolism of the carcinogen 1,2-dibromoethane, *Cancer Res.,* 38, 2438, 1978.

175. **Banerjee, S. and Van Duuren, B. L.,** Binding of carcinogenic halogenated hydrocarbons to cell ma-cromolecules, *J. Natl. Cancer Inst.,* 63, 707, 1979.

176. **Nachtomi, E. and Sarma, D. S. R.,** Repair of rat liver DNA *in vivo* damaged by ethylene dibromide, *Biochem. Pharmacol.*, 26, 1941, 1977.

177. **Banerjee, S., Van Duuren, B. L., and Kline, S. A.,** Interaction of potential metabolites of the carcinogen ethylene dibromide with protein and DNA *in vitro, Biochem. Biophys. Res. Commun.*, 90, 1214, 1979.

178. **Sattsangi, P. D., Leonard, N. J., and Frihart, C. R.,** 1,N^2-Ethenoguanine and N^2,3-ethenoguanine. Synthesis and comparison of the electronic spectral properties of these linear and angular triheterocycles related to the Y bases, *J. Org. Chem.*, 42, 3292, 1977.

179. **Kayasuga-Mikado, K., Hashimoto, T., Negishi, T., Negishi, K., and Hayatsu, H.,** Modification of adenine and cytosine derivatives with bromoacetaldehyde, *Chem. Pharm. Bull.*, 28, 932, 1980.

180. International Agency for Research on Cancer, *IARC Monographs on the Evaluation of the Carcinogenic Risk of Chemicals to Man*, Vol. 12, IARC, Lyon, 1976, 77.

181. **Nelson, N.,** The carcinogenicity of chloro ethers and related compounds: a brief note, in *Incidence of Cancer in Humans*, Proc. Cold Spring Harbor Laboratory Conference on Cell Proliferation, Watson, J. D. and Winsten, J. A., Eds., Cold Spring Harbor Laboratory, Cold Spring Harbor, N.Y., 1977, 115.

182. **Mukai, F. and Hawryluk, I.,** The mutagenicity of some halo-ethers and haloketones, *Mutat. Res.*, 20, 228, 1973.

183. **Mukai, F.,** unpublished results.

184. **Van Duuren, B. L., Goldschmidt, B. M., Katz, C., and Seidman, I.,** Brief communication. Dimethylcarbamoyl chloride, a multipotential carcinogen, *J. Natl. Cancer Inst.*, 48, 1539, 1972.

185. **Sellakumar, A. R., Laskin, S., Kuschner, M., Rusch, G., Katz, G. V., Snyder, C. A., and Albert, R. E.,** Inhalation carcinogenesis by dimethylcarbamoyl chloride in Syrian Golden hamsters, *J. Environ. Pathol. Toxicol.*, 4, 107, 1980.

186. **Dulak, N. C. and Snyder, C. A.,** The relationship between the chemical reactivity and the inhalation direct carcinogenic potency of direct-acting chemical agents, *Proc. Am. Assoc. Cancer Res.*, 21, 106, 1980.

187. **Segal, A., Mate, U., Solomon, J. J., and Van Duuren, B. L.,** Formation of O^6-acyl guanine derivatives following *in vitro* reactions between dimethyl- and diethylcarbamyl chloride with calf thymus DNA, *Proc. Am. Assoc. Cancer Res.*, 22, 84, 1981.

188. **Thiess, A. M., Hey, W., and Zeller, H.,** Zur Toxikologie von Dichloromethyläther — Verdacht auf carcinogene Wirkung auch beim Menschen, *Zentralbl. Arbeitsmed.*, 23, 97, 1973.

189. International Agency for Research on Cancer, IARC Monographs on the Evaluation of the Carcinogenic Risk of Chemicals to Humans, Vol. 4, IARC, Lyon, 1974, 231.

190. **Albert, R. E., Pasternack, B. S., Shore, R. E., Lippmann, N. N., and Ferris, B.,** Mortality patterns among workers exposed to chloromethyl ethers. A preliminary report, *Environ. Health Perspect.*, 11, 209, 1975.

191. **Pasternack, B. S., Shore, R. E., and Albert, R. E.,** Occupational exposure to chloromethyl ethers, *J. Occup. Med.*, 19, 741, 1977.

192. **Kuschner, M., Laskin, S., Drew, R. T., Cappiello, V., and Nelson, N.,** Inhalation carcinogenicity of alpha halo ethers. III. Lifetime and limited period inhalation studies with bis(chloromethyl)ether at 0.1 ppm, *Arch. Environ. Health*, 30, 73, 1975.

193. **Leong, B. K. J., MacFarland, H. N., and Reese, W. H., Jr.,** Induction of lung adenomas by chronic inhalation of bis(chloromethyl) ether, *Arch. Environ. Health*, 22, 663, 1971.

194. **Van Duuren, B. L., Goldschmidt, B. M., Katz, C., Langseth, L., Mercado, G., and Sivak, A.,** Alpha-haloethers: a new type of alkylating carcinogen., *Arch. Environ. Health*, 16, 472, 1968.

195. **Van Duuren, B. L., Katz, C., Goldschmidt, B. M., Frenkel, K., and Sivak, A.,** Carcinogenicity of halo-ethers. II. Structure-activity relationships of analogs of bis(chloromethyl)-ether, *J. Natl. Cancer Inst.*, 48, 1431, 1972.

196. **Zajdela, F., Croisy, A., Barbin, A., Malaveille, C., Tomatis, L., and Bartsch, H.,** Carcinogenicity of chloroethylene oxide: an ultimate reactive metabolite of vinyl chloride, and bis(chloromethyl)-ether after subcutaneous administration and in initiation-promotion experiments in mice, *Cancer Res.*, 40, 352, 1980.

197. **Yao, C. C. and Miller, G. C.,** Research study of bis(chloromethyl) ether formation and detection in selected work environments, DHEW (NIOSH) Publ. No. 79-118, 1979, 151.

198. **Goldschmidt, B. M., Van Duuren, B. L., and Frenkel, K.,** The reaction of ^{14}C-labelled bis(chloromethyl)-ether with DNA, *Proc. Am. Assoc. Cancer Res.*, 16, 66, 1975.

199. American Chemical Society, Key chemicals: vinyl chloride, *Chem. Eng. News*, 58, 9, 1980.

200. International Agency for Research on Cancer, *IARC Monographs on the Evaluation of the Carcinogenic Risk of Chemicals to Humans*, Vol. 19, IARC, Lyon, 1979, 377.

201. **Watanabe, P. G., McGowan, G. R., Madrid, E. O., and Gehring, P. J.,** Fate of [^{14}C]-vinyl chloride following inhalation exposure in rats, *Toxicol. Appl. Pharmacol.*, 37, 49, 1976.

202. **Green, T. and Hathway, D. E.,** The chemistry and biogenesis of the S-containing metabolites of vinyl chloride in rats, *Chem. Biol. Interact*, 17, 137, 1977.

203. **Barbin, A., Brésil, H., Croisy, A., Jacquignon, P., Malaveille, C., Montesano, R., and Bartsch, H.,** Liver microsome-mediated formation of alkylating agents from vinyl bromide and vinyl chloride, *Biochem. Biophys. Res. Commun.,* 67, 596, 1975.

204. **Laib, R. J. and Bolt, H. M.,** Alkylation of RNA by vinyl chloride metabolites *in vivo:* formation of 1,N^6-etheno-adenosine, *Toxicology,* 8, 185, 1977.

205. **Laib, R. J. and Bolt, H. M.,** Formation of 3,N^4-ethenocytidine moieties in RNA by vinyl chloride metabolites *in vitro* and *in vivo, Arch. Toxicol.,* 39, 235, 1978.

206. **Hathway, D. E.,** Mechanisms of vinyl chloride carcinogenicity/mutagenicity, *Br. J. Cancer,* 44, 557, 1981.

207. **Van Duuren, B. L., Goldschmidt, B. M., Katz, C., Seidmann, I., and Paul, J. C.,** Carcinogenic activity of alkylating agents, *J. Natl. Cancer Inst.,* 53, 695, 1974.

208. **Enterline, P. E. and Henderson, V. L.,** Updated mortality in workers exposed to epichlorohydrin, *J. Occup. Med.,* in press.

209. **Preussmann, R., Schneider, H., and Epple, F.,** Untersuchungen zum Nachweis alkylierender Agentien, II. Der Nachweis verschiedener Klassen alkylierender Agentien mit einer Modifikation der Farbreaktion mit 4-(4'-Nitrobenzyl)pyridin, *Arzneim.-Forsch.,* 19, 1059, 1969.

210. National Academy of Sciences, Board of Toxicology and Environmental Health Hazards, *Formaldehyde — An Assessment of Its Health Effects,* National Academy of Sciences, Washington, D.C., 1980, 38.

211. U.S. Department of Health, Education and Welfare, Smoking and Health. A Report of the Surgeon General, DHEW Publ. No. (PHS) 79-50066, 1979, chap. 11.

212. **Yodaiken, R. E.,** The uncertain consequences of formaldehyde toxicity, *JAMA,* 246, 1677, 1981.

213. **Horten, A. V., Tye, R., and Stemmer, K. L.,** Experimental carcinogenesis of the lung. Inhalation of gaseous formaldehyde or an aerosol of coal tar by C_3H mice, *J. Natl. Cancer Inst.,* 30, 31, 1963.

214. **Nettesheim, P.,** unpublished data.

215. **Swenberg, J. A., Kerns, W. D., Mitchell, R. I., Gralla, E. J., and Pavkov, K. L.,** Induction of squamous cell carcinoma of the rat nasal cavity by inhalation exposure to formaldehyde vapor, *Cancer Res.,* 40, 3398, 1980.

216. **Kerns, W. D.,** Long-term inhalation toxicity and carcinogenicity studies of formaldehyde in rats and mice, presented at the Chemical Industry Institute of Toxicology, November 20 to 21, 1980, Raleigh, N.C., 1980.

217. National Institute for Occupational Safety and Health, Formaldehyde-Evidence of Carcinogenicity, U.S. Department of Health and Human Services, NIOSH Current Intelligence Bull. 34, 1981, 14.

218. **Akabane, J.,** Aldehydes and related compounds, *Int. Encycl. Pharmacol. Therap. Sect. 20,* 2, 523, 1970.

219. **Williams, R. T.,** *Detoxification Mechanisms: The Metabolism and Detoxification of Drugs, Toxic Substances and Other Organic Compounds,* 2nd ed., John Wiley & Sons, New York, 1959, 88.

220. **Neely, W. B.,** The metabolic fate of formaldehyde-^{14}C intraperitoneally administered to the rat, *Biochem. Pharmacol.,* 13, 1137, 1964.

221. **Feldman, M. Y.,** Reactions of formaldehyde with bases, nucleosides and nucleotides, *Progr. Nucleic Acid Res. Mol. Biol.,* 13, 1, 1973.

222. National Academy of Sciences, Committee on Medical and Biological Effects of Environmental Pollutants, *Nickel,* National Academy of Sciences, Washington, D.C., 1975, 277.

223. International Agency for Research on Cancer, *IARC Monographs on the Evaluation of the Carcinogenic Risk of Chemicals to Humans,* Nickel Compounds. Vol. 11, IARC, Lyon, 1976, 75.

224. U.S. Department of Health and Human Service, Smoking and Cancer. A Report of the Surgeon General, U.S. Department of Health Service Office on Smoking and Health 1982, U.S. Public Health Service No. DHHS(PHS) 82-50179, Washington, D.C., 1982.

225. **Doll, R., Morgan, L. G., and Speier, F. E.,** Cancers of the lung and nasal sinuses in nickel workers, *Br. J. Cancer,* 24, 622, 1970.

226. **Sunderman, F. W., Jr. and Donnelly, A. J.,** Studies of nickel carcinogenesis. Metastasizing pulmonary tumors in rats induced by the inhalation of nickel carbonyl, *Am. J. Clin. Pathol.,* 46, 1027, 1965.

227. **Ottolenghi, A. D., Haseman, J. K., Payne, W. W., Falk, H. L., and MacFarland, H. N.,** Inhalation studies of nickel sulfide in pulmonary carcinogenesis of rats, *J. Natl. Cancer Inst.,* 54, 1165, 1975.

228. **Hueper, W. C.,** Experimental studies in metal carcinogenesis. IX. Pulmonary lesions in guinea pigs and rats exposed to prolonged inhalation of powdered metallic nickel, *Arch. Pathol.,* 65, 600, 1958.

229. **Sunderman, F. W., Jr.,** Inhibition of induction of benzopyrene hydroxylase by nickel carbonyl, *Cancer Res.,* 27, 950, 1967.

230. **Sunderman, F. W., Jr.,** Mechanisms of metal carcinogenesis, *Biol. Trace Element Res.,* 1, 63, 1979.

231. **Witschi, H. P.,** A comparative study of *in vivo* RNA and protein synthesis in rat liver and lung, *Cancer Res.,* 32, 1686, 1972.

232. **Sunderman, F. W., Jr. and Esfahani, M.,** Nickel carbonyl inhibition of RNA polymerase activity in hepatic nuclei, *Cancer Res.,* 28, 2565, 1968.

233. International Agency for Research on Cancer, *IARC Monographs on the Evaluation of the Carcinogenic Risk of Chemicals to Humans,* Vol. 15, IARC, Lyon, 1977, 223.

234. National Institute for Occupational Safety and Health, Criteria for Recommended Standard Occupational Exposure to Isopropyl Alcohol, U.S. Department of Health, Education and Welfare Publ. No 76, 1976, 142.

235. **Weil, C. S., Smyth, H. F., Jr., and Nale, T. M.,** Quest for a suspected industrial carcinogen, *Arch. Ind. Hyg. Occup. Med.,* 5, 535, 1952.

236. **Howell, J. S.,** Intranasal administration of 9,10-dimethyl-1,2-benzanthracene to rats: the development of breast and lung tumours, *Br. J. Cancer,* 15, 263, 1961.

237. **Jerina, D. M., Lehr, R., Schaefer-Ridder, M., Yagi, H., Kale, J. M., Thakker, D. R., Wood, A. W., Lu, A. Y. H., Ryan, D., West, S., Levin, R., and Conney, A. H.,** Bay region epoxides of dihydrodiols: a concept which explains mutagenic and carcinogenic activity of benzo(a)pyrene and benz(a)anthracene, in *Origins of Human Cancer,* Hiatt, H., Watson, J. D., and Winsten, I., Eds., Cold Spring Harbor, N.Y., 1977, 639.

238. **Melikan, A. A., La Voie, E. J., Hecht, S. S., and Hoffmann, D.,** Influence of a bay region methyl group on formation of 5-methylchrysene dihydrodiol epoxide: DNA adducts in mouse skin, *Cancer Res.,* 42, 1239, 1982.

239. **Weinstein, I. B., Jeffrey, A. M., Jenette, K. W., Blotstein, S. M., Harvey, R. G., Harris, C., Autrup, H., Kasai, H., and Nakanishi, K.,** Benzo(a)pyrene diol epoxides as intermediates in nucleic acid binding *in vitro* and *in vivo, Science,* 193, 592, 1976.

240. **Schoental, R. and Gibbard, S.,** Nasal and other tumors in rats given 3,4,5-trimethoxy-cinnamaldehyde, a derivative of sinapaldehyde and other α,β-unsaturated aldehydic wood lignin constituents, *Br. J. Cancer,* 26, 504, 1972.

241. **Miller, J. A., Swanson, A. B., and Miller, E. C.,** The metabolic activation of safrole and related naturally occurring alkenylbenzenes in relation to carcinogenesis by these agents, in *Naturally Occurring Carcinogens — Mutagens and Modulations of Carcinogenesis,* Miller, E. C., Ed., Japan Sci. Soc. Press, Tokyo, 1979, 111.

242. **Van Duuren, B. L., Orris, L., and Nelson, N.,** Carcinogenicity of epoxides lactones and peroxy-compounds. II, *J. Natl. Cancer Inst.,* 35, 707, 1965.

243. **Laskin, S., Sellakumar, A. R., Kuschner, M., Nelson, N., LaMendola, S., Rusch, G. M., Katz, G. V., Dulak, N. C., and Albert, R. E.,** Inhalation carcinogenicity of epichlorohydrin in noninbred Sprague-Dawley rats, *J. Natl. Cancer Inst.,* 65, 751, 1980.

244. **Feron, V. J. and Kroes, R.,** One-year time sequence inhalation toxicity of vinyl chloride in rats. II. Morphological changes in the respiratory tract, ceruminous glands, brains, kidneys, heart and spleen, *Toxicology,* 13, 131, 1979.

245. **Dahl, A. R., Hadley, W. M., Hahn, F. F., Benson, J. M., and McClellan, R. O.,** Cytochrome P-450-dependent monooxygenases in olfactory epithelium of dogs: possible role in tumorigenicity, *Science,* 216, 57, 1982.

246. **Hadley, W. M. and Dahl, A. R.,** Cytochrome P-450 dependent monooxygenase activity in rat nasal epithelial membranes, *Toxicol. Lett.,* 10, 417, 1982.

247. **Brittebo, E. B., Castonguay, A., Furuya, K., and Hecht, S. S.,** Metabolism of tobacco-specific nitrosamines by cultured rat nasal mucosa, *Cancer Res.,* submitted.

Chapter 11

METABOLISM OF N-NITROSAMINES BY THE NASAL MUCOSA

Eva B. Brittebo and Hans Tjälve

TABLE OF CONTENTS

I.   Background 234

II.   Tissue Distribution of *N*-Nitrosamines 234

III.   Tissue Specificity of *N*-Nitrosamine Metabolism..............................235

IV.   The Nasal Mucosa as a Site of *N*-Nitrosamine Metabolism 236

V.   Comments..244

Acknowledgments..247

References..249

I. BACKGROUND

A notable feature of the *N*-nitrosamines is the organ specificity of their carcinogenic effects. It is generally accepted that reactive metabolic products of the compounds are the initiators of the tumor production, but the basis for the organ specificity has not been clearly established. However, of importance in this respect may be the ability of the organs to metabolize the different *N*-nitrosamines.

A frequent finding in the carcinogenicity studies with *N*-nitrosamines is the presence of tumors in the nasal cavity.[1,2] In a series of whole body autoradiographic studies we have observed a localization of *N*-nitrosamine metabolites in the nasal mucosa and in other extrahepatic tissues. This stimulated our interest in exploring the possibility that a metabolism of the *N*-nitrosamines might occur *in situ* in these extrahepatic tissues. On the basis of the autoradiographic data, various tissues were therefore selected and tested for their ability to metabolize the *N*-nitrosamines in vitro. The results from the experiments indicated that a metabolism of the *N*-nitrosamines occurs in several tissues and that the nasal mucosa is a site with a marked *N*-nitrosamine metabolizing capacity. This chapter will survey some of the obtained results.

The investigations have been performed mainly in mice and rats, but in some instances hamsters have also been studied. The *N*-nitroso compounds investigated include *N,N*,-dialkyl nitrosamines, such as *N*-nitrosodimethylamine, *N*-nitrosodiethylamine, and *N*-nitrosodibu-tylamine and cyclic *N*-nitrosamines, such as *N*-nitrosopyrrolidine, *N,N*-dinitrosopiperazine, *N*-nitrosopiperidine, and *N'*-nitrosonornicotine.[3-10] Some of the studied *N*-nitrosamines are volatile and in these instances low temperature autoradiography and autoradiography with heated tape sections were used to distinguish the tissue localization of the volatile nonme-tabolized *N*-nitrosamines from the distribution of the nonvolatile metabolites. Previous studies have indicated that at the metabolism of the *N*-nitrosamines, unstable metabolites are formed which spontaneously decompose to reactive toxic products.[11] The metabolism may also yield aldehydes and alcohols and these are further oxidized and subsequently join the one- and two-carbon pool of the body.[11,12] They may then serve as precursors of endogenous substances or they may be oxidized to CO_2. This means that when /^{14}C/-labeled *N*-nitrosamines are studied, some of the radioactive metabolites may be used to form one- or two-carbon fragments. Thus, to distinguish the part of the radioactivity which is used in the biosynthetic activities of the body, the distribution of metabolites formed from /^{14}C/-formaldehyde, /^{14}C/-acetaldehyde, and /^{14}C/-acetate was also studied by whole body autoradiography.[3,13] In the in vitro experiments it was sometimes possible to use the [14]CO_2-production as an index of the *N*-nitrosamine metabolism. It should be observed, however, that in these instances the [14]CO_2-production is dependent on the intermediary metabolism and that some steps in this pathway may be rate-limiting.

II. TISSUE DISTRIBUTION OF *N*-NITROSAMINES

Many *N*-nitrosamines are volatile and nonpolar substances. Our results have indicated that these compounds (e.g., *N*-nitrosodimethylamine, *N*-nitrosodiethylamine, *N*-nitrosodi-butylamine, and *N*-nitrosopyrrolidine) are evenly distributed in the body and thus they are able to pass the cellular membranes freely.[3-8] This implies that the nonmetabolized compounds must be relatively innocuous to the tissues and that the injurious effects are due to metabolites.

N'-nitrosonornicotine is also distributed throughout the whole body, but since it is a weak base it will be trapped in areas with a low pH, such as in the lumen of the stomach.[9,10] *N'*-nitrosonornicotine is also localized in pigmented tissues.[9]

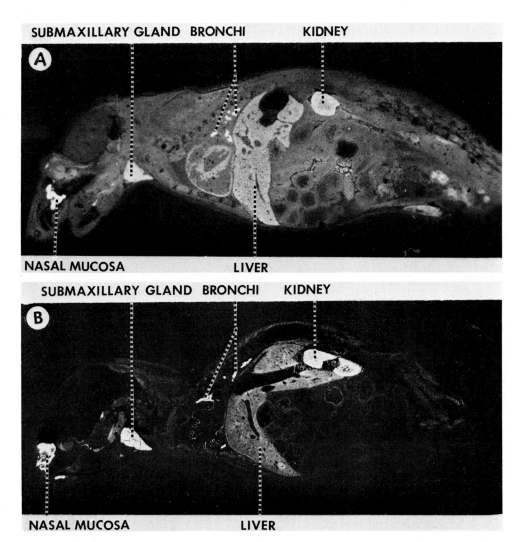

FIGURE 1.   Autoradiograms of a C57BL-mouse 1 min after an i.v. injection of *N*-/^{14}C/nitrosodiethylamine (sagittal section). (A) Exposure of a section at $-70°C$. (B) Exposure of a heated tape section from the same mouse at $-20°C$. In (A) a considerable radioactivity is present in the nasal and bronchial mucosa, the submaxillary gland, the liver and the kidney; in the other tissues, there is a uniform distribution of radioactivity. In (B) the volatile radioactivity has disappeared, whereas the nonvolatile metabolites remain in the above-mentioned tissues. (From Brittebo, E., Löfberg, B., and Tjälve, H., *Chem.-Biol. Interact.*, 34, 209, 1981. With permission.)

III. TISSUE SPECIFICITY OF *N*-NITROSAMINE METABOLISM

The in vivo autoradiography showed a rapid localization of metabolites in specific tissues after the administration of the /^{14}C/-labeled *N*-nitrosamines (Figure 1).[4] The tissues accumulating metabolites sometimes showed variations between the different compounds and also, when more than one animal species was studied, species variations in the distribution pattern of the metabolites could be observed. There were also features which were common to most of the studied *N*-nitrosamines. A consistent finding was a strong and rapid localization of metabolites in the nasal mucosa. In fact, with the exception of *N*-nitrosodimethylamine (which was studied in mice) this has been observed for all the *N*-nitrosamines so far investigated.[3-10] The tracheobronchial mucosa and the mucosa of the esophagus and the tongue, the liver and the kidneys, are tissues which in addition often showed considerable levels of metabolites. Other tissues, such as the salivary and lacrimal glands, Zymbal's gland, and the preputial glands, were in some instances found to accumulate metabolites. A few examples of tissue localizations of metabolites will be given below. The liver dominated the distribution picture after the administration of N-/^{14}C/nitrosodimethylamine to mice, but after the administration of N-/^{14}C/nitrosodiethylamine, metabolites were also found in several extrahepatic tissues, such as the nasal and bronchial mucosa, the salivary and lacrimal glands, and the mucosa of the esophagus and tongue (Figure 1B).[3-5] After the injection of N-/^{14}C/ nitrosopyrrolidine, the tracheobronchial mucosa strongly accumulated metabolites in mice, but not in rats, whereas in both species metabolites were detected in the nasal mucosa, the liver, and the kidneys.[7,8]

In some instances, the "biosynthetic distribution pattern", due to the incorporation of one- or two-carbon fragments into endogenous materials, could be observed at 30 min or at later intervals after the administration of the /^{14}C/-labeled N-nitrosamines.[3-8] This distribution pattern was characterized by a strong labeling of tissues with a high cell turnover and/or protein synthesis, such as in the gastrointestinal mucosa and the lymphomyeloid system.

As mentioned previously, the in vivo results formed the basis for in vitro experiments. The purpose was to establish whether the observed localization of metabolites was due to a local degradation in the tissues or might be due to metabolites which were formed by the liver and had reached the tissues via the blood. The results indicated that in most instances metabolites were formed locally in the tissues. Thus, the in vivo localization of metabolites in tissues such as the bronchial and esophageal mucosa and in the mucosa of the nose could be correlated with a local formation of metabolites in these tissues in vitro. In many, although not all, instances there are reports of cancer induction in the tissues capable of N-nitrosamine metabolism, suggesting that *in situ* metabolic activation plays an important role in the pathogenesis of the N-nitrosamine-induced tumors. This is the case with the nasal mucosa, on which we will now focus our attention.

IV. THE NASAL MUCOSA AS A SITE OF N-NITROSAMINE METABOLISM

After the administration of the radioactive N-nitrosamines, there was usually a high level of metabolites in the nasal mucosa already at the shortest survival intervals (1 to 5 min). A retention of the radioactivity in this tissue could be seen for more than 24 hr. The highest labeling was usually present in the region of the ethmoturbinates. This was the case after the administration of N-/^{14}C/nitrosodiethylamine to mice and rats (Figures 2 and 3). Autoradiography of /^{14}C/-acetate, which illustrates the "biosynthetic labeling", showed the highest radioactivity in the area of the naso- and maxilloturbinates (Figure 3B), which may indicate that the labeling in the ethmoturbinates after the N-/^{14}C/nitrosodiethylamine administration is due to a large extent to alkylating metabolites. After the administration of N'-/^{14}C/nitrosonornicotine, whole body autoradiography showed a similar labeling of the nasal mucosa as after the N-/^{14}C/nitrosodiethylamine injections (Figure 4).[9,10] When the tissue sections were fixed and washed with organic solvents, firmly bound radioactivity was still present in the nasal mucosa, whereas in some other tissues (e.g., the salivary glands) the radioactivity was removed (Figure 4B).[10] Experiments with N-/^{14}C/nitrosopiperidine in rats and in Chinese hamsters (Figure 5) and N,N-nitrosopiperazine in rats (Figure 6) gave similar distribution pictures as described for N-nitrosodiethylamine and N'-nitrosonornicotine.

Microautoradiographic studies have indicated the precise localization of tissue-bound radioactivity in the nose of the Sprague-Dawley rat after the administration of N'-/^{14}C/ nitrosonornicotine (Figures 7 and 8). The microautoradiograms showed a labeling of both the olfactory and the respiratory epithelium. There was also a strong labeling of the subepithelial glands (Bowman's glands) in the olfactory area. In fact, the subepithelial glands

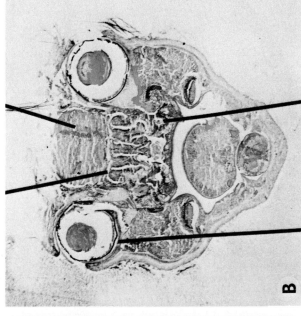

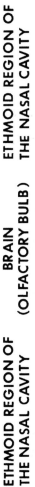

ETHMOID REGION OF   BRAIN
THE NASAL CAVITY   (OLFACTORY BULB)

CONJUNCTIVAL PART   MAXILLARY
OF THE EYELID   SINUS

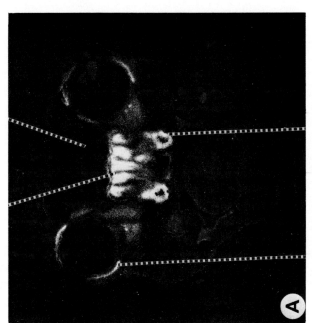

ETHMOID REGION OF   BRAIN
THE NASAL CAVITY   (OLFACTORY BULB)

CONJUNCTIVAL PART   MAXILLARY
OF THE EYELID   SINUS

FIGURE 2. (A) Detail of an autoradiogram of a C57BL-mouse 5 min after an i.v. injection of *N*-/¹⁴*C*/nitrosodiethylamine (transversal section). (B) Corresponding hematoxylin-eosin stained section. A high level of nonvolatile metabolites is present in the mucosa of the ethmoid region of the nasal cavity and in the mucosa of the maxillary sinuses. Radioactivity is also present in the conjunctival parts of the eyelids. (From Brittebo, E., Löfberg, B., and Tjälve, H., *Chem.-Biol. Interact.*, 34, 209, 1981. With permission.)

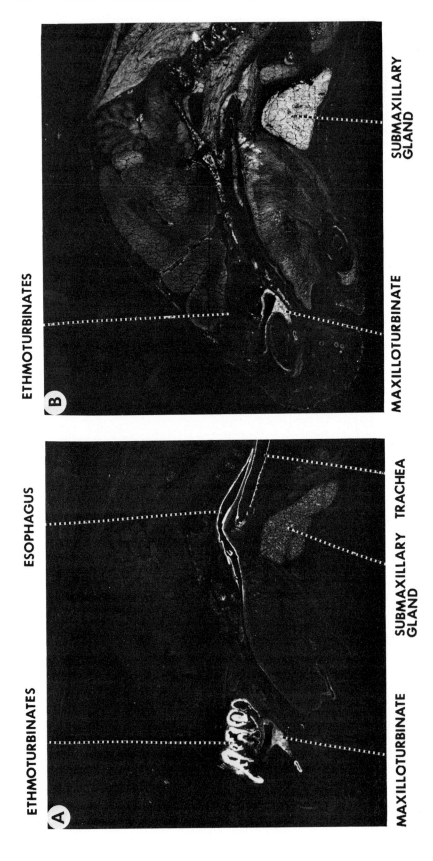

FIGURE 3.   Autoradiogram of Sprague-Dawley rats 5 min after an i.v. injection of (A) N-/^{14}C/nitrosodiethylamine and (B) /^{14}C/-acetate.   A high level of nonvolatile metabolites is present in the mucosa of the ethmoid region of the nasal cavity in (A), whereas no such labeling is present in (B).   In the mucosa of the maxilloturbinate, radioactivity is present both in (A) and (B).

MUCOSA OF THE
ETHMOTURBINATES   ESOPHAGEAL MUCOSA

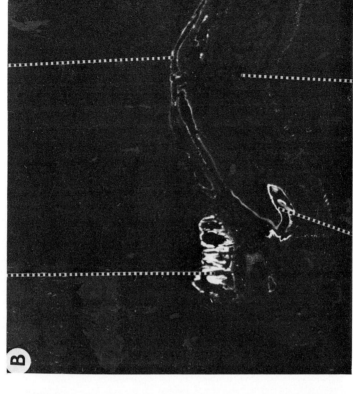

MUCOSA OF THE TONGUE   SALIVARY GLAND

FIGURE 4.   Details of autoradiograms of a Sprague-Dawley rat 30 min after an i.v. injection of N'-$[^{14}C]$/nitrosonornicotine.   (A):   Nonextracted tissue section.   (B):   An adjacent tissue section — fixed and organic solvent extracted. In (A), a high radioactivity can be seen in the nasal and esophageal mucosa, the mucosa of the tongue and in the submaxillary gland, whereas a lower uniformly distributed radioactivity is present in the other tissues. In (B), tissue-bound radioactivity can be seen in the nasal and esophageal mucosa and in the mucosa of the tongue, whereas the radioactivity in the submaxillary gland and in the other tissues has disappeared. (From Brittebo, E. B. and Tjälve, H., *Carcinogenesis*, 2, 952, 1981. With permission.)

ETHMOTURBINATES   **BRONCHI**

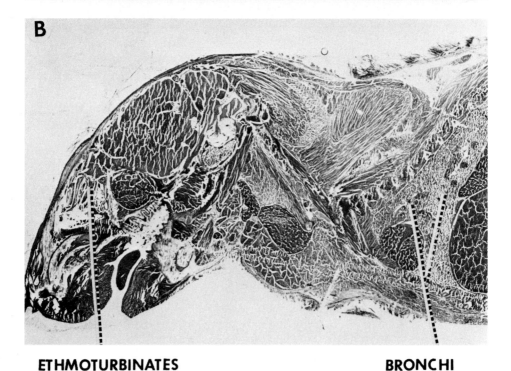

ETHMOTURBINATES   **BRONCHI**

FIGURE 5.   (A) Detail of an autoradiogram of a Chinese hamster 1 min after an i.v. injection of *N*-/^{14}C/ nitrosopiperidine. (B) Corresponding hematoxylin-eosin stained section. A high level of nonvolatile metabolites is present in the mucosa of the ethmoid region of the nasal cavity and of the bronchi.

**ETHMOID REGION OF
THE NASAL CAVITY**   **ESOPHAGUS**

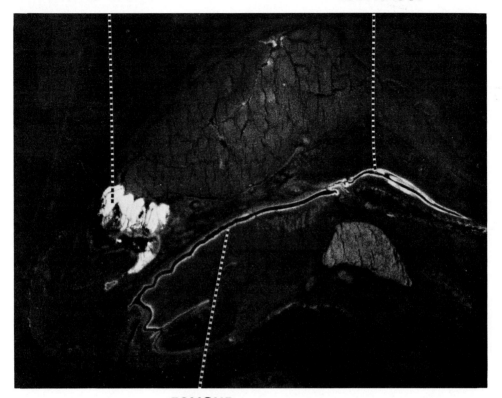

TONGUE

FIGURE 6.   Detail of an autoradiogram of a Sprague-Dawley rat 5 min after an i.v. injection of *N,N,*-
/^{14}C/dinitrosopiperazine. A high level of radioactivity is present in the mucosa of the ethmoid region of the nasal
cavity and in the mucosa of the tongue and esophagus.

usually showed the strongest tissue labeling in the nose. The epithelium of the nasolacrimal
duct was in addition labeled. In contrast to other epithelial areas, the epithelium of the
vomeronasal organ was nonlabeled, and this applied both to the olfactory and the respiratory
parts of the epithelium.

The ability of the nasal mucosa to metabolize the *N*-nitrosamines was also studied in in
vitro experiments, using either the [14]CO$_2$-production or the formation of tissue-bound metabolites as measures of the metabolism.[4-6,8,10] Results of such experiments are seen in Table
1 and Figures 9 and 10. It can be seen that the nasal mucosa in mice has a very high capacity
to degrade *N*-nitrosodiethylamine (Table 1).[4] In rats, the nasal mucosa was much more active
than the liver in forming tissue-bound metabolites from *N'*-/^{14}C/nitrosonornicotine (Figure
9).[10] In contrast, the liver in mice had a higher capacity than the nasal mucosa to form
tissue-bound radioactivity from *N*-/^{14}C/nitrosopyrrolidine (Figure 10).[8] The liver in mice and
rats also had a higher capacity than the nasal mucosa to form [14]CO$_2$ from *N*-/^{14}C/nitroso-
pyrrolidine.[8] Autoradiography was sometimes performed in vitro by incubation of the nasal
area in a buffer containing a /^{14}C/-labeled *N*-nitrosamine. Figure 11 shows the labeling of
the nasal mucosa of the rat after in vitro incubation with *N*-/^{14}C/nitrosodibutylamine.[6] There
is a higher level of metabolites in the naso- and maxilloturbinates than of the ethmoturbinates.

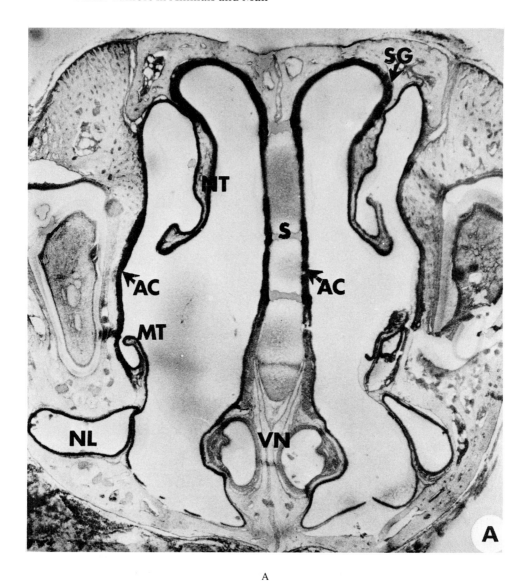

A

FIGURE 7.   Microautoradiograms of the nose of a Sprague-Dawley rat killed 4 hr after an i.v. injection of N' -/^{14}C/nitrosonornicotine. The nasal area was fixed in formalin, decalcified in formic acid and via an alcohol series embedded in paraffin. Sections were then taken in a microtome, deparaffinized in an alcohol series, and dipped in a liquid film emulsion (NTB-2, Eastman-Kodak®). After exposure, the films were developed and fixed and the sections were stained with hematoxylin-eosin. Since the tissues have been extensively exposed to formalin, formic acid, and ethanol, it is assumed that only the tissue-bound metabolites are retained. (A) Transversal section through the entire nose: a strong labeling (black silver grains) is present in the mucosa of the nasal cavity, including the turbinates and the septum. There is also a strong labeling of subepithelial glands, situated dorsally in the olfactory area. In addition, a labeling is present in the mucosa of the nasolacrimal duct. In contrast, the mucosa of the vomeronasal organ is nonlabeled. Magnification × 25; (B) Detail of the dorsal area of the nose, showing radioactivity in the subepithelial glands and in the mucosal linings. Magnification × 95. S = nasal septum; SG = subepithelial glands; VN = vomeronasal organ; NL = nasolacrimal duct; NT = nasoturbinate; MT = maxilloturbinate; AC = acinous glands; OL = olfactory epithelium; RE = respiratory epithelium. (From Löfberg, B., Brittebo, E. and Tjälve, H., *Cancer Res.*, 42, 2877, 1982. With permission.)

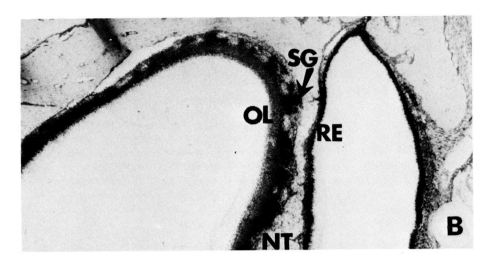

FIGURE 7B

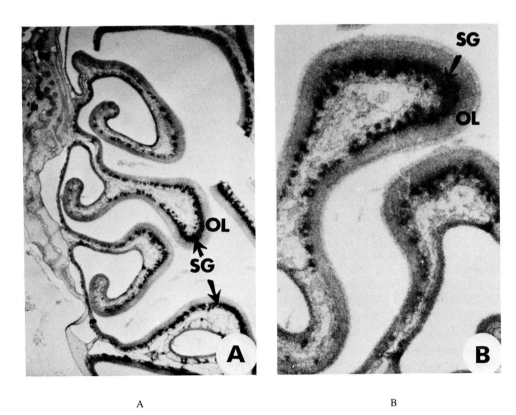

A   B

FIGURE 8.   Microautoradiograms from the nose of a Sprague-Dawley rat killed 4 hr after an i.v. injection of
N'-/^{14}C/nitrosonornicotine. The autoradiograms were obtained as described in Figure 7. (A,B) Ethmoturbinates
with strongly labeled subepithelial glands and more weakly labeled olfactory epithelium. (Magnification (A) ×
30; (B) × 70). (C) The septum with strongly labeled subepithelial glands and more weakly labeled olfactory
epithelium. (Magnification × 180). (D) The vomeronasal organ. The olfactory and respiratory epithelia of the
vomeronasal organ are nonlabeled, whereas the respiratory epithelium of the septum is labeled. Acinous glands
localized laterally and dorsally to the vomeronasal organ are nonlabeled. (Magnification × 160). SG = subepithelial
glands; OL = olfactory epithelium, RE = respiratory epithelium; AC = acinous glands. (From Löfberg, B.,
Brittebo, E. and Tjälve, H., *Cancer Res.*, 42, 2877, 1982. With permission.)

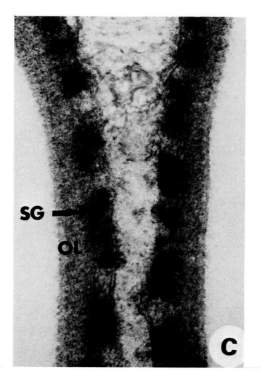

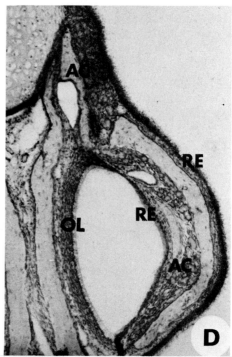

FIGURE 8C   FIGURE 8D

V. COMMENTS

It appears from our studies that the nasal mucosa is a tissue with a marked capacity to metabolize several *N*-nitrosamines. Since the nasal mucosa is one of the preferential target tissues for the *N*-nitrosamine carcinogenesis, our results are consistent with the view that the tissue-specific toxicity of the *N*-nitrosamines is caused by metabolites produced *in situ* within the tissue. Incubations with rat nasal mucosa produced a higher level of tissue-bound *N'*-nitrosonornicotine metabolites than ay of the other tissues studied, and the nasal mucosa is also the major site of tumor formation after *N'*-nitrosonornicotine treatment.[14,15] Studies by Singer and Taylor have indicated that the *N'*-nitrosonornicotine-induced tumors originate from the olfactory epithelium of the turbinates.[14] The tumors were suggested to arise from both the surface epithelium and the subepithelial glands of the mucosa, in which tissue-bound *N'*-nitrosonornicotine metabolites were found in our microautoradiographic study. *N,N*-dinitrosopiperazine induces tumors of the nasal cavity in rats, and this has also been shown for *N*-nitrosopiperidine in rats, and Chinese hamsters.[16-18] Our results indicate that the nasal mucosa metabolizes these *N*-nitrosamines, and thus it appears that the susceptibility of the nasal mucosa is related to its capacity for *N*-nitrosamine metabolism. However, a metabolism of *N*-nitrosodiethylamine, *N*-nitrosopyrrolidine, and *N*-nitrosodibutylamine was also observed in experiments with the nasal mucosa of the rat, but in this species *N*-nitrosodiethylamine and *N*-nitrosopyrrolidine have only a weak carcinogenic effect towards the nasal mucosa, and for *N*-nitrosodibutylamine nasal cavity tumors have not been reported.[19-21]

These data indicate that although a metabolism of the *N*-nitrosamines may be a necessary prerequisite for tumor production, other factors, e.g., the DNA-repairing capacity, may ultimately determine the presence or absence of tumors. It is also possible that in some instances the observed *N*-nitrosamine metabolism may involve a detoxification rather than a metabolic activation.

Table 1
PRODUCTION OF $^{14}CO_2$ AND INCORPORATION OF RADIOACTIVITY IN THE ACID-INSOLUBLE MACROMOLECULES FROM *N*-/^{14}C/NITROSODIETHYLAMINE BY VARIOUS TISSUES OF C57BL MICE IN VITRO

Tissue	$^{14}CO_2$-Production (dpm/mg tissue/wet weight/)	Radioactivity incorporated in the acid-insoluble material (dpm/mg acid-insoluble protein)
Region of nasal cavities (3)	349.9 ± 35.1	146.7 ± 11.1
Sublingual gland (3)	174.8 ± 29.9	326.4 ± 16.6
Liver (4)	150.0 ± 24.6	150.0 ± 23.0
Submaxillary gland (4)	101.7 ± 7.2	179.0 ± 14.9
Lung (5)	82.5 ± 10.1	168.0 ± 28.8
Intraorbital lacrimal gland and conjunctival part of the eyelid (3)	71.2 ± 9.7	279.1 ± 14.1
Trachea and larynx (4)	61.0 ± 10.9	125.5 ± 41.2
Parotid gland (3)	37.8 ± 5.1	94.8 ± 12.8
Esophagus (4)	23.0 ± 2.0	217.0 ± 21.3
Tongue (4)	18.7 ± 3.0	60.1 ± 7.7
Adrenal (3)	12.3 ± 2.6	—[a]
Ovary (3)	10.4 ± 0.2	—
Forestomach (3)	6.0 ± 0.6	—
Kidney (3)	5.8 ± 0.5	—
Harderian gland (3)	3.7 ± 0.3	—
Diaphragm (3)	3.5 ± 0.4	—
Spleen (4)	2.9 ± 0.1	—
Pancreas (4)	2.8 ± 0.3	—
Heart muscle (4)	2.5 ± 0.1	—
Thymus (3)	2.4 ± 0.1	—
Glandular stomach (3)	2.4 ± 0.2	—
Small intestine (3)	2.3 ± 0.2	—
Testis (3)	2.3 ± 0.1	—
Control (TCA-denaturated liver) (10)	2.1 ± 0.1	—

Note: Tissue slices were incubated in Warburg respiratory vessels in Krebs-Ringer phosphate solution to which 0.1 μCi of *N*-/^{14}C/-nitrosodiethylamine was added (2.5 μ*M)*.Incubations were performed for 60 min under an atmosphere of oxygen at 37°C. The incubations were terminated by the addition of trichloroacetic acid. Formed $^{14}CO_2$ trapped on filter papers moistened with KOH, and radioactivity incorporated in the acid-insoluble tissue precipitates, were determined. The results show the radioactivity trapped on filter paper expressed as disintegrations per minute (dpm) per milligram incubated tissue slices, and in the precipitates expressed as dpm/mg acid-insoluble protein (mean ± S.E.). The figures in parentheses denote the number of incubations.

[a]   Dash indicates no detectable radioactivity.

From Brittebo, E., Löfberg, B., and Tjälve, H., *Chem. Biol. Interact.,* 34, 209, 1981. With permission.

Our studies have indicated that the enzymes engaged in the *N*-nitrosamine metabolism have an expressed organ specificity, and in addition to the liver, are localized in extrahepatic tissues such as the mucosa of the respiratory system and the mucosa of the esophagus. Recently it has become clear that the mucosa of the bronchi and bronchioles possesses an enzymatic system capable of metabolizing exogenous chemicals such as the pulmonary toxin 4-ipomeanol.[22] These studies have led to the view that the damage of the Clara cell in the

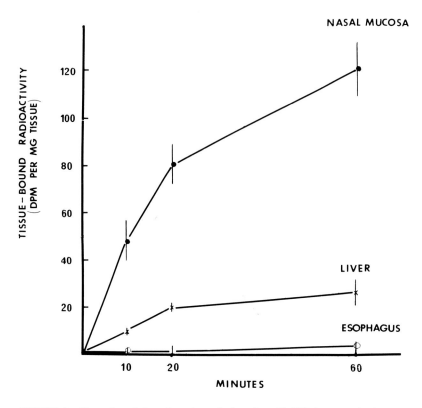

FIGURE 9.   Formation of tissue-bound metabolites from N'-/^{14}C/nitrosonornicotine as a function of time. Incubation flasks containing slices of the nasal mucosa, liver, and esophagus of Sprague-Dawley rats were incubated with N'-/^{14}C/nitrosonornicotine (3 μM). The incubations were performed under an atmosphere of oxygen at 37°C and were terminated at various time intervals by the addition of trichloroacetic acid. After extraction of the precipitate with organic solvents, the nonextractable radioactivity in the precipitate was determined. (Mean ± S.E.; n = 4). (From Brittebo, E. B. and Tjälve, H., *Carcinogenesis*, 2, 959, 1981. With permission.)

bronchiolar mucosa caused by this compound is due to reactive metabolites formed *in situ* in this cell type. The nonciliated bronchiolar (Clara) cells have been implicated as a site of cytochrome P-450-dependent mixed-function oxidase activity in the respiratory mucosa.[23,24] Autoradiographic studies with labeled nitrosamines in hamsters[25] indicate that Clara cells are also involved in metabolism of these compounds.

There is evidence that in the liver the metabolism of N-nitrosamines is cytochrome P-450 dependent and that an initial hydroxylation of a carbon in α-position to the N-nitroso group is an important metabolic activation step.[26,27] In considering the nasal mucosa as a site of metabolism of N-nitrosamines, it therefore appears as if cytochrome P-450 is also present in specific cells in the nasal mucosa.

A labeling of the nasal mucosa has previously been observed in several whole body autoradiographic studies. Thus, after inhalation of volatile organic solvents such as styrene, methylene chloride, chloroform, carbon tetrachloride, and trichloroethylene, a localization of metabolites was registered in the nasal mucosa.[28] After i.v. injections of dimethyl mercury and mustard gas, metabolites have also been found in the nasal mucosa.[29,30] An uptake of radioactivity in the nasal mucosa has also been observed after i.v. injections of several /^{14}C/-labeled chlorinated hydrocarbons, such as polychlorinated biphenyls and the sulfur-containing metabolites thereof.[31,32]

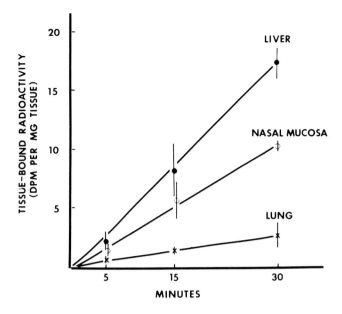

FIGURE 10. Production of tissue-bound metabolites from N-/^{14}C/nitrosopyrrolidine by tissues from C57BL-mice in vitro: tissue slices were incubated in Krebs-Ringer phosphate solution to which 0.1 μCi of N-/^{14}C/ nitrosopyrrolidine (3 μM) was added. The incubations were performed under an atmosphere of oxygen at 37°C and were terminated at various time intervals by the addition of trichloroacetic acid. After extraction of the precipitates with organic solvents, the nonextractable radioactivity in the precipitates was determined. (Mean ± S.E., n = 3). (From Brittebo, E., Löfberg, B., and Tjälve, H., *Xenobiotica*, 11, 619, 1981. With permission.)

In this paper we have discussed some recent results which have demonstrated an ability of the nasal mucosa to metabolize N-nitrosamines. However, there are still a number of questions to be answered. For example, a detailed description of the cell types which are responsible for the metabolism of different N-nitrosamines is of importance. No information is currently available about the metabolic pathways of the N-nitrosamines in the nasal mucosa, or of the nature of the reactive metabolite formed by this tissue. Additional studies are also needed to define the reactions of the N-nitrosamine metabolites with the tissue macromolecules in the nasal mucosa. It would also be of interest to examine whether the nasal mucosa has an ability to metabolize compounds other than the N-nitrosamines.

ACKNOWLEDGMENTS

The studies were supported with grants from the National Swedish Environment Protection Board, the Swedish Tobacco Company, and the Swedish Work Environment Fund.

NASO-
TURBINATE   **MAXILLO-**
TURBINATE   **ETHMO-**
TURBINATES

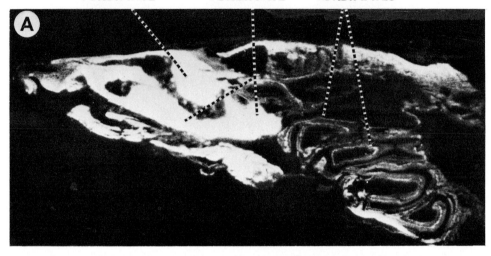

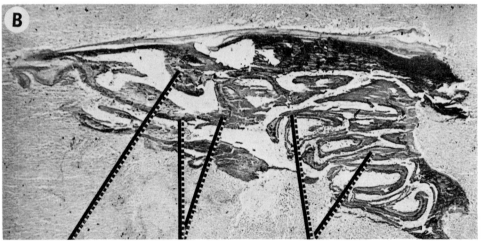

NASO-
TURBINATE   **MAXILLO-**
TURBINATE   **ETHMO-**
TURBINATES

FIGURE 11.   (A) Autoradiogram of the nasal region of a Sprague-Dawley rat which was incubated with N-/^{14}C/ nitrosodibutylamine (0.2 mM) for 60 min (sagittal section). (B) Corresponding hematoxylin-eosin stained section. A high level of nonvolatile metabolites is present in the mucosa of the naso- and maxilloturbinates, whereas the labeling of the mucosa of the ethmoturbinates is considerably lower. (From Brittebo, E. B. and Tjälve, H., *Chem.-Biol. Interact.*, 38, 231, 1982. With permission.)

REFERENCES

1. **Druckrey, H., Ivankovic, S., Mennel, H. D., and Preussmann, R.,** Selektive Erzeugung von Carcinomen der Nasenhöhle bei Ratten durch *N,N'*-di-Nitrosopiperazin, Nitrosopiperidin, Nitrosomorpholin, Methylallyl-, Dimethyl-, und Methyl-vinyl-nitrosamin, *Z. Krebsforsch.*, 66, 138, 1964.
2. **Thomas, C.,** Zur Morphologie der Nasenhöhlentumoren bei der Ratte, *Z. Krebsforsch.*, 67, 1, 1965.
3. **Johansson, E. and Tjälve, H.,** The distribution of ^{14}C-dimethylnitrosamine in mice. Autoradiographic studies in mice with inhibited and noninhibited dimethylnitrosamine metabolism and a comparison with the distribution of ^{14}C-formaldehyde, *Toxicol. Appl. Pharmacol.*, 45, 565, 1978.
4. **Brittebo, E., Löfberg, B., and Tjälve, H.,** Sites of metabolism of *N*-nitrosodiethylamine in mice, *Chem.-Biol. Interact.*, 34, 209, 1981.
5. **Brittebo, E., Lindgren, A., and Tjälve, H.,** Foetal distribution and metabolism of *N*-nitrosodiethylamine in mice, *Acta Pharmacol. Toxicol.*, 48, 355, 1981.
6. **Brittebo, E. B. and Tjälve, H.,** Tissue-specificity of *N*-nitrosodibutylamine metabolism in Sprague-Dawley rats, *Chem.-Biol. Interact.*, 38, 231, 1982.
7. **Johansson-Brittebo, E. and Tjälve, H.,** Studies on the distribution and metabolism of *N-/*^{14}*C/nitrosopyrrolidine* in mice, *Chem.-Biol. Interact.*, 25, 243, 1979.
8. **Brittebo, E., Löfberg, B., and Tjälve, H.,** Extrahepatic sites of metabolism of *N*-nitrosopyrrolidine in mice and rats, *Xenobiotica*, 11, 619, 1981.
9. **Brittebo, E. and Tjälve, H.,** Autoradiographic observations on the distribution and metabolism of *N'-/*^{14}*C/nitrosonornicotine* in mice, *J. Cancer Res. Clin. Oncol.*, 98, 233, 1980.
10. **Brittebo, E. B. and Tjälve, H.,** Formation of tissue-bound *N'*-nitrosonornicotine metabolites by the target tissues of Sprague-Dawley and Fischer rats, *Carcinogenesis*, 2, 959, 1981.
11. **Heath, D. F.,** The decomposition and toxicity of dialkylnitrosamines in rats, *Biochem. J.*, 85, 72, 1962.
12. **Brouwers, J. A. J. and Emmelot, P.,** Microsomal *N*-demethylation and the effect of the hepatic carcinogen dimethylnitrosamine on amino acid incorporation into the proteins of rat livers and hepatomas, *Exp. Cell Res.*, 19, 467, 1960.
13. **Johansson-Brittebo, E. and Tjälve, H.,** Studies on the tissue-disposition and fate of *N-/*^{14}*C/ethyl-N-*nitrosourea in mice, *Toxicology*, 13, 275, 1979.
14. **Singer, G. M. and Taylor, H. W.,** Carcinogenicity of *N'*-nitrosonornicotine in Sprague-Dawley rats, *J. Natl. Cancer Inst.*, 57, 1275, 1976.
15. **Hecht, S. S., Chen, C. B., Ohmori, T., and Hoffmann, D.,** Comparative carcinogenicity in F344 rats of the tobacco-specific nitrosamines, *N'*-nitrosonornicotine and 4-(*N*-methyl-*N*-nitrosamino)-*1*-(3-pyridyl)-*1*-butanone, *Cancer Res.*, 40, 298, 1980.
16. **Lijinsky, W. and Taylor, H. W.,** Carcinogenicity of methylated dinitrosopiperazines in rats, *Cancer Res.*, 35, 1270, 1975.
17. **Lijinsky, W. and Taylor, H. W.,** Tumorigenesis by oxygenated nitrosopiperidines in rats, *J. Natl. Cancer Inst.*, 55, 705, 1975.
18. **Reznik, G., Mohr, U., and Kmoch, N.,** Carcinogenic effects of different nitroso-compounds in Chinese hamsters. II. *N*-nitrosomorpholine and *N*-nitrosopiperidine, *Z. Krebsforsch.*, 86, 95, 1976.
19. **Lijinsky, W. and Taylor, H. W.,** Relative carcinogenic effectiveness of derivatives of nitrosodiethylamine in rats, *Cancer Res.*, 38, 2391, 1978.
20. **Lijinsky, W. and Taylor, H. W.,** The effect of substituents on the carcinogenicity of *N*-nitrosopyrrolidine in Sprague-Dawley rats, *Cancer Res.*, 36, 1988, 1976.
21. **Rogers, A. E., Sanchez, O., Feinsod, F. M., and Newberne, P. M.,** Dietary enhancement of nitrosamine carcinogenesis, *Cancer Res.*, 34, 96, 1974.
22. **Boyd, M. R., Burka, L. T., Wilson, B. J., and Sasame, H. A.,** In vitro studies on the metabolic activation of the pulmonary toxin, 4-ipomeanol, by rat lung and liver microsomes, *J. Pharmacol. Exp. Ther.*, 207, 677, 1978.
23. **Boyd, M. R.,** Evidence for the Clara cell as a site of cytochrome P450-dependent mixed-function oxidase activity in lung, *Nature (London)*, 269, 713, 1977.
24. **Serabjit-Singh, C. J., Wolf, C. R., Philpot, R. M., and Plopper, C. G.,** Cytochrome P-450: localization in rabbit lung, *Science*, 207, 1469, 1979.
25. **Reznik-Schüller, H. and Reznik, G.,** Experimental pulmonary carcinogenesis, *Int. Rev. Exp. Pathol.*, 20, 211, 1979.
26. **Czygan, P., Greim, H., Garro, A. J., Hutterer, F., Schaffner, F., Popper, H., Rosenthal, O., and Cooper, D. Y.,** Microsomal metabolism of dimethylnitrosamine and cytochrome P-450 dependency of its activation to a mutagen, *Cancer Res.*, 33, 2983, 1973.
27. **Chen, C. B., Hecht, S. S., and Hoffmann, D.,** Metabolic α-hydroxylation of the tobacco-specific carcinogen, *N'*-nitrosonornicotine, *Cancer Res.*, 38, 3639, 1978.

28. **Bergman, K.,** Whole-body autoradiography and allied tracer techniques in distribution and elimination studies of some organic solvents, *Scand. J. Work Environ. Health,* 5(Suppl. 1), 1, 1979.

29. **Östlund, K.,** Studies on the metabolism of methyl mercury and dimethyl mercury in mice, *Acta Pharmacol. Toxicol.,* 27(Suppl. 1), 1, 1969.

30. **Clemedson, C.-J., Kristoffersson, H., Sörbo, B., and Ullberg, S.,** Whole body autoradiographic studies of the distribution of sulphur 35-labelled mustard gas in mice, *Acta Radiol.,* 1, 314, 1963.

31. **Brandt, I.,** Tissue-localization of polychlorinated biphenyls. Chemical structure related to pattern of distribution, *Acta Pharmacol. Toxicol.,* 40(Suppl. 2), 1, 1977.

32. **Brandt, I. and Bergman, Å.,** Bronchial mucosal and kidney cortex affinity of 4- and 4,4′-substituted sulphur-containing derivatives of 2,2′,5,5′-tetrachlorobiphenyl in mice, *Chem.-Biol. Interact.,* 34, 47, 1981.

Chapter 12

SUMMARY AND CONCLUSIONS

Sherman F. Stinson and Gerd Reznik

In this book, we have attempted to compile a comprehensive review of topics relevant to nasal cavity and nasopharyngeal cancer (NPC). The anatomical, epidemiological, and pathological aspects of the subject have been presented and discussed. It seems pertinent, in summary, to draw some generalizations that will help to provide an overall understanding of the importance of the field and point to directions in need of further investigation.

First it must be reemphasized that nasal cavity cancer and NPC are separate entities. Not only are the embryological origins and the types of tumors observed in each region different, but the etiologic agents involved in carcinogenesis of the respective areas are also distinct.

Several occupational groups have shown a predisposition for developing nasal cavity carcinoma. All have heavy nasal exposure to locally acting physical or chemical agents in the form of dusts, chemicals, or chemicals adsorbed to dusts. These groups include nickel, wood, and shoe workers. Possible mechanisms include a primary effect causing mucostasis and impaired clearance, resulting in chronic sinusitis or rhinitis. Direct chemical effects such as alkylation have also been proposed.

NPC, on the other hand, has not been tied to a particular occupational group, but shows strong regional or ethnic concentration. Some regions of China, Southeast Asia, Africa, and Alaska show particularly high incidences of NPC. A strong association of this disease with herpesvirus (Epstein-Barr virus) has been shown, and other environmental agents such as nitrosamines or smoke, coupled with a genetic predisposition, may also be involved.

Several excellent animal models are available for the study of the various aspects of nasal cavity carcinogenesis, as rodents and larger animals appear to be much more susceptible to the development of these neoplasms than humans. Nasal cancer has been observed in several domestic species and may be environmentally related. Although "spontaneous" nasal tumors are rare in laboratory rodents, they are easily induced by nitrosamines and various environmental substances. The sensitivity of animals for the development of nasal cancer may be related to the design of their nasal cavities, providing increased epithelial surface area for exposure, and a more tortuous course for the air to follow, allowing increased deposition of airborne compounds.

No suitable animal model for human NPC has been described, as most animals lack a region analogous to the human nasopharynx. Further, although some chemical agents related epidemiologically to human NPC have induced nasal cavity tumors in animals, and animal tumors histologically similar to human NPC have occasionally been described, viral effects have not been implicated (or studied to any great extent), so a similar mechanism cannot be postulated.

Though much is known concerning nasal cavity and nasopharyngeal carcinogenesis, information on some areas is deficient. More study is required of the normal ultrastructural anatomy of the nasal epithelium to clearly define the cell types present, especially in the olfactory regions. This is necessary to delineate origins and differences between neuroepithelial and epithelial tumors arising in these regions. The relative roles of chemical, physical, and viral agents in carcinogenesis need to be examined, epidemiologically as well as experimentally, and synergistic effects between these agents should be studied. The significance of early reactions associated with nasal carcinogenesis, such as chronic sinusitis and rhinitis, should be characterized if the mechanisms of nasal carcinogenesis are to be fully understood. Finally, further carcinogenesis bioassays must be conducted to detect environmental compounds or groups of compounds which require further study as potential nasal carcinogens.

With the current high level of contaminants to which people are continually exposed, both occupationally and environmentally, and with the vulnerable position occupied by the nasal epithelium, nasal carcinogenesis is not a field that should be neglected. Although reported incidences of nasal cancer are low, we have seen that many sensitive occupational and regional or ethnic groups have much higher frequencies. Further, inadequate sampling techniques at autopsy, both in experimental animals as well as humans, make it likely that many nasal cancers are not detected, so actual incidences could be much higher than reported.

INDEX

A

Acetaldehyde
  carcinogenicity, 36
  respiratory tract lesions caused by, 129
Acetaminophen, *N*-hydroxylation, 210
Acrolein, respiratory tract lesions caused by, 129
Acrylic molds, for aerosol deposition measurement,
  21
Adenocarcinoma of nasal cavity
  environmental compounds causing, 162—163
  nitrosamine-induced
    in Chinese hamster, 70, 71
    in European hamster, 67—69
    in hamster, 56—58, 65—66
    in mouse, 71, 72
    in rat, 49—50, 53, 54, 56
  N-nitrosodiethylamine and, 56—58
Adenoma
  nasal cavity
    environmental compounds causing, 162—164
    nitrosamine-induced, in rat, 51, 52
  pulmonary, *N*-nitrosonornicotine-induced, 80
Aerosol clearance, 19—20
Aerosol deposition, 18—23
  anatomic factors affecting
    in animals, 20
    in humans, 21
  animals and 21—23
  Brownian diffusion and, 19
  cigarette smoke, 117
  electrostatic attraction, 18, 19
  gravitational settling, 19
  humans and, 22—23
  impaction, 19
  interception, 18, 19
  physical factors affecting, 18—19
Aflatoxin B$_1$
  carcinogenicity, 162
  in monkey, 160
Airflow, and aerosol deposition in airways, 20—21
Aldehydes
  carcinogenicity, 36, 38—40
  in cigarette smoke, 129
Alkaloids, tobacco, 80, 86
Alpha particles, 140
Aluminosilicate particles, fused (FAP), as vehicle
  for radionuclides, 146
Anabasine, 80
  structure, 86
Anatabine, 80
  structure, 86
Animal model
  carcinogenesis bioassays, 158—160
  inhalation toxicology, 116—118
Antibody(ies)
  anti-EBV, 178, 181
  complement-fixing, 191

  monoclonal, 173
  neutralizing, 178
Antibody-dependent cellular cytotoxicity assay
  (ADCC), EB virus membrane antigen, 174
Anticomplement immunoenzymatic (ACIE) test, in
  nasopharyngeal carcinoma, 193
Antigens, EBV-associated, 173, 181
Aromatic amines, metabolic activation, 209—210
Autoradiography
  nitrosamine-induced nasal cavity tumors, 64, 67
  nitrosamine metabolism in nasal mucosa, 236—
    241
  (2′-^{14}C)NNN and (2′-^{14}C)NNK, 209
  tissue distribution of *N*-nitrosodimethylamine in
    mouse, 234—236

B

Basal cells
  nitrosamine-induced olfactory neoplasms and, 61,
    63, 64, 67
  response to nitrosamines, 51—52
  TSNA-induced nasal cavity tumors and, 84
BCME, see Bis(chloromethyl)ether
Beagles, see also Dogs
  cobalt-60-induced nasal cavity tumors, 150
  nasal cavity characteristics, 25
  nasal-pharyngeal airway, 13—14
    cross-section of cast, 9, 13
    silicone rubber cast, 4
  radiation-induced sinonasal tumors, 143
  respiratory tract, silicone rubber cast, 6
Beta particles, 140
Bioassay
  carcinogenicity of environmental compounds, see
    also Carcinogenesis bioassay of environmen-
    tal compounds, 158—166
  sensitivity, 159
  tobacco-specific nitrosamines, 80—82
Bis(chloromethyl)ether (BCME), 217
  carcinogenicity, 34—36, 162, 217
  formation from formaldehyde and hydrogen chlo-
    ride, 38, 217
  nasal cavity tumors in rodents and, 159
Blot hybridization, for detection of EB virus DNA
  repeats, 193—194
Bone-related neoplasms
  radiation-induced, in dogs, 143—150
  radium and, 141
Bowman's glands, 54
  adenocarcinoma, 58
  nitrosamine activation, 67
  rat nasal cavity, 119, 121
Brain, invasion by olfactory tumors, 97, 106
Bromoacetaldehyde, 215
Brownian diffusion, and particle deposition in airways, 19

Burkitt's lymphoma, 172
Bushbabies, nitrosamine-induced nasal cavity tumors in, 72—73
Butenolide, respiratory tract lesions caused by, 129

C

Calcium-45 (^{45}Ca), and cancer in mice, 142
Cantonese salted fish, carcinogenicity, 163, 164, 166
α-Carbon hydroxylation
    N-nitrosonornicotine, 208
    NNK, 209
Carcinogenesis bioassay of environmental compounds, 158—166
    animal model, 158—160, 251
    relevance of animal bioassays to human nasal cancer, 165—166
    route of exposure, 164
    sacrifice times, 161
    sampling procedures, 160—161
    sensitivity, 159
    sex susceptibility, 164
Carcinoma, see specific type, e.g, Adenocarcinoma
Casts/casting, see also Acrylic molds; Epoxy casts; Silicone rubber casts
    cross-sectioning, 3
        beagle, 9, 13
        guinea pig, 8, 12
        rat, 7, 11
        rhesus monkey, 10, 14,
    epoxy, 2
    gross examination, 3
    nasal-pharyngeal airway, 4—15
    silicone rubber, 2—3
Cerium-144
    chloride
        bone-related and nasal cavity tumors in dogs and, 147—149
        carcinogenicity, 162
        inhalation toxicology, 146, 147
    fused aluminosilicate particles and, inhalation toxicology, 146
    sinonasal tumors and, 151
    in rats, 142
Cervical carcinoma, 172
China
    EB virus and nasopharyngeal carcinoma in, 186—197
    serological mass surveys for EB virus VCA/IgA antibody, 194
Chinese hamster, see Hamster, Chinese
Chloroacetaldehyde, 217
Chloromethyl methyl ether, carcinogenicity, 162
Choana, human adult, 15
C$_3$H$_6$ONCl, see Dimethylcarbamoyl chloride (DMCC)
Chondrosarcoma, radiation-induced, in dogs, 143—145
Chromosome marker, in nasopharyngeal carcinoma, 195

Cigarette smoke(ing)
    cancer and, 80, 162
        in humans, 166
    constituents, respiratory tract lesions caused by, 129
    inhalation toxicology, 116—118, 122—127
    nickel concentration in, 220
    particulate deposition in airways, 117
    radon exposure and, in respiratory carcinogenesis in dogs, 148
Clara cells, 246
Cobalt-60 (^{60}Co), carcinogencity in beagles, 150
Complement-fixing antibody, to EB virus, 191
p-Cresidine, 209
    carcinogenicity, 209
    nasal cavity tumors in rodents and, 159
    uses, 209
Cribriform plate, tumor invasion, 54, 56
Curie, 140
Cytochrome P-450
    in nitrosamine metabolism, 208, 246
    in phenacetin metabolism, 210
Cytochrome P-450 dependent monooxygenases, in metabolic activation of nasal cavity carcinogens, 222—223
Cytomegalovirus, in nasopharyngeal carcinoma, 195

D

N-Deacylation, of phenacetin, 210
Deethylation, oxidative, of phenacetin, 210
Demethylation, of hexamethylphosphoramide, 213
Deposition, see Aerosol deposition
Diazohydroxide, 206
Dibromochloropropane
    carcinogencity, 162
    nasal cavity tumors in rodents and, 159
Dibromoethane, 215
    carcinogenicity, 162, 215
    metabolism, 215
    nasal cavity tumors in rodents and, 159
    uses, 215
Dichlorobutene, carcinogenicity, 162
2,6-Dimethyl aniline, carcinogenicity, 163, 164
Dimethylcarbamoyl chloride (DMCC), 215—217
    carcinogenicity, 28—33, 162, 216
    metabolism, 217
    species differences in susceptibility to, 33
    uses, 215
Dimethyl sulfate, carcinogenicity, 162
N,N'-Dinitroso-2,6-dimethylpiperazine, and nasal cavity tumors in rats, 50
N,N'-Dinitrosopiperazine, and nasal cavity tumors in rats, 50
Dioxane, 211—212
    carcinogenicity, 162, 211
    metabolism, 211—212
    nasal cavity tumors in rodents and, 159
Dissection, nasal airways, 2
DMCC, see Dimethylcarbamoyl chloride

DNA
  bis(chloromethyl)ether reaction with, 217
  dimethylcarbamoyl chloride reaction with, 217
  synthesis, nickel and, 220
DNA adducts
  formaldehyde, 220
  N-nitrosodiethylamine, 202
  vinyl chloride, 219
DNase enzyme, EB virus-associated, 178
Dogs, see also Beagles
  nitrosamine-induced nasal cavity tumors, 73, 74
  radiation-induced sinonasal tumors, 142—150
  thio-TEPA metabolism in, 214
Douglas fir, pyrolysis products and olfactory lesions
      in mice, 129, 130

                    E

Electron microscopy, nitrosamine-induced nasal cav-
      ity tumors in Syrian Golden hamster, 59—64
Electrostatic attraction, and particle deposition in
      airways, 18, 19
Environmental compounds, see also specific com-
      pound, 162—163
  carcinogenesis bioassay, 158—166
  carcinogenicity of, 161—165
  nasopharyngeal carcinoma and, 190
Epichlorhydrin, 218—219
  carcinogenicity, 33—34, 162, 219
Epidermoid carcinoma, radiation-induced, in dogs,
      143, 144
Epiglottis
  beagle, 14
  guinea pig, 12
  rhesus monkey, 15
Epithelial cells, EB virus association with, 174—
      176
Epithelioid cell line, from NPC patients, 195
Epithelium of nasal cavity
  carcinogenesis bioassay of environmental com-
      pounds, 158—166
  nasopharyngeal, histologic changes and EB virus
      antibody, 194
  olfactory, 54
    basal cells, 61, 63
    cell types, 118
    nitrosamine effect on, 55, 57—59
    nitrosamine-induced carcinoma, 61—64
    radiation-induced tumors of, 142
    rat nasal cavity, 118—120, 125
  respiratory
    cell types, 118
    hyperplasia (in rat), cigarette smoke and, 126,
      127
    hypertrophy (in rat), cigarette smoke and, 126
    rat nasal cavity, 118—120, 123, 126—127
    squamous metaplasia (in rat), cigarette smoke
      and, 126, 127, 129
    ulcerations, pyrolysis products and, 129—130
  stratified squamous

necrosis, 130, 132
  rat nasal cavity, 118—120, 125
Epoxy casts, 2
  nasal-pharyngeal airway of guinea pig, 5
Epstein-Barr (EB) virus
  antibody to, 178
    complement fixation tests of, 191
    histologic changes in nasopharyngeal mucosa
      and, 194
    immunoautoradiography, 193
    immunoenzymatic test, 192—193
    immunofluorescent tests, 191—192
  association with epithelial cells, 174—176
  biology, 172—174
  DNA repeats, blot hybridization for, 193—194
  early antigen (EA), 173
    antibody against, 178
  history, 172
  HR-1, 173
  latent infection, 173
  lymphocyte detectable membrane antigen, 173
  membrane antigen (MA), 173
  nasopharyngeal carcinoma and, 172—182
    causative role, 195—196
    in China, 188—197
  nuclear antigen (EBNA), 173, 1974
    ACIE test for, 193
  replication, 173
    in epithelial hybrid cell lines, 176
  retinoids and, 197
  VCA/IgA antibody, and histologic changes of na-
      sopharyngeal mucosa, 194
  virus capsid antigen (VCA), 173
    antibody against, 178
Esophageal tumors
  N'-nitrosoanabasine-induced, 80
  N'-nitrosonornicotine-induced, 81
Esthesioneuroblasts, in TSNA-induced olfactory tu-
      mors, 84
Esthesioneuroepithelioma
  following BCME exposure, 35—37
  environmental compounds causing, 162—163
  hamster nasal cavity, nitrosamine-induced, 65, 66
  rat nasal cavity, nitrosamine-induced, 49—50
  Syrian Golden hamster, 58—59
Ethanol, and carcinogenicity of NNN and NPYR, in
      Syrian Golden hamsters, 82
Ethmoturbinate region
  beagle, 9, 13
  guinea pig, 8, 12
  rat, 5, 7
  rhesus monkey, 10, 15
O⁶-Ethylguanine, 202
European hamster, see Hamster, European
Eustachian tube openings
  in guinea pig, 12
  in rat, 5

                    F

Fallout, see Radioactive fallout

Formaldehyde, 219—220
  biotransformation, 220
  carcinogenicity, 36, 39—40, 162, 219
  hydrogen chloride and, carcinogenicity, 38—40,
    162, 219
  nasal cavity tumors in rodents and, 159
  sources, 219
Formulated oil products, and nasal cavity lesions in
  rats, 130, 131
Frontal sinuses
  beagle, 9, 14
  radiation-induced epidermoid carcinoma, 143,
    144

G

Gamma rays, 140
Genetic factors, in nasopharyngeal carcinoma, 189
Gerbil
  diethylnitrosamine-induced nasal carcinoma, 160
  nitrosamine-induced nasal cavity tumors, 70—72
Gingival carcinoma, radiation-induced, in dogs,
    143, 145
Glutathione, in 1,2-dibromoethane metabolism, 215
Glycidal, 222
Goblet cell
  density estimation, 123
  hyperplasia, cigarette smoke and, 123—128
  rat nasal epithelium, 119, 121
Gravitational settling, and aerosol deposition in air-
    ways, 19
Group A marker chromosome, in NPC lymphoblas-
    toid cell lines, 195
Guinea pig
  nasal cavity
    acrylic mold, aerosol deposition in, 21, 22
    characteristics, 25
  nasal-pharyngeal airway, 11—13
    cross-section of cast, 8, 12
    epoxy cast, 5

H

Hamster
  cigarette smoke-induced respiratory lesions in,
    129
  nasal cancer, spontaneous occurrence, 159
  nitrosaminoketone-induced nasal cavity tumors,
    89, 107—111
Hamster, Chinese
  nasal cavity distribution of N-/^{14}C/nitrosopiperi-
    dine, 240
  nitrosamine-induced nasal cavity tumors, 70—72
Hamster, European
  nitrosamine-induced nasal cancer, 160
  nitrosamine-induced nasal cavity tumors, 67—70
Hamster, Syrian Golden
  carcinogenicity of NNN, NAB, and NNK, 81—
    82

dimethylcarbamoyl chloride-induced nasal tumors
    in, 29, 31—33, 216
  nasal effects of cigarette smoke, 126
  nitrosamine-induced nasal tumors in, 56—67, 129
  N-nitrosodiethanolamine-induced respiratory tract
    tumors, 203
  N-nitrosodiethylamine-induced respiratory tract tu-
    mors, 202
  N-nitrosomorpholine carcinogenicity in nasal cav-
    ity, 204
  N-nitrosopyrrolidine carcinogenicity, 205
  N-nitrosopyrrolidine metabolism in, 206
  NNN- and NNK-induced nasal cavity tumors, 207
HCHO, see Formaldehyde
Hemangiosarcoma
  radiation-induced, 146, 147
  in dogs, 143, 144
Herpes simplex virus II, 172
Herpesviruses, nonhuman, and malignant disease in
    animals, 172
Hexamethylphosphoramide (HMPA), 212
  carcinogenicity, 162, 213
  metabolism, 213
  uses, 212
Homer-Wright pseudorosettes, 84, 105
HR-1 EBV, 173
Humans
  aerosol deposition in airways, 22—23
  bis(chloromethyl)ether carcinogenicity, 217
  cigarette smoking and cancer, 166
  isopropyl oil carcinogenicity, 220
  leukemia and thio-TEPA therapy, 214
  nasal cancer, relevance of animal bioassays to,
    165—166
  nasal cavity, 15
    characteristics, 25
    dimensions, 15—16
    sagittal section, 17
    structure, 116
  nasopharyngeal carcinoma, see also Nasopharyn-
    geal carcinoma, 159
  nickel carcinogenicity, 220
  oat cell carcinoma of lung, 165—166
  radiation-induced sinonasal cancer, 140—141
  respiratory tract, 16
  thio-TEPA anti-cancer therapy, 214
  vinyl chloride carcinogenicity, 217
  wood dust hazards, 221—222
Hydrolysis
  bis(chloromethyl)ether, 217
  dimethylcarbamoyl chloride, 217
Hydrogen chloride plus formaldehyde, carcinogenic-
    ity, 38—40
α-Hydroxylation
  N-nitrosodiethylamine, 202
  N-nitrosomorpholine, 204
  N-nitrosopyrrolidine, 205, 206
β-Hydroxylation, N-nitrosomorpholine, 204
N-Hydroxylation
  acetaminophen, 210
  phenacetin, 211

I

IgA antibody, to EBV antigens, 191
IgG antibody, to EBV early antigens, 191
Image-analyzing computer, in nasal cavity measurements, 4
Immunoautoradiography, in nasopharyngeal carcinoma, 193
Immunoenzymatic tests, in nasopharyngeal carcinoma, 192—193
Immunofluorescent test
  antibodies to EB virus, 191—192
  EBV antigens, 173
Immunosuppression, cigarette smoke and, 127
Impaction, and aerosol deposition in airways, 19
Inertia, and particle deposition in airways, 18—19
Infection, respiratory
  effect on interpretation of experimental pulmonary pathology, 117—118
  opportunistic, and cigarette smoke immunosuppression, 127
Infectious mononucleosis, 172
Inflammatory cell, mononuclear, in rat nasal cavity, 119
Inflammatory (suppurative) reaction, in nasal cavity, cigarette smoke and, 126, 127
Inhalation toxicology
  aldehydes, 36, 38—40
  animal model, 116—118
    microbiological status, 117—118
    nasal cavity structure and function, 116—117
    particulate deposition, 117
  beta-emitting radionuclides, 143, 146—149
  bis(chloromethyl)ether, 34—36, 217
  cerium-144, 146—149
  cigarette smoke, 116—118, 122—127
    animal model, 116—118
    long-term studies, 126
    methodology, 122—123
    results, 123—127
    short-term studies, 126
  cigarette smoke constituents, 127, 129
    1,2-dibromoethane, 215
    dimethylcarbamoyl chloride, 28—29, 216
    epichlorhydrin, 34, 35, 219
    factors in, 131
    formaldehyde, 219
    formulated industrial products, 130
    hexamethylphosphoramide, 213
    irritants, 127, 129—132
    nickel compounds, 220
    nitrosamines, 48—74, 129
    pyrolysis products, 129—130
    strontium-90, 146—149
    subchronic toxicity studies, 161
      1,2-dibromoethane, 215
    sulfur dioxide, 129
    vinyl chloride, 217
      monomer, 129
    yttrium-91, 146—149

Interception, and particle deposition in airways, 18, 19
Interferon, for nasopharyngeal carcinoma, 196—197
Ionizing radiation, see Radiation, ionizing
Irritants, nasal, see also Cigarette smoke
  cigarette smoke components, 127, 129
  formulated industrial products, 130
  nitrosamines, see Nitrosamines
  pyrolysis products, 129—130
  respiratory tract lesions caused by, 127, 129—132
  sulfur dioxide, 129
Isopropyl oils, 220—221
  carcinogenicity, 221
Isosafrole, 222

K

Kulschitsky cell, and oat cell carcinoma of lung, 165—166

L

Lamina propria, rat nasal cavity, 118—119
Laryngopharynx
  beagle, 9, 14
  guinea pig, 8, 12
  rat, 5, 7
  rhesus monkey, 10, 15
Larynx
  beagle, 9, 14
  guinea pig, 8, 12—13
  rat, 5, 7, 11
  rhesus monkey, 10, 15
Leukemia, and thio-TEPA therapy, 214
Leukocytes, globule, in rat nasal cavity, 119
Linear energy transfer (LET), 140, 150
Liver
  nitrosamine metabolism, 241
  tumors, nitrosamine-induced, 81
Lucké adenocarcinoma of frog, 172
Lung tumors, nitrosamine-induced, 81
Lymphoblastoid cell line, from NPC patient, 195
Lymphocyte(s)
  in rat nasal cavity, 119
    effect of cigarette smoke on, 125
Lymphocyte detectable membrane antigen (LYDMA), 173
Lymphoma, Burkitt's, 172

M

Man, see Humans
Marek's disease of fowl, 172
Maxillary sinus
  beagle, 9, 14
  effect of cigarette smoke on, in rat, 125

guinea pig, 12
Maxilloturbinates
  beagle, 9, 13
  guinea pig, 8, 12
  rat, 5, 7
  rhesus monkey, 10, 15
Mesenchymal neoplasms of nasal cavity, environ-
    mental compounds causing, 162—163, 165
Metastases, from nasal carcinoma, 162—163, 165
2-Methoxy aniline, carcinogenicity, 163, 164
2-Methoxy-5-methyl aniline, carcinogenicity, 163,
    164
2-Methoxy-5-methylbenzenamine, 209
1-Methoxy-4-nitro-2,3,5,6-tetrachlorobenzene, car-
    cinogenicity, 163, 164
Methyl hydroxylation, NNK, 209
4-(Methylnitrosamino)-1-(3-pyridyl)-1-butanone
    (NNK), 207
  autoradiography, 209
  carcinogenesis, 207
  metabolic deactivation, 209
  metabolism, 209
  methyl hydroxylation, 209
  nasal cavity tumors in rats, 49
  oxidation, 209
  reduction, 209
  sources, 207
Methyl oxidation, hexamethylphosphoramide, 213
Metyrapone, and *N*-nitrosodibutylamine metabolism,
    208
Mice
  1,2-dibromoethane-induced nasal cavity tumors
    in, 215
  hydrogen chloride-induced olfactory lesions in,
    129
  isopropyl oil carcinogenicity, 221
  nasal cancer, spontaneous occurrence, 159
  nitrosamine-induced nasal cavity tumors, 71, 72
  nitrosaminoketone (NNK) carcinogenicity, 81
  nitrosaminoketone-induced nasal cavity tumors,
    95, 96
  N-/¹⁴C/nitrosodiethylamine distribution in nasal
    cavity, 237
  N-nitrosonornicotine (NNN) carcinogenicity in,
    80, 81
  NNN and NNK-induced nasal cavity tumors, 207
  olfactory lesions due to pyrolysis products of po-
    lyurethane foam, polyvinyl chloride, and
    Douglas fir, 129
  radiation-induced nasal cavity tumors, 141—142
  sulfur dioxide-induced nasal cavity lesions, 129
  thio-TEPA metabolism, 214
Microautoradiography, nitrosamine metabolism in
    nasal mucosa, 236, 241—244
Microcomplement fixation test, in nasopharyngeal
    carcinoma, 191
Monkey
  nasal carcinogenesis, 160
  respiratory tract, silicone rubber cast, 6
Monkey, rhesus
  aerosol deposition in airways, 20

nasal cavity characteristics, 25
nasal-pharyngeal airway, 15
  cross-section of cast, 10, 14
  silicone rubber cast, 4
Monoclonal antibody, to EBV membrane antigen,
    173
Mouse, see Mice
Mouthbreaking, 116, 117
Mucociliary clearance rate, 20
Mucoepidermoid carcinoma, nitrosamine-induced, in
    canine nasal cavity, 73, 74
Mucous cells, response to nitrosamines, 52
Mucus hypersecretion, cigarette smoke and, 126,
    127
Myeloproliferative disorders, in strontium-90-fed
    beagles, 143

N

Nares
  beagle, 9, 13
  guinea pig, 8, 11
  human adult, 15
  rat, 5, 7
  rhesus monkey, 10, 15
Nasal airways (cavity)
  aerosol clearance from, 19—20
  aerosol deposition in, 18—23
  anatomy
    casting, 2—4
    computed tomography, 2
    dissection study, 2
    methods of study, 2—4
  carcinogens, 202—223
  dimethylcarbamoyl chloride-induced tumors, 28—
    33
  histopathology after cigarette smoke exposure,
    122—127
  human adult, 15
    dimensions, 15
    sagittal section, 17
  interspecies comparison, 25
  mucociliary clearance rate, 20
  nitrosamine-induced tumors, 48—74
  radiation-induced cancers
    in animals, 141—150
    in humans, 140—141
    pathogenesis, 150—152
  rat, microanatomy, 118—121
  sampling procedures, 160—161
  structure and function in choosing animal model,
    116—117
TSNA-induced tumors
  anatomy and histogenesis, 82—85
  carcinogenicity assays in animals, 80—82
  early stages, 83
volume, 3
  in beagle, 14
  in guinea pig, 12
  in human adult, 15

in rat, 5
in rhesus monkey, 15
Nasal septum, effect of cigarette smoke on (in rat),
123—125
Nasal turbinates, effect of cigarette smoke on (in
rats), 125
Nasolacrimal duct, effect of cigarette smoke on (in
rats), 125
Nasopharyngeal carcinoma (NPC), 159
age-specific mortality in China, 188—190
anticomplement immunoenzymatic (ACIE) test in,
193
anti-EBV antibody in, 178
blot hybridization for detection of DNA repeats
in, 193—194
in China, 188—197
control and prevention, 196—197
cytomegalovirus in, 195
detection through use of antibody and other markers, 178—181
EA/IgA antibody levels, 191
EA/IgG antibody levels, 191
environmental carcinogens and, 190
epidemiology in China, 188—190
epithelioid cell line from, 195
Epstein-Barr virus and, 172—182
causative role, 195—196
in China, 188—197
EBV antibody and mucosal histology, 194
genetic factors in China, 189
geographic distribution in China, 188
group A marker chromosome in, 195
histological classification, 177
immunoautoradiography in, 193
immunoenzymatic test in, 192—193
immunofluorescence test in, 191
incidence rate, 188
interferon for, 196—197
in vitro model, 175—177
lymphoblastoid cell lines with giant group A
marker chromosome, 195
microcomplement fixation test, 191
radiotherapy for, 196
serological mass surveys in China, 194
urinary nucleosides in, 179—181
VCA/IgA antibody levels, 191, 193
Nasopharynx
beagle, 9, 14
guinea pig, 8, 12
rat, 5, 7
rhesus monkey, 10, 15
Neuroblast, in nitrosamine-induced nasal cavity tumors, 60—62, 67
Neuroblastoma, olfactory, see
Esthesioneuroepithelioma
Neuroendocrine cells, in olfactory epithelium, 58
Neuroepithelial carcinoma, nasal cavity, environmental compounds causing, 162—164
Neuroepithelial tumors, olfactory, *N*-nitrosodiethy-
lamine and, 58—59
Neutralizing antibody, to EBV DNase, 178

Neutrons, 140
Nickel/nickel compounds, 220
carcinogenicity, 220
sources, 220
Nicotine, 80
structure, 86
Niridazole, carcinogenicity, 162
Nitrosamines, see also specific nitrosamines
biosynthetic distribution pattern, 236
carcinogenicity, 48—74
in rats, 48—56
in Syrian Golden hamster, 56—57
metabolism, 234
in nasal mucosa, 236—247
tissue specificity, 235—236
tissue distribution, 234
tobacco-specific, see also Tobacco-specific nitrosamines, 80—111
Nitrosaminoaldehyde (NNA), 80
structure, 86
Nitrosaminoketone (NNK)
carcinogenicity assays, 81
levels in tobacco and tobacco smoke, 80
nasal cavity tumors and
in hamster, 89, 107—111
in mouse, 95, 96
in rat, 90, 92, 93, 97—101, 105
organospecificity, in Syrian Golden hamster, 82
structure, 86
N'-Nitrosoanabasine (NAB), 80
carcinogenicity assays, 80
structure, 86
N-Nitroso-*N*-bis(2-acetoxypropyl)amine, and nasal
cavity tumors in mice, 71, 72
N-Nitroso-bis(2-hydroxypropyl)amine, and nasal
cavity tumors in rats, 50
N-Nitroso-*N*-bis(2-hydroxypropylamine), and nasal
cavity tumors in mice, 71, 72
N-Nitroso-bis(2-hydroxypropyl)amine nasal cavity
tumors in rats and, 49
nasal cavity tumors in Syrian Golden hamsters
and, 65
N-Nitrosodibutylamine (DBN)
^{14}C-labeled, nasal cavity distribution in rat, 241,
248
nasal cavity tumors and
in Chinese hamster, 71
in European hamster, 68—70
N-Nitroso-3,4-dichloropiperidine, and nasal cavity
tumors in rats, 50
N-Nitroso-3,4-dichloropyrrolidine, and nasal cavity
tumors in rats, 50
N-Nitrosodiethanolamine, 203—204
carcinogenicity, 203
metabolism, 204
nasal cavity tumors in Syrian Golden hamster
and, 65
sources, 203
N-Nitrosodiethylamine, 202—203
^{14}C-labeled, nasal cavity distribution in rodents,
237—238

carcinogenicity, 202
  in monkey, 160
α-hydroxylation, 202
metabolism, 202—203
nasal cavity tumors and
  in bushbabies, 72, 73
  in Chinese hamsters, 71
  in dogs, 73, 74
  in European hamsters, 68, 69
  in gerbils, 71, 160
  in mice, 71
  in rats, 49, 51
  in Syrian Golden hamsters, 56—64, 67, 129
sources, 202
N-Nitroso-O,N-diethylhydroxylamine, and nasal
    cavity tumors in rats, 49
N-Nitroso-di-isopropanolamine
  nasal cavity tumors in European hamster and, 69
  nasal cavity tumors in rats and, 49
N-Nitrosodi-isopropylamine, and nasal cavity tumors
    in rats, 49
N-Nitrosodimethylamine
  ^{14}C-labeled, tissue distribution in mice, 235—236
  nasal cavity tumors and
    in Chinese hamster, 71
    in rats, 49
    in Syrian Golden hamster, 65, 129
N-Nitroso-2,6-dimethylmorpholine
  nasal cavity tumors in rats and, 49
  nasal cavity tumors in Syrian Golden hamster,
    and, 65
N-Nitroso-di-n-propylamine
  nasal cavity tumors in rats and, 49
  nasal cavity tumors in Syrian Golden hamsters
    and, 65
N-Nitrosodipropylamine, and nasal cavity tumors in
    mice, 71, 72
N-Nitrosoethyl-n-butylamine, and nasal cavity tu-
    mors in rats, 49
N-Nitrosoheptamethyleneimine
  nasal cavity tumors and
    in European hamsters, 69
    in rats, 50
    in Syrian Golden hamsters, 66
N-Nitrosohexamethyleneimine
  nasal cavity tumors in rats and, 50
  nasal cavity tumors in Syrian Golden hamsters
    and, 66
N-Nitroso-(2-hydroxypropyl)(2-oxopropyl)amine,
    and nasal cavity tumors in Syrian Golden
    hamsters, 65
N-Nitroso-hydroxypropyl-n-propylamine
  nasal cavity tumors in rats and, 49
  nasal cavity tumors in Syrian Golden hamsters
    and, 65
N-Nitrosomethylallylamine, and nasal cavity tumors
    in rats, 49
N-Nitrosomethyl-n-amylamine, and nasal cavity tu-
    mors in rats, 49
N-Nitrosomethylbenzylamine, distribution in rat, 53
N-Nitrosomethylethylamine, and nasal cavity tumors
    in rats, 49

N-Nitrosomethyl piperazine, and nasal cavity tumors
    in rats, 50, 51, 53, 55—56
N-Nitrosomethyl-n-propylamine
  nasal cavity tumors in rats and, 49
  nasal cavity tumors in Syrian Golden hamster
    and, 65
N-Nitrosomethylpropylamine, and nasal cavity tu-
    mors in mice, 71, 72
N-Nitrosomethylvinylamine, and nasal cavity tumors
    in rats, 49
N-Nitrosomorpholine, 204—205
  carcinogenicity, 204
  hydroxylation, 204
  metabolism, 204
  nasal cavity tumors
    in Chinese hamster, 71
    in European hamster, 69
    in rats, 49
    in Syrian Golden hamster, 65
  sources, 204
N-Nitrosonornicotine (NNN), 80, 207—209
  autoradiography, 209
  α-carbon hydroxylation, 208
  carcinogenicity, 207
    assays, 80—81
  ^{14}C-labeled, nasal cavity distribution in rat, 239,
    242—244
  levels in tobacco, tobacco smoke, and snuff-dip-
    per's saliva, 80
  metabolic activation, 208
  metabolism, 207—208
    in rat nasal mucosa, 239, 242—244
  nasal cavity effects, in rat, 87—88, 91, 102—
    104, 106
  nasal cavity tumors and
    in rats, 50
    in Syrian Golden hamster, 66
  organospecificity
    in rat, 81
    in Syrian Golden hamster, 82
  sources, 207
  structure, 86
  tissue distribution, 234
N-Nitroso-β-oxopropyl-n-propylamine, and nasal
    cavity tumors in Syrian Golden hamster, 65
N-Nitroso-1-oxopropylpropylamine, and nasal cavity
    tumors in Syrian Golden hamster, 65
N-Nitrosopiperazine, and nasal cavity tumors in
    rats, 50
N-Nitrosopiperidine
  ^{14}C-labeled, nasal cavity distribution in Chinese
    hamster, 240
  nasal cavity tumors and
    in Chinese hamster, 71
    in dogs, 73, 74
    in European hamster, 69
    in rats, 50
    in Syrian Golden hamster, 66
N-Nitroso-3-piperidinol, and nasal cavity tumors in
    rats, 50
N-Nitroso-4-piperidinol, and nasal cavity tumors in
    rats, 50

N-Nitroso-4-piperidinone, and nasal cavity tumors in rats, 50
N-Nitrosopyrrolidine (NPYR), 205—206
  carcinogenicity, 205
  ethanol and, 82
  α-hydroxylation, 205, 206
  metabolism, 205—206
  nasal cavity tumors and
    in rats, 50
    in Syrian Golden hamster, 66
  sources, 205
N-Nitroso-3-pyrroline, and nasal cavity tumors in rats, 50
NNK, see 4(Methylnitrosamino)-*1*-(3-pyridyl)-*1*-butanne; Nitrosaminoketone
NNN, see *N*-Nitrosonornicotine
Nornicotine, 80
  structure, 86
NPYR, see *N*-Nitrosopyrrolidine
Nucleosides, in urine of cancer patients, 179—181

O

Occupational risk
  bis(chloromethyl)ether, 217
  epichlorhydrin, 219
  isopropyl oils, 220
  nasal cavity carcinoma, 251
  nickel, 220
  wood workers, 221
Organotin biocide, experimental, and nasal cavity lesions in rats, 130, 132
Oropharynx
  beagle, 9, 14
  guinea pig, 8, 12
  rat, 5, 7
  rhesus monkey, 10, 15
OSPA, metabolism, 214
Osteosarcoma
  radiation-induced
    in dogs, 143—145, 147
    in rodents, 141—142
  radium and, 141
  strontium-90 and, 139
Oxidation
  1,2-dibromoethane, 215
  hexamethylphosphoramide, 213
  NNK, 209

P

Papilloma
  DMCC inhalation and, 29
  nitrosamine-induced
    in European hamster, 67, 69
    in mouse, 72
    in rat, 49—51
  squamous cell, see Squamous cell papilloma
Paranasal sinuses, 116

radiation-induced cancer, 140—152
  in animals, 141—150
  in humans, 140—141
  pathogenesis, 150—152
Particle deposition, see Aerosol clearance; Aerosol deposition
Pharyngeal isthmus
  guinea pig, 8, 12
  rat, 5
  rhesus monkey, 10, 15
Phenacetin
  carcinogenecity, 163, 210
  metabolic activation, 211
  metabolism, 210—211
Phenylglycidil ether, carcinogenicity, 162
Plutonium 239 (^{239}Pu)
  bone-related and nasal cavity neoplasms in dogs, 143—144
  sinonasal carcinoma and, 150
  tumors in mice and, 141
Polynuclear aromatic hydrocarbons (PAH), metabolic activation, 221
Polyps, papillary, nitrosamine-induced, 67, 69
Polyurethane foam, pyrolysis products and olfactory lesions in mice, 129, 130
Polyvinyl chloride (PVC), pyrolysis products and olfactory lesions in mice, 129
Primates, nonhuman, nitrosamine-induced nasal cavity tumors in, 72—73
Procarbazine
  carcinogenicity, 162
  nasal carcinogenesis in rats and, 160
  nasal cavity tumors in rodents and, 159
Pseudorosettes, in TSNA-induced olfactory tumors, 104
Pulmonary carcinoma, radiation-induced, 146, 147

Q

Quinoxaline-1,4-dioxide, carcinogenicity, 162

R

Rad, 140
Radiation
  age-related sensitivity study, 150
  dose, 138—139
    terminology, 140
  dose distribution, 139—140
  dose rate, 139
  dose-response relationships, 138
  ionizing, 138, 140
  types, 140
Radiation carcinogenesis, 138—152
  cancer of nose and paranasal sinuses
    in animals, 141—150
    in humans, 140—141
    pathogenesis, 150—152
  promotion factors, 138

terminology, 140
threshold dose, 138
Radioactive fallout, 139
Radionuclides
  alpha-emitters, 141, 150
  beta-emitters, 141, 150
    inhalation toxicology, 143, 146—149
  bone-seeking, 141
    bone-related and nasal cavity neoplasms in
      dogs and, 143—145
    sinonasal cancer and, 150—152
  carcinogenicity
    in dogs, 142—150
    in rodents, 141—142
  fused aluminosilicate particles, 146
  half-life, 140
    tumor induction and, 146
  internally deposited, radiation dose distribution,
    139—140
  organospecificity, 139
    tumor induction and, 146
  soluble, inhalation studies, 146, 147
Radiotherapy, for nasopharyngeal carcinoma, 196
Radium, carcinogenicity in humans, 141
Radium-226 (^{226}Ra)
  bone-related and nasal cavity neoplasms in dogs,
    143—145
  osteosarcoma in mice and, 141
  sinonasal cancer and, 150
Radon daughters, and cigarette smoke, in respiratory carcinogenesis in dogs, 148
Raji cells, HR-1 EBV infected, 174
Rat
  bis(chloromethyl)ether-induced nasal cavity tu-
    mors in, 34—36, 217
  p-cresidine-induced nasal cavity tumors in, 209
  1,2-dibromoethane-induced nasal cavity tumors
    in, 215
  1,2-dibromoethane metabolism, 215
  dimethylcarbamoyl chloride-induced nasal tumors
    in, 28—29
  dioxane-induced nasal cavity tumors, 211
  dioxane metabolism, 211—212
  epichlorhydrin-induced nasal tumors, 33—34, 219
  formaldehyde-hydrogen chloride-induced nasal tu-
    mors in, 38—40
  formaldehyde-induced nasal cavity carcinoma,
    219
  formulated oil product fumes and respiratory le-
    sions, 130, 131
  hexamethylphosphoramide-induced nasal cavity
    tumors, 213
  nasal cancer, spontaneous occurrence, 159
  nasal cavity
    acrylic mold, aerosol deposition in, 21, 22
    anatomy, microscopic, 118—121
    characteristics, 25
    lamina propria, 118—119
    N-/^{14}C/nitrosodibutylamine distribution, 241,
      248
    N-/^{14}C/nitrosodiethylamine distribution, 238

    N-/^{14}C/nitrosonornicotine distribution, 239,
      242—244
    olfactory epithelium, 118—120
    respiratory epithelium, 118—120
    response to *N*-nitrosonornicotine, 87—88, 91,
      102—104, 106
    stratified squamous epithelium, 118—120
    transverse section, 120
    tumors, 159
  nasal histopathology after cigarette smoke expo-
    sure, 122—127
    method of study, 122—123
    results, 123—127
  nasal-pharyngeal airway, 5—7, 11
    cross-section of cast, 7, 11
    silicone rubber cast, 4
  nickel carcinogenicity, 220
  nitrosamine-induced nasal cavity tumors in, 48—
    56, 244
  nitrosaminoketone carcinogenicity, 81
  nitrosaminoketone-induced nasal cavity tumors,
    90, 92, 93, 97—101, 105
  nitrosaminoketone metabolism, 209
  N-nitrosoanabasine carcinogenicity, 80, 81
  N-nitrosodiethanolamine metabolism, 204
  N-nitrosomorpholine metabolism, 204, 205
  N-nitrosonornicotine carcinogenicty, 81
  N-nitrosonornicotine metabolism, 207—208
  N-nitrosopyrrolidine metabolism, 205
  organotin biocide-induced olfactory lesions, 130,
    132
  particulate deposition in cigarette smoke, 177
  phenacetin carcinogenicity, 210
  radiation-induced nasal cavity tumors, 142
  respiratory tract, silicone rubber cast, 6
  thio-TEPA-induced nasal carcinoma, 214
  thio-TEPA metabolism, 214
  trimethoxycinnamaldehyde-induced nasal cavity
    tumors, 222
  vinyl chloride-induced olfactory epithelial carci-
    noma, 217
  vinyl chloride-induced olfactory lesions, 129
Reduction, NNK, 209
Relative bioloical effectiveness (RBE), 140, 150
Respiratory tract
  bis(chloromethyl)ether-induced tumors, 35
  DMCC-induced tumors, 29
  human, 16
Retinoids, for NPC prevention, 197
Reynolds number, 20
Rhinitis
  effect on interpretation of experimental pulmonary
    pathology, 117—118
  nasal carcinogenesis and, 165
  necrotizing, cigarette smoke and, 129
RNA synthesis, nickel and, 220
Ro 10-7359, see Retinoids
Roentgen (R), 140
Rosettes, in TSNA-induced olfactory tumors, 84,
  85, 87—103, 106

S

Sebaceous carcinoma, external ear canal, radiation-induced, 142
Sectioning
  skull, 160—161
  transverse, nasal cavity study, 2
Sensory cells, olfactory
  nitrosamine effect on, 62
  toxic degeneration, 55
Serous glands and ducts, in rat nasal cavity, 119, 121
Sex susceptibility, in carcinogenesis bioassays, 164
Silicone rubber casts, 2—3
  nasal-pharyngeal airways, 4
  respiratory tract, 6
Sinonasal cancer, radiation-induced
  in animals, 141—150
  in humans, 140—141
  pathogenesis, 150—152
Sinusitis, and nasal carcinogenesis, 165
Skull sectioning, 160—161
Squamous carcinoma, radiation-induced, in dogs, 143, 145
Squamous cell carcinoma of nasal cavity
  bis(chloromethyl)ether exposure and, 35
  DMCC and, 29
    in Syrian Golden hamster, 216
  environmental compounds causing, 162—163
  epichlorhydrin and, 219
  formaldehyde exposure and (in rat), 40—43
  hexamethylphosphoramide and (in rat), 213
  nitrosamine-induced
    in Chinese hamster, 70, 71
    in dog, 73, 74
    in European hamster, 67—70
    in mouse, 71, 72
    in rat, 49—50, 52, 54, 55
  radiation-induced (in dog), 148, 149
Squamous cell papilloma of nasal cavity
  environmental compounds causing, 162—164
  nitrosamine-induced
    in hamster, 65
    in mouse, 71
  N-nitrosodiethylamine and (in hamster), 56
Strontium-90 (^{90}Sr)
  bone-related and nasal cavity neoplasms in dogs, 143—148
  cancer in mice and, 142
  chloride
    bone-related and nasal cavity neoplasms in dogs, 147
    inhalation toxicology, 146, 147
    sinonasal tumors, 151
  epidermoid carcinoma of nasal cavity in dogs and, 143
  in fused aluminosilicate particles, carcinogenicity, 146
  ingestion of, bone-related and nasal cavity neoplasms in dogs, 143, 145

osteosarcoma and, 139
sinonasal cancer and, 150
Sulfur dioxide, respiratory tract lesions caused by, 129
Sustentacular cells, 61
  in nitrosamine-induced olfactory neoplasms, 61, 62, 64
Syrian Golden hamster, see Hamster, Syrian Golden

T

Tetrachlorodibenzo dioxin, carcinogenicity, 163
Thio-TEPA, 214
  carcinogenicity, 163, 163, 214
  metabolism, 214
  nasal cavity tumors in rodents and, 159
  uses, 214
Tobacco-specific nitrosamines (TSNA), 80
  bioassay, 80—82
  formation and occurrence, 80
  metabolic activation, 207—209
  nasal cavity tumors and, microscopic anatomy and histogenesis, 82—85
  structure, 86
o-Toluidine, metabolism, 210
Tomography, computed
  human nasal airways, tracings from, 17
  nasal airways, 2
Trachea
  beagle, 9, 14
  guinea pig, 8, 13
  papillomas, TSNA-induced, 81—82
  rat, 7, 11
Transverse sections, rat nasal nasal cavity, 119, 120
3,4,5-Trimethoxycinnamaldehyde, 221—222
  carcinogenicity, 163, 166
TSNA, see Tobacco-specific nitrosamines
Tumorigenesis
  aldehydes, 36, 38—40
  bis(chloromethyl)ether, 34—36
  dimethylcarbamoyl chloride, 28—33
  environmental compounds, 162—163
  epichlorhydrin, 33—35
  nitrosamines, 48—74
  radiation in, see also Radiation carcinogenesis, 138
Turbulence, airflow, and particle deposition in airways, 20, 21

U

Ulcers, respiratory epithelium, pyrolysis products and, 129—130

V

Ventricles, laryngeal

beagle, 9, 14
rat, 7, 11
rhesus monkey, 10, 15
Vinyl chloride, 217
    carcinogenesis, 217
    metabolism, 217—218
    monomer, and olfactory lesions in rats, 129
    use for, 217
Virus capsid antigen (VCA), 173

W

Wood dust, 221
World Health Organization (WHO), classification of
    nasopharyngeal carcinoma, 177

X

X-rays, 140

carcinogenicity, 142

Y

Yttrium-91 (^{91}Y)
    chloride
        bone-related and nasal cavity neoplasms in
            dogs, 147
    inhalation toxicology, 146, 147
    in fused aluminosilicate particles, carcinogenicity,
        146
    sinonasal cancer and, 151

Z

Zymbal gland, 142